PLANT-BASED SPORTS NUTRITION

Expert Fueling Strategies for Training, Recovery, and Performance

D. Enette Larson-Meyer, PhD, RDN
Matt Ruscigno, MPH, RDN

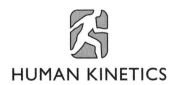

HUMAN KINETICS

Library of Congress Cataloging-in-Publication Data

Names: Larson-Meyer, D. Enette, 1963- author.
Title: Plant-based sports nutrition : expert fueling strategies for training, recovery, and performance / D. Enette Larson-Meyer and Matt Ruscigno.
Description: Champaign, IL : Human Kinetics, [2020] | Includes bibliographical references and index.
Identifiers: LCCN 2018059516 (print) | LCCN 2019001559 (ebook) | ISBN 9781492588863 (epub) | ISBN 9781492568650 (PDF) | ISBN 9781492568643 (print)
Subjects: LCSH: Athletes--Nutrition. | Veganism--Health aspects. | Physical fitness.
Classification: LCC TX361.A8 (ebook) | LCC TX361.A8 L365 2020 (print) | DDC 613.7/11--dc23
LC record available at https://lccn.loc.gov/2018059516

ISBN: 978-1-4925-6864-3 (print)

Senior Acquisitions Editor: Michelle Maloney; **Managing Editor:** Miranda K. Baur; **Copyeditor:** Annette Pierce; **Indexer:** Nancy Ball; **Permissions Manager:** Martha Gullo; **Graphic Designer:** Denise Lowry; **Cover Designer:** Keri Evans; **Cover Design Associate:** Susan Rothermel Allen; **Photograph (cover):** t_trifonoff/iStockphoto/Getty Images, zi3000/iStockphoto/Getty Images; **Photographs (interior):** © Human Kinetics, unless otherwise noted; **Photo Asset Manager:** Laura Fitch; **Photo Production Manager:** Jason Allen; **Senior Art Manager:** Kelly Hendren; **Illustrations:** © Human Kinetics, unless otherwise noted; **Printer:** Sheridan

Human Kinetics books are available at special discounts for bulk purchase. Special editions or book excerpts can also be created to specification. For details, contact the Special Sales Manager at Human Kinetics.

Printed in the United States of America   10 9 8 7 6 5 4 3 2

The paper in this book is certified under a sustainable forestry program.

Human Kinetics
P.O. Box 5076
Champaign, IL 61825-5076
Website: www.HumanKinetics.com

In the United States, email info@hkusa.com or call 800-747-4457.
In Canada, email info@hkcanada.com.
In the United Kingdom/Europe, email hk@hkeurope.com.

For information about Human Kinetics' coverage in other areas of the world, please visit our website: **www.HumanKinetics.com**

E7339

Tell us what you think!
Human Kinetics would love to hear what we can do to improve the customer experience. Use this QR code to take our brief survey.

ELM: This book was written in memory of Dr. Roland L. Weinsier, MD, DrPH, a wonderful teacher, mentor, and scientist who lived an active vegetarian lifestyle. It is also dedicated to my three young athletes, Lindsey, Marlena, and Ian, who have proven at every level how easy it is to be a plant-based athlete.

MR: Dedicated to everyone working to improve their performance, and the world.

CONTENTS

ACKNOWLEDGMENTS

ELM: I would like to thank all my mentors over the years, including Dr. Gary Hunter, Dr. JP Flatt, Dr. Brad Newcomer, Dr. Eric Ravussin, Dr. Ron Maughan, and Dr. Melinda Manore. Each of you has helped me grow in understanding the science and appreciating the challenge. This book would not be possible without your mentorship. I would also like to acknowledge all of the athletes, coaches, trainers, research volunteers, and training partners who I have worked and trained with over the years. Thank you for your friendship and your dedication. Finally, I would like to acknowledge my husband, Mike, for his patience during the grinding times while writing both editions of this book. Thank you and go green.

MR: All of my dietitian colleagues from the Vegetarian Nutrition Practice Group of the Academy of Nutrition and Dietetics—thank you for your continued support and guidance. Also Enette and the entire team at Human Kinetics for having me contribute to this wonderful project. All of my plant-based / vegan friends and colleagues striving to create a new world: You inspire me to do better. And of course my fabulous partner, Laura, whose support has been life changing. Lastly, you, the reader. We wouldn't have done this work if it wasn't for you; take this info and be your best self!

INTRODUCTION

Everyone is an athlete. The only difference is that some of us
are in training, and some are not.

—*George Sheehan*

Enette's Story

I never liked meat as a kid. Somewhat fortunately, I grew up in the era of casseroles, skillet dishes, and Hamburger Helper, so it was easy to "hide" the meat or chicken amid the pasta, rice, potatoes, and other veggies. My mother tells me that my favorite thing to order at restaurants was either three scoops of mashed potatoes or coconut encrusted shrimp if it was available. Admittedly, the potatoes were served with a meat-based gravy.

I did not officially become vegetarian until my junior year of college. I remember the day like it was yesterday. I returned from my first anatomy lab to a sit-down Monday-night dinner at my sorority and made the connection that the piece of meat on my plate looked exactly like my own skeletal muscle. My journey after that was not as easy as it might have been today. Grocery stores did not carry veggie burgers, tofu dogs, or hummus, and tofu was known only as bean curd on the menu at Chinese restaurants. The dogma at the time was that vegetarians had to eat complementary proteins at every meal. I put sunflower seeds and peanut butter or cheddar cheese on everything in attempts to "complement" my plant proteins. Despite running and an intense weight training program, I gained over 7 pounds (3 kg) my first semester as a vegetarian, and if I am being honest, it was not muscle.

My options opened up when I moved to Boston for my dietetic internship. Massachusetts General Hospital had a great collection of meatless heart-healthy recipes, and I was exposed to cooking with beans and tofu. It has been a journey—becoming a foodie and learning how to cook healthy, tasty, and satisfying meals for busy days and special dishes for holidays and special occasions (hoping family and friends wouldn't miss the meat). It has been a journey sifting through the scientific literature in attempts to understand how nutrition influences human and environmental health and the advantages and potential pitfalls of vegetarian-based diets—particularly for athletes. And, it has also been a journey of learning how to share my knowledge and excitement about plant-based diets with athletes, clients, fellow health and exercise professionals, and the public.

I am happy to have the opportunity to update *Vegetarian Sports Nutrition* and reflect back on the journey. Since its initial publishing in 2007, interest in plant-centered diets—including both vegan and semivegetarian diets—for athletes and the general population has grown and continues to grow. This has included the emergence of more commercially available vegetarian products, trends toward demand for more plant-based options in college cafeterias, and vegan menu options now offered at some high schools. Current mainstream interest in the environmental aspects of plant-based eating and sustainable agriculture has paralleled the increased push for higher-protein diets and a growing industry supporting commercial products for vegans and vegetarians. I am also thankful that I am joined in this updated edition by my colleague, Matt Ruscigno, a fellow dietitian and athlete who follows a plant-based diet. I know you will find that Matt brings character to this edition, along with extensive experience with vegan diets for athletes. Look for his contributions throughout, labeled "Vegan View." Together, we will share what we understand to be the plant-based advantage.

Matt's Story

As a young kid I'd move snails off of the sidewalk after a rain so they wouldn't be stepped on, and my days were spent adventuring with the family dog, my beloved Samantha. Soon after, I connected that food came from animals. My parents, born and raised in New York City where they hadn't given much thought to the origin of the chicken in chicken Parmesan, didn't know what to do with me. I flirted with vegetarianism on and off and then at 17 years old, influenced by mid-1990s punk bands who espoused veganism, I gave up animal products for good. It timed well with going off to college where, after giving up on studying physics in order to become a stuntman, I switched to nutrition. Two degrees and certification as a registered dietitian later, I've dedicated my life to helping people eat more plant-based foods in a way that is healthy and satisfying.

I have always struggled with calling myself an athlete; I quit all team sports when I was a high school freshman and instead spent my time skateboarding and BMXing—endeavors that take significant athletic ability and skill, but are outside of what we think of as traditional sports. This eventually turned into mountain biking, commuting by bike, and road riding. Then after college I headed out from Huntington Beach, California, on a $100 road bike with my front wheel pointed toward my hometown of Bethlehem, Pennsylvania. Two months on the road in rural parts of the United States riding 85 miles (137 km) a day, mostly alone, taught me a lot about vegan nutrition, food access, and athleticism. I was hooked, and when I moved to California, I got involved in double centuries, which are 200-mile (322 km) road bike events. The progression then to Ironman, ultrarunning, and a 500-mile (805 km) nonstop bike race I did solo three times, was based more on adventure than being an athlete.

Around this time, in the mid-2000s, I witnessed Scott Jurek win the Badwater 135 (217 km) ultrarun twice, as a vegan, and realized that a vegan athlete was going to become a thing. The interest in the past decade has skyrocketed, and I believe that arrow is still pointing up. Way up.

Therefore it's an honor to bring my experience to this much-needed book. As I travel the world talking about vegan sports nutrition, people ask me an abundance of specific questions, and now we have all of the answers in one place. It's a tremendous undertaking and I cannot thank Enette enough for her expertise, attention to detail, and tremendous knowledge and experience. Our desire is for it to be useful and effective for many, many people. The evidence that one can eliminate or reduce animal products and still compete at a high level is there; the limiting factors are having the knowledge and applying it. Therefore you will find useful, practical steps alongside the charts, graphs, and research studies. For my contributions look for the "Vegan View" sections, along with a few stories here and there about vegan athletes I have worked with.

The Story of This Edition

This book is dedicated to vegetarian and vegan athletes in all sports and adventures, and of all ages and abilities—from the casual and recreational athlete to the world-class competitor—as well as to athletes who eat a plant-based diet and those contemplating a shift to one that is more plant-centered. It is also dedicated to Armed Forces and military personnel who serve through athletic endeavors. Its purpose is to help athletes gain or maintain optimal nutrition for peak performance as well as health. The advice is based on the latest scientific knowledge combined with practical experience from Enette's 30-plus years as a sport dietitian, scientist, and vegetarian recreational runner, cyclist, and now kayaker and yogi. It is enhanced by Matt's 15 years of experience as a public health dietitian, athlete, and vegan for over two decades.

As with the first edition, this book is designed to help you optimize your training, performance, and health through better food choices. The book reviews the latest information on fueling athletic performance and offers suggestions on how you—as a busy athlete—can easily meet your energy, carbohydrate, protein, fat, fluid, and vitamin and mineral needs through a plant-based diet. It contains sections that allow you to assess your current diet and tailor your food choices according to your training and wellness goals.

The book also ventures into many topics that periodically trouble athletes, including questions about muscle gain, vitamin and mineral supplements and ergogenic aids, the need for a translation of the latest nutrition lingo (including omega-3s, FODMAPs, anti-inflammatory foods, and the ketogenic diet), and the struggles associated with losing weight, gaining muscle, avoiding fatigue, and remaining injury free. In addition, the last two chapters focus on athletes who eat a plant-based diet while living and cooking in the real world (and a real kitchen). In fact, new to this edition is chapter 15, where we share our favorite simple but tasty and satisfying mostly-vegan recipes. In a nutshell, the book provides athletes who eat a vegetarian, vegan, or plant-based diet with the tools for making consistent food choices to optimize training, peak performance, and good health.

Keep the training and the faith!

1 | Gaining the Plant-Based Advantage

> I met my husband on a hilly century ride—a 100-mile (160 km) bicycle ride—in the mining country just north of Phoenix. After riding with him and his buddy for a few miles, he asked me—out of the blue—if I was vegetarian. I was taken aback at first and was almost offended. I nearly snapped back, "Do I look like a vegetarian?" He skirted the question at first, explaining that he, as a physician, had been reading some of Dean Ornish's work and that he was interested in the health aspects of vegetarian diets. He then told me that he had never known a vegetarian and finally replied, "Yes, you do look like someone who is healthy and might be vegetarian."
>
> The rest is history. I ended up dropping him somewhere around the 70-mile (112 km) mark and—after our first date at a vegetarian restaurant—he gave up flesh foods and despite getting older still kicks my butt in most athletic endeavors. I often wonder to this day, however, if it was just a lucky guess or if I somehow looked like I had the plant-based advantage.
>
> – Enette

Scientific evidence collected over the last 40 to 50 years has noticeably changed our understanding of the role of plant-based diets in human health and disease prevention. Vegetarian, or plant-based, diets appear to be advantageous over omnivorous, or meat-containing, diets for promoting health and longevity, suggesting that indeed there may be an advantage to eating more plant foods and eating little to no animal foods. Although our knowledge is far from complete regarding the benefits of vegetarian eating on the health and performance of athletes, it is clear that athletes at all levels can gain an advantage from following a plant-based diet (see box 1.1 for a definition of plant-based diet).

The topic of plant-based sports nutrition is becoming increasingly popular. It appears that ever since the publication of the first edition of this book, more and more athletes and active people are adopting plant-based diets. Many more are probably intrigued by the potential health and environmental benefits but may not know how or whether a plant-based diet is compatible with peak performance. Although we don't know exactly how many athletes are vegan, vegetarian, or semivegetarian, we do know that many well-known (and even not-so-well-known) athletes follow plant-based diets, including vegan ultramarathoner and seven-time winner of the Western States Endurance Run Scott Jurek; Olympic champion snowboarder Hannah Teter; six-time Ironman triathlon champion Dave Scott (vegan); former National Football League tight end Tony Gonzalez; former National Basketball Association center Robert Parish; former Mr. Universe Bill Pearl; mixed martial arts fighter Mac Danzig; tennis champions Martina Navratilova, Billie Jean King, and Venus and Serena Williams; and baseball legend Hank Aaron, just to name a few (for lists of other well-known vegetarian athletes, see www.therichest.com/sports/other-sports/top-10-vegetarian-or-vegan-athletes and https://vegetarian.procon.org/view.resource.php?resourceID=004527). New England Patriots quarterback Tom Brady also reports following a plant-based diet that contains small amounts of lean meat and poultry.[79]

We also have an idea that the percentage of athletes who follow plant-based diets is likely similar to that reported for the general population. Recent polls have estimated that approximately 3.3 percent of American adults are vegetarian (report never eating meat, fish, seafood, or poultry) or vegan (never eat eggs, dairy, or flesh foods),[1] whereas approximately 5 percent of high school students (grades 9-12) are vegetarian, which includes approximately 1 percent who are vegan.[2] The numbers for athletes are likely even higher when people who are mostly vegetarian—but eat fish or poultry on occasion—are included. For example, according to the estimates of the Vegetarian Resource Group,[1] an additional 14 percent of American adults eat vegetarian at more than half of their meals and 15 percent eat vegetarian at many of their meals but less than half of the time.[3] Furthermore, an estimated 36 percent of the U.S. population reports always or sometimes ordering vegetarian meals when eating out.[1] These results suggest that many more Americans may fall in the semivegetarian category. Many may even be contemplating vegetarianism. The numbers in the United States, however, are low compared to worldwide estimates. A household survey of budgets, expenditure, and living standards conducted in 29 countries suggested that about 22 percent of the world population is vegetarian.[4] One of the only published surveys of athletes found that as many as 8 percent of athletes participating in the 2010 Commonwealth Games reported following vegetarian diets and 1 percent reported following vegan diets.[5] These numbers are likely higher if we include those who consume a little bit of fish, poultry, and lean red meat.

Box 1.1

What Is Really Meant by Plant-Based Diet?

The use of the term *plant-based* diet has become popular over recent years along with other terms such as *plant-centered* or *plant-forward* nutrition. Like a lot of emerging nutrition and health terms, however, plant-based diet has no explicit definition and may mean anything from vegan to semivegetarian (or flexitarian). According to a recent article published in *Vegetarian Journal*,[12] the term "plant-based diet" evokes various ideas and images to different people, to different researchers, and to the media. In a recent One Poll Survey by the Vegetarian Resource Group, respondents were asked to state what plant-based diet means.[12] The survey found that 20 percent of respondents thought it referred to a vegetarian diet, 17 percent thought it referred to a vegan diet, 13 percent thought it referred to a whole-foods diet that could contain animal products, and 24 percent admitted to not knowing what this term meant. An evaluation of the research literature produced a similar array of definitions, with 74 percent of 80 research studies published within the past 10 years not explicitly defining the term.[12]

In writing this book, Matt and I define plant-based diet as an eating pattern and philosophy that is heavily or exclusively based on plant foods, such as cereals, grains, fruits, vegetables, legumes, nuts, and seeds, but it may include limited amounts of animal foods, including fish, poultry, and even more-sustainably raised red meat. We heavily emphasize that plant-based nutrition also means more whole foods. We do this for two reasons. First, we recognize that the need to be a "pure" vegan or vegetarian is a top reason many former vegetarians reverted back to meat eating. Second, we understand that placing greater emphasis on reductions in animal consumption by the public is likely to have a greater impact on human and environmental health and animal welfare than complete omission of all animal foods by only a few.[8] Within this context, we encompass a spectrum of plant-based patterns, as outlined in box 1.2, that ranges from vegan to vegetarian to semivegetarian. Our hope is that we support you in your athletic journey fueled by exclusively or mostly plant foods.

This chapter introduces the concept of plant-based eating, reviews the potential benefits of plant-based diets on health and performance, and offers tips—for those interested in a more vegetarian diet—on making the first steps toward gaining the plant-based advantage. For both veteran vegans and those who are new to following a diet free of animal-based food, this chapter is also intended to help strengthen your beliefs and practices—whether they can be documented scientifically or simply felt spiritually or intuitively. The ensuing chapters are intended to help you understand and overcome potential nutritional challenges and further you along your path to gaining the plant-based advantage. This advantage will help you feel and perform your best in your chosen sport or activity—whether it be running, cycling, swimming, soccer, tennis, golf, Olympic lifting, dancing, walking, or skateboarding. *Is* there a plant-based advantage? Matt and I truly believe there is. (See Matt's additional thoughts on the vegan advantage in this and later chapters.)

Vegan View: Ultrarunners Leading the Pack

In 2011, I attended the Javelina Jundred, a 100-mile (160 km) trail race in Arizona, to shoot a video project documenting vegan athletes. We were there to film Donovan Jenkins at his first attempt at the distance, but we quickly discovered he wasn't the only vegan at the event. As it turned out, the race organizers are also vegan and were more than happy to help our project! At the start, we ran into Catra Corbett, an ultrarunner who has run more than 100 races over 100 miles and has logged over 100,000 lifetime running miles (160,934 km). She's also been a vegan for more than two decades. Out on the trail, the third-place runner wore a "go vegan" shirt. Wow, we thought, veganism is huge among ultrarunners!

When we interviewed these runners, we found that many of them came to eating this way not for an athletic advantage, but for concern about animals and the environment. The positive impact that vegan eating had on their performance was an added, surprising bonus. Every runner we spoke to that weekend who ate a plant-based diet (I had a little time as I paced Donovan on the course for 26 miles [42 km].) spoke about quicker recovery times, an easier time keeping weight down, feeling lighter, and the most exciting benefit: getting to eat more food!

Since then, several running teams focused on plant-based diets have popped up, including the Strong Hearts Vegan Power team based in Syracuse, New York, the Humane League runners, and the No Meat Athlete chapters around the country. These runners are showing that a plant-focused diet and athleticism can go hand in hand.

Types of Athletes Who Eat Plant-Based Diets

The motivations for following a plant-based diet are numerous—for both athletes and nonathletes—and include health, environmental, ethical, ecological, religious, spiritual, economical, aesthetic, and other reasons that could include a meat allergy[6] brought on perhaps by a tick bite.[7] Yes, this is indeed a real occurrence! The most common reasons, however, are health benefits, animal protection, disgust of meat and animal products, and environmental concern.[8] Environmental concern in particular is becoming widespread as more and more people recognize that raising meat requires more land and natural resources than planting crops, and contributes more to the production of greenhouse gasses, including methane and carbondioxide.[9,10] A growing interest in the planet also appears to be true among athletes.[9] Not surprisingly, however, the variety in rationales means that athletes who eat plant-based diets do not hold the same beliefs or make the same food choices. Although it is common to categorize athletes who eat vegetarian or plant-based diets into groups based on food choices (see box 1.2), these categories don't always fit and may unnecessarily label people. This is because athletes who eat plant-based diets fall into a spectrum of eating philosophies and practices that aren't easily categorized. For example, two lacto-ovo vegetarian runners may have different philosophies about dairy products. One may consume several servings of dairy products per day, and the other may consume dairy only when it is found as an ingredient in prepared foods or offered as a dish of ice cream. These individuals may also elect to omit foods for quite different reasons, including animal welfare, acne, or lactose intolerance. Similarly, some vegans may be extremely strict, eliminating all commercially prepared foods that are processed with or contain animal derivatives (e.g., commercial bread or granulated sugar), and some will simply avoid foods of obvious animal origin and still train in leather athletic shoes. All are athletes who eat plant-based diets and all have unique beliefs, practices, and needs that are independent of arbitrary classification.

Although categorizing can serve its purposes—for example, in the food labeling of vegan products—I think it is more important that athletes understand how their individual philosophies and food preferences potentially influence their nutrient intake. That said, I also think it is important to include occasional fish and poultry eaters and semivegetarians in the ranks of vegetarian athletes. I wonder whether Tom Brady would agree, and I hope this will not rankle purists. In my experience training with and professionally counseling fellow vegetarian athletes, I have found that many elect to occasionally eat fish or poultry during holidays, when attending social events, or even if feeling

Types of Vegetarian and Plant-Based Diets

The following are the four major groups, according to the Vegetarian Resource Group:

- Lacto-ovo vegetarian: Does not eat meat, fish, or fowl; eats dairy and egg products.
- Ovo vegetarian: Does not eat meat, fish, fowl, or dairy; eats eggs.
- Lacto vegetarian: Does not eat meat, fish, fowl, or eggs; eats dairy products.
- Vegan: Does not eat any animal products, including meat, fish, fowl, eggs, dairy, and honey; most vegans also do not use animal products such as silk, leather, and wool.

In addition, the following categories can be considered plant based:

- Macrobiotic vegetarian: Avoids most animal-derived foods and emphasizes unprocessed organic foods.
- Pesco vegetarian: Does not eat red meat or fowl; eats dairy and egg products and fish occasionally.
- Pollo vegetarian: Does not eat red meat or fish; eats dairy and egg products and fowl occasionally.
- Semivegetarian (also called Flexitarian): Tries to limit meat intake.

insecure about their nutrient intake. One study of vegetarians living in Vancouver, British Columbia, found that 57 percent admitted to occasional intake of fish and 18 percent admitted to occasional intake of chicken.[11] Interestingly, a recent study of more than 11,000 adults in the United States found that 86 percent of individuals who had adopted a vegetarian diet at some point in their lives went back to eating meat, with nearly half claiming it was because it was too difficult to be "pure" in their diet choices.[8] On the other hand, many vegetarian athletes may want to move toward more strict practices. According to the study of the Vancouver vegetarians, 62 percent, including four of six vegans, reported that their diets had become more restrictive over time, and 53 percent planned additional changes that most frequently targeted a reduction in the use of dairy products.[11]

The Plant-Based Advantage

Many have felt the vegetarian, or shall we say plant-based, advantage. I felt it that first spring semester I gave up meat immediately after my first anatomy lab. Despite a nearly 7 pound (3.2 kg) weight gain, I felt better than I ever had. I noticed an improvement in my general well-being after changing to a vegetarian diet. Many of my clients over the years have also felt this, but, as you can imagine, it is difficult to pinpoint and is rarely mentioned in scientific literature. One study of Israeli athletes found that 60 percent of the female athletes reported an improvement in their general well-being after changing to a vegetarian diet.[13] This included experiencing fewer headaches.

Daniel, as described in the Bible, also felt it. After it was determined he was handsome, intelligent, and well trained enough to serve in the royal court, Daniel made up his mind that he did not want to become ritually unclean by eating the food and drinking the wine of the royal court. He went to the guard in charge of him and his three friends and said, "Test us for 10 days. Give us vegetables to eat and water to drink. Then compare us to the young men who are eating the food of the royal court, and base your decision on how we look." Ten days later, Daniel and his friends were described as looking "healthier and stronger than all those who had been eating the royal food" and were then allowed to "eat vegetables instead of what the king provided" (Dan. 1:8-16 Good News Bible). The feeling noted by Daniel perhaps summarizes why many major religions, excluding Christianity in general, emphasize vegetarian practices for spiritual reasons, healing, or meditation.

Historical records also tell us that many of the athletes of the ancient Olympics[14,15] as well as the Roman gladiators[16]—all images of strength, power, and endurance—may also have felt a vegetarian or plant-based advantage. Despite the fact that the most widely quoted account of an athlete of antiquity is that of the legendary wrestler Milo of Croton, who reportedly ate a gargantuan amount of meat, the diet of most ancient-Olympic athletes was most likely vegetarian.[14] Their diets, like that of most Greeks and Romans of the time, consisted mostly of cereals, fruits, vegetables, legumes, and wine diluted with water. When meat was consumed, it consisted mostly of goat (in Greece) and pig (in Rome) flesh.[17] In fact, the earliest Greek athlete whose special diet was recorded was Charmis of Sparta, whose training diet is said to have consisted mostly of dried figs.[15]

What Science Says

Unfortunately, we can't measure the full aspect of the plant-based advantage and prove, for example, that switching to a vegetarian diet will promote a greater sense of well-being or improve health in its full definition. This definition—derived from the Old English word for *hale*—includes being whole and hearty and of sound mind, body, [and spirit] and having the capacity to live, work, and interact joyfully with [nature] and other human beings.[18] We can, however, look at the scientific evidence supporting the advantage of plant-based diets compared to the typical Western diet on both physical health (from the perspective of disease risk) and performance. Admittedly, the evidence is much stronger for health advantages than for performance advantages. While this should be motivating by itself, there are also interesting indications that plant-based diets may aid in training and exercise recovery. This of course is no surprise to us!

Potential Health Benefits

Research has shown time and time again that vegetarians living in affluent countries enjoy remarkably good health, exemplified by less obesity,[19] high blood pressure, hyperlipidemia (elevated total and LDL cholesterol), heart disease, diabetes, dementia, and many cancers,[20-23] including colon and breast cancers. Some, but not all, studies suggest even greater health benefits of vegan diets (see table 1.1). Vegetarians also appear to live longer and healthier lives.[24] The reasons for these positive health effects, however, are difficult to pinpoint and may be related to the absence of meat, the greater variety and amount of plant foods, or other lifestyle practices associated with vegetarianism. Undeniably, evidence suggests that all three may be involved in the vegetarian advantage.[25]

Numerous studies have found that meat intake—particularly red and processed meat—is associated with increased risk for a variety of chronic diseases, including heart disease,[24,26-28,] diabetes,[27-29] and certain cancers,[24,30] including colon cancer.[31-33] In contrast, an abundant consumption of fruits and vegetables,[34-36] legumes,[21,37] unrefined grains,[36,38-41] and nuts [21,37] is consistently associated with a lower risk for many chronic degenerative diseases and, in some cases, even with increased longevity. In addition, research indicates that consumption of plant foods can dampen the negative effects of animal products. A recent study in rats, for example, observed that chlorophyll—found in green, leafy, and other vegetables—prevents tumor growth and toxic effects on cells that red meat has on colon cancer generation.[42]

TABLE 1.1   Key Findings From the Adventist Health Studies Conducted in Seventh-Day Adventists (SDA) in the United States and Canada

Cancer	Vegetarians have an 8% lower risk for all cancers and a 24% lower risk for gastrointestinal (GI) cancers; vegans have particularly lower risk (16%) for all cancers and a 34% lower risk for female-specific cancers, whereas lacto-ovo vegetarians have a 25% lower risk for GI cancer. In the Adventist 1 study, nonvegetarians have a 54% greater risk for prostate cancer and 88% greater risk for colon cancer.
	Frequent beef consumption increases risk for bladder cancer.
	Legume consumption reduces risk for colon and pancreatic cancers.
	Higher consumption of all fruit (and dried fruit) lowers risk of lung, prostate, and pancreatic cancers.
Dementia	Meat consumption increases the risk for dementia. People who eat meat are more than twice as likely to develop dementia. People who have eaten meat for many years are more than three times as likely to develop signs of dementia (AHS-1).
Diabetes	Vegetarian diets appear to lower risk for type 2 diabetes compared to nonvegetarian diets (AHS-1 and AHS-2). Self-reported diabetes among SDAs is less than half that reported by the general population (ADH-1). The prevalence of diabetes is lowest among vegans and vegetarians (2.9% and 3.2%) compared to pesco vegetarians (4.8%), semivegetarians (6.1%), and nonvegetarians (7.6%) (AHS-2). Risk of developing diabetes over a two-year follow up is 62% lower in vegans, 38% in vegetarians, 21% in pesco vegetarians, and 51% in semivegetarians.
Heart disease	Following a vegetarian, vegan, or fish-containing diet reduces the risk of heart disease. Vegetarian men have a 37% reduced risk of developing ischemic heart disease compared with nonvegetarians (AHS-1). Mortality from ischemic heart disease is 20% lower in occasional meat eaters, 34% lower in people who eat fish (but not meat), 34% lower in lacto-ovo vegetarians, and 26% lower in vegans compared to regular meat eaters.
	Beef consumption increases heart disease risk in men but not necessarily in women. Men who eat beef three or more times a week are more than twice as likely to have fatal ischemic heart disease than are vegetarians.
	Eating nuts and whole grains provides a protective effect against fatal and nonfatal ischemic heart disease in both men and women. People who eat nuts five or more times a week have approximately half the risk of those who eat nuts less than once a week.
	People who consume mainly whole-wheat bread have 59% lower risk for nonfatal coronary heart disease, and 89% lower risk for fatal heart disease compared to those who mainly consume white bread.
Hypertension	Following a vegetarian diet lowers the risk for hypertension. Vegans are 47% less likely than nonvegetarians to develop hypertension after adjusting for body weight and other confounders, whereas vegetarians are 14% less likely. Results are similar among black and white Adventists (AHS-2). SDA semivegetarians are 50% more likely to have hypertension than SDA vegetarians (AHS-1).
Metabolic syndrome (elevated serum triglycerides, elevated blood sugar, low HDL [good] cholesterol, elevated diastolic and systolic blood pressure, abdominal fat)	Vegetarians are less likely to have all of the components of metabolic syndrome except for lower HDL compared to nonvegetarians. The prevalence of metabolic syndrome is 25.2% in vegetarians, 37.6% in semivegetarians, and 39.7% in nonvegetarians (AHS-2).
Arthritis	Following a vegetarian diet lowers risk for arthritis. SDA vegetarians are at a lower risk for arthritis than nonvegetarians are (AHS-1).
Longevity and all-cause mortality	A longitudinal advantage is noted for those who follow vegetarian diets (AHS-1). Pesco vegetarians have a 19% reduced risk of all-cause mortality over the six-year period, followed by vegans (15% reduced risk), lacto-ovo vegetarians (9%), and semivegetarians (8%), with stronger effects seen in men than in women (AHS-2).

Combined data from the Adventist Health Study 1 (AHS-1) and the Adventist Health Study 2 (AHS-2) (23,24,28,45,46).

Another consideration is that meat-containing diets are probably not as safe as vegetarian diets when it comes to food poisoning, found commonly in undercooked or improperly processed or undercooked meats, and exposure to environmental contaminants, which can be concentrated in animal flesh. A recent study in France found that exposure to persistent organic pollutants, including polychlorinated biphenyls, polychlorinated dibenzodioxins, and polychlorinated dibenzofurans, was dramatically lower in the vegetarian population because of the nonconsumption of food of animal origin.[43] This is not to say vegetarians are immune to contaminants: E. coli and salmonella can be found in raw vegetables and sprouts grown with animal-based fertilizers and other toxins. In the French study, exposure to mycotoxins (e.g., found in peanuts), plant estrogens, and some heavy metals (aluminum, cadmium, selenium, nickel) was higher in vegetarians.[43]

The most recent evidence against red meat has revealed a link between heart disease risk through gut bacteria.[77,78] In a clinical trial, participants had 3 times higher levels of a molecule called TMAO (trimethylamine N-Oxide) when given red meat as the major protein source for 1 month compared to when provided either poultry or plant-based protein diets for the same amount of time.[78] TMAO is known to alter blood platelets and raise risk of developing blood clots, but recent research also suggests its production by gut bacteria

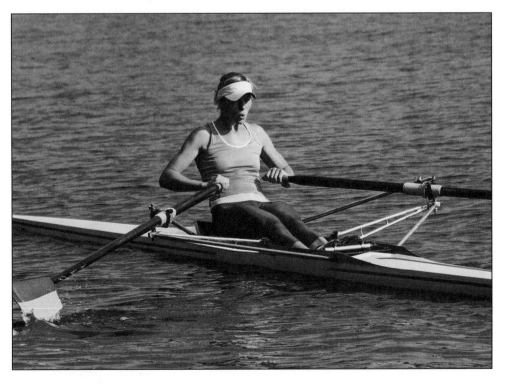

One of the most common reasons for eating vegetarian, especially among athletes, is general health benefits.

Anton Hlushchenko/fotolia.com

is increased and elimination by the kidney is dampened with diets high in red meat. Gut production of TMAO was lowered and kidney production higher when individuals followed plant-based protein diets high in legumes, nuts and grains, as well as when white meat was the main source of protein.

The beneficial effects of plant foods in the prevention of chronic diseases are, on their own merit, more definite than the detrimental effects of meat. In fact, large-scale studies among vegetarians and nonvegetarian Seventh day-Adventist populations have observed that more health benefits are linked to the protective effect of plant foods than the hazardous effects of animal foods.[24] In support of this thinking, findings from the Oxford Vegetarian Study and the Health Food Shoppers Study that were conducted throughout England and Wales found that vegetarians shared similarly lower mortality rates with health-conscious omnivores who regularly shopped at health food stores.[44]

Factoring out the lifestyle factors is a bit more difficult because vegetarians as a group tend to be more physically active, less overweight and obese, more health conscious, and perhaps less stressed than their meat-eating counterparts. They also are less likely to smoke and drink excessively. This presents a challenge for researchers assessing the relationships between diet and disease risk, because studies must adjust research data to account for these and other differences between vegetarians and nonvegetarians. Although major epidemiological studies attempt to statistically control for such confounding factors, study results are still often criticized because it is not possible to fully adjust for all lifestyle differences between vegetarian and nonvegetarian populations.

Fortunately, much data is available from two important long-term studies conducted by researchers at Loma Linda University in California. The Adventist Health Study I and II explored the links between diet, lifestyle, and disease among Seventh-day Adventists in California and Canada. What is particularly noteworthy about the Adventist Health Studies is that they were able to compare the health risks of vegetarians (who make up approximately 40% of the Adventist population), occasional meat eaters, and nonvegetarians in a population with generally similar lifestyle habits. Adventists, for example, attend religious services regularly and are health conscious. They do not smoke or drink alcoholic beverages and most avoid coffee and tea. Hence, findings for the study provide more powerful (or should we say less murky) evidence supporting the benefits of plant-based diets because the lifestyles of the vegetarians and meat eaters tend to be quite similar. The large number of participants studied—approximately 96,000 in Adventist Health Study 2—also allows for distinguishing small differences among vegetarians, vegans, and semivegetarians and between black and white individuals.[23] Of the cohort, 29 percent were lacto-ovo vegetarian, 8 percent vegan, 10 percent pesco vegetarian, 5 percent semivegetarian, and 48 percent nonvegetarian. Approximately 27 percent were black, and the majority of participants were white.

The findings from the Adventist Health Studies are summarized in table 1.1 on page 8. Collectively, the findings indicate that both increased plant foods and decreased animal flesh offer positive health advantages. Intriguingly, the Adventists believe that it is no coincidence that results independently emphasize the protective qualities of seeds such as nuts, beans, whole grains, and fruits because in the first chapter of the Bible, it reads that God said, "I have provided all kinds of grain and all kinds of fruit for you to eat but for all the wild animals and all the birds I have provided leafy plants for food" (Gen. 1:29 Good News Bible).

Potential Performance Benefits

Much less is known about whether plant-based diets offer training or sport performance advantages. Although a handful of studies in the early 1900s investigated the value of a vegetarian diet as a means of increasing physical capacity, most of these studies were not scientifically rigorous[47] (for example, they did not involve random assignment to a vegetarian or a meat-containing diet, or blinding the researchers to the study group) and in a few cases may have produced the answers the investigator or athlete desired, which was that a vegetarian diet is superior to a flesh-containing diet.

One of these studies, conducted by a professor of political economy at Yale University in the early 1900s, consisted of a series of endurance tests conducted on 49 men classified as flesh-eating athletes, flesh-abstaining athletes (vegetarian athletes), and sedentary flesh abstainers (vegetarians).[48] The endurance tasks involved holding the arms horizontally, performing deep knee bending, and doing leg raises (lying on the back) for as long as possible. The investigators found that vegetarian athletes had considerably more endurance than the flesh-eating athletes and that many of the untrained vegetarians were also able to out endure the flesh-eating athletes. In a similar type of experiment a few years later, a Belgian researcher determined that vegetarian students had greater endurance of the forearm than meat-eating students.[49] Forearm endurance was determined by measuring the maximum number of times the students could lift a weight on a pulley by squeezing a handle. The vegetarians performed an average of 69 reps, and the meat eaters performed 38 reps. [47]

The early research may have been provoked by reports that vegetarian athletes living in Europe and America were outperforming their meat-eating rivals and setting records in cycling, distance footraces, swimming, tennis, and the marathon[47] (see table 1.2). The United States' Will Brown, for example, who in the late 1890s switched to a vegetarian diet for health reasons, thrashed all records for the 2,000-mile (3,218 km) bicycle race. About 20 years later in 1912, a runner named Hannes Kolehmainen, one of the "Flying Finns," became one of the first men to run a marathon (26.2 miles [42 km]) in less than 2 hours, 30 minutes.[47]

Why the vegetarians seemed to demonstrate superior endurance performance is certainly intriguing, but, as the early investigators themselves noted, it may have been partially explained by grit and partially explained by the motivation of the vegetarians to outdo their meat-eating rivals.[47] This is probably something many of you reading this book fully understand. Another reason for the increased endurance of the vegetarians—which was not yet understood

TABLE 1.2 Early Feats of Vegetarian Athletes

Year	Athletic feat
1896	James Parsley led the London Vegetarian Cycling Club to victory over two nonvegetarian clubs. A week later he won the most prestigious hill-climbing race in England, breaking the hill-climbing record by nearly a minute. Other members of the club also performed remarkably.
1890s	Will Brown thrashed all records for the 2,000-mile (3,218 km) bicycle race, and Margarita Gast established a women's record for the 1,000-mile (1,609 km) race.
1893	The first two competitors to racewalk the 372 miles (599 km) from Berlin to Vienna were vegetarians.
1890s (late)	Eleven of the first 14 finishers in the 62-mile (100 km) foot race across Germany were vegetarian.
1912	Hannes Kolehmainen was one of the first men to complete the marathon in less than 2 hours, 30 minutes.
Early 1900s	The West Ham Vegetarian Society fielded an undefeated tug-of-war team.

Data from D.C. Nieman, 1999, "Physical Fitness and Vegetarian Diets: Is There a Relation?" *American Journal of Clinical Nutrition* 70 (1999): 570S-575S.

in the early 1900s—was that the carbohydrate content of the vegetarians' diet was most likely much higher than that of the meat eaters.[47] Higher carbohydrate intake (as will be discussed in chapter 3) would give the vegetarians an endurance advantage over their opponents. Other plausible reasons include the high phytochemical content of vegetarian diets in general and the potential of these diets to induce a slight serum alkalinity, which could be of benefit during intense exercise bouts.[50] Depending on food choices, a higher intake of magnesium[51,52] and dietary nitrates[53] may offer further performance benefits. Additional information on these factors is presented in chapters 8 and 11.

In recent years, however, the advantage in endurance performance noted in the early vegetarians has been less evident. Better-controlled comparisons have found that male and female athletes following vegetarian diets have aerobic, anaerobic, and strength capacities that are similar to their equally trained meat-eating counterparts.[13,54] One recent study of 46 vegetarian endurance athletes and their matched omnivorous teammates, however, revealed higher cardiorespiratory fitness in female but not male vegetarian athletes.[54] Randomized control trials—although few and far between—have also failed to find a benefit or detriment to aerobic or anaerobic performance as a result of switching to a vegetarian diet for as long as 12 weeks.[50] In one of these studies, the strength and endurance performance of eight male omnivorous athletes was unaltered when the athletes were randomly assigned to a lacto-ovo vegetarian diet for six weeks compared to their performance on a macronutrient-matched, meat-rich diet for six weeks.[55,56]

Indeed, even though science lacks proof that a vegetarian diet offers short-term advantage to athletic performance, this should not dissuade you from sticking to or starting a plant-based diet. Most of the studies have been short term and have focused simply on the completion of an exercise task under the controlled conditions of a laboratory. As athletes, we know that peak performance on the field or during a race draws on many things and often takes years of training (and eating) to achieve. We also know that well-being drives peak performance. Hence, to truly prove a benefit to athletic performance, scientists would have to somehow clone a group of athletes and compare how they performed over a lifetime as a vegetarian (or near vegetarian) and as a meat eater. Alternately, scientists could follow closely matched athletes who ate either meat or a plant-based diet to determine which group was more likely to perform better over the long run, and similar to the Adventist Health Studies, adjust for known confounding variables such as training, motivation, injury, and overall nutrition. Despite the elusiveness of this concept, however, we can focus on the potential benefits of a plant-based diet on recovery and, as mentioned earlier, its role in keeping us healthy as we train.

Potential Benefits During Recovery

Plant-based diets are abundant in vitamins and other plant chemicals called phytochemicals. Many of these compounds function as antioxidants and may protect against more than just cancer and heart disease.[57,58] Many are able to sequester reactive by-products—called free radicals—that are produced in muscle during strenuous exercise. While small amounts of these reactive by-products may serve as a signal to trigger various exercise-induced adaptations, excess radicals may promote exercise-induced injury to muscle proteins and contribute to muscle fatigue[59,60] and muscle soreness. The body has a complex defense mechanism that aids in eliminating free radicals; however, dietary antioxidants interact cooperatively with this system to help control and sequester free radicals. Theoretically, higher antioxidant intake on a plant-based diet may reduce exercise-associated oxidative stress and modulate immune function and inflammation.[61] Furthermore, the vegetarian diet is likely to promote higher intakes of the antioxidant vitamins (vitamin C, vitamin E, and beta-carotene) and other phytochemicals.[57,58,61] Studies have noted convincingly that vegetarians have higher circulating concentrations of the antioxidant vitamins[57,58,61] and possibly also higher levels of other beneficial phytochemicals. To this end, studies have also found that vegetarians experience less damage from free radicals to DNA (our body's genetic material) in the blood[62] and less lipid peroxidation, or damage by free radicals to lipid-containing structures.[63] Although research has not yet shown whether a vegetarian diet[61] protects against free-radical damage in muscle (as it does in blood), several studies have found that supplementation with certain antioxidants reduces damage to the lipid components in the muscle cell.[60,64] In agreement, several studies have found that consuming various fruit and vegetable juices, including tart cherries,[65-67] pomegranate,[68,69] black currant,[70] and a combination of black grape, raspberry, and red currant[71] as juice or concentrates, reduced exercise-induced oxidative stress and possibly also muscle soreness and damage. This does not mean that other fruits don't offer similar effects, just that they have yet to be studied.

Hence—although additional studies are needed—high levels of dietary anti-oxidant vitamins or phytochemicals may protect the muscles against free-radical damage[61] or assist in reducing inflammation.[72,73] This idea has been around for quite some time. In fact, in my days as a postdoctoral student at the University of Alabama at Birmingham, we were interested in the exercise-overstress response.[74] With exercise overstress, the muscle becomes damaged and is temporarily unable to produce high levels of energy using oxidative processes until recovery, which can take several weeks to several months depending on the severity of the initial performance effort.[74] While attempting to re-create this overstress response, we measured many athletes before and after a marathon race or a bout of strenuous up and down jumping in the laboratory and found that we were able to induce overstress only in the nonvegetarian subjects. The vegetarians were somehow protected, which we hypothesized was caused by the high levels of antioxidants in their diets.

Do Only Purists Gain the Advantage?

Perhaps a final lingering question is whether athletes have to be purists to gain the vegetarian advantage. I think not. Although in some areas, an exclusively plant-based diet appears to produce a health advantage over dairy-containing diets, there are also cases—as will be reviewed in this book—in which con-suming dairy or small amounts of other animal foods, such as fish, may make it easier to meet daily nutrient requirements without the need for dietary supplements. In fact, in the previously mentioned U.S. survey, pressure to be "pure" was the most common reason former vegetarians had gone back to eating meat.[8] Additionally, a health benefit from consuming a little fish often emerges in the literature, particularly related to all-cause mortality[23] and colon cancer.[75] Most of the potential health risks of red meat do not appear to hold true for poultry,[30,31] (other than the potential for developing antibiotic-resistant bacteria from conventionally raised chicken[76]), and studies looking at wild game consumption are lacking. This thinking, however, does not imply that animal foods are needed in any way, shape, or form for athletes to meet their nutri-ent needs. It does mean, though, that athletes who choose to eat a little fish, chicken, or even red meat now and again are probably just as likely to reap the major advantages of vegetarianism as the purists are. The important thing is simply that you eat a diet containing ample cereals, grains, fruits, vegetables, and legumes and limit the consumption of animal foods to fit your health and personal philosophy. The careful selection of animal foods raised locally and in a more sustainable and humane fashion should also be a consideration for athletes opting to eat some dairy or meat.

To further illustrate the need for flexibility and the downside to striving for purity, I know for certain that there are times when many vegetarian athletes have to decide whether to pick the pepperoni off the pizza. I remember returning from my first double-century bicycle race (320 km) and finding that what I was most craving—hot vegetable soup—contained floating specks of beef. I also remember my racing partners eating hot chili after a rainy March 10K, which prompted me to drive for miles in search of a vegetarian bowl, which I never found. Most notably, I remember asking the race director of a local bike ride to order vegetarian pizza, only to find that the faster guys had devoured it, leaving only pepperoni, before I crossed the finish line. Although many of us swear we would never eat meat-contaminated pizza, others would pick those pieces of pepperoni off the pizza when driven by hunger (although they might dab the pizza with a napkin to remove any remaining highly saturated pepperoni fat). Yes, the world would be much better for athletes who eat a plant-based diet if race directors just ordered vegetarian for everyone, but in the real world, our decision to occasionally eat meat-contaminated pizza does not make us less-healthy athletes even though we eat plant-based diets. Indeed, some flexibility may help us socialize better with our nonvegetarian teammates, as long as we draw the line when they are headed to Bubba's Pork House for breakfast.

Going and Staying Meatless

Although many readers have been vegetarian for some time, others may be new to plant-based eating or just at the point of contemplating going completely meatless. If you are not yet experiencing the benefits of a vegetarian diet and are ready to move in this direction, the information presented in box 1.3 may be helpful for making an easy and gradual transition. The slow transition—which is generally recommended by dietitians—provides a comfortable progression that allows you time to find new ways to meet nutrient needs without meat. The goal is to make changes that you can live with and that are nutritionally sound. The alternative is the "become-vegetarian-overnight" approach that I jumped into years ago. Although this approach works for some, it often does not give athletes enough time to educate themselves on plant-based food choices and patterns. Interestingly, the aforementioned study of former vegetarians[8] found that an abrupt transition (over days or weeks) to vegetarianism was a likely reason many reverted back to meat eating, with some not having time to develop full buy-in to the vegetarian philosophy or not understanding how to cook and replace the flavor and texture of meat. Box 1.3 may also be help-ful if you choose the abrupt transition; however, you will have to be diligent in assessing your daily diet and finding ways to satisfy your nutrient needs. If you don't, you may experience a decline in your health and performance caused by poor nutritional choices, not the vegetarian or vegan diet. Remember that to gain the plant-based advantage, you have to eat soundly.

The remaining chapters of this book are packed with information and practical how-tos, whether you are an athlete new to, or transitioning to, or a veteran of, a plant-based diet. They are designed to help you gain the vegetar-ian advantage, avoid common (and even not-so-common) dietary pitfalls and

Box 1.3

Steps for an Easy Transition to a Vegetarian Diet

1. Take stock of your current diet.

- Make a list of the foods and meals that you normally eat.
- Identify the foods and meals that are vegetarian, and build from these as a foundation. Examples include spaghetti with marinara sauce, bean burritos, and cheese sandwiches.
- Plan to eat a vegetarian meal several times a week using foods you know and enjoy.

2. Add more vegetarian meals by revising favorite recipes that are meat based.

For example, chili can be made using beans, textured vegetable protein (TVP), or tofu in place of ground beef. The beef in spaghetti sauce can be replaced with TVP or sautéed vegetables.

3. Expand your options by finding new recipes in cookbooks and online and trying different products from the store.

Many vegetarian meals can be made without a recipe and without much time in the kitchen. Try seasoned-rice mixes, spaghetti with sauce from a jar, vegetable chow mein, burritos with canned refried beans, and vegetarian baked beans with rice or quinoa. Try various brands of vegetarian burgers and meatless hot dogs. Also check out chapters 14 and 15 for additional ideas.

4. Make a list of vegetarian meals that you can eat away from home.

Inventory your options at the cafeteria, nearby restaurants, and convenience stores. Look for vegetarian soups, salads, pasta salads, pasta primavera, vegetable pizza, and baked potatoes. Chinese, Thai, Indian, and Middle Eastern restaurants offer numerous vegetarian entrees. Choices from a convenience store may include a bean burrito or a microwavable frozen entree supplemented with fresh fruit or veggies.

Plan vegetarian meals to go using leftovers from a home-cooked or restaurant meal. Other ideas for portable vegetarian meals include bean or vegetable soup in a thermos, peanut butter and banana sandwiches, bean dip with pita bread or crackers, and cheese with bread and fruit.

5. Eliminate meat at breakfast.

Try some of the meat analogues that look and taste like bacon or sausage to make the change easier.

6. Take stock of your menu once again.

Do your meals include . . .

- a variety of grains, legumes and soy products, vegetables, and fruits?
- some fresh fruits and vegetables daily? (Aim for at least 5 servings per day.)
- primarily whole grains with little processing? (Aim for 6-11 servings per day.)

© 2001, Vegetarian Nutrition Dietetic Practice Group, a Dietetic Practice Group of the Academy of Nutrition and Dietetics. Adapted with permission.

fine-tune your diet so that you can feel and train your best. Only then can you perform optimally. The last two chapters focus on guiding you as you learn to prepare simple and flavorful vegan or vegetarian recipes to fuel your training, performance, and health. We know that taste and cooking skills are important for gaining and keeping the plant-based advantage. Eat on!

2 | Getting Adequate Calories From a Plant-Based Diet

Nathan is a recreational mountain biker who is married and has two kids. He stumbled on plant-based eating for disease prevention after listening to a popular athlete's podcast. He decided to go all in by completely removing animal products and oil from his diet and limiting calorically dense plant foods like nuts and seeds. He saw fast results, losing 20 pounds (9 kg) in two months. His family got on board and was happy to be eating healthier and exploring new foods.

But after the initial bump in his fitness that came with the weight loss, his output plateaued. His energy levels dropped and he started to second guess his dietary change. Was it a lack of protein, like his friends teased him about? Or low iron levels?

It turns out that Nathan simply was not consuming enough calories to fuel his workouts. His dietary switch created a caloric deficit that enabled weight loss but hindered physical output. This negative balance affected his training, but fortunately, the solution was not technical: just needed to eat more food. Nathan loved huge salads made with a variety of raw veggies, but his salads did not contain many calories despite the large volume of food. The first adjustment was adding nuts, seeds, and homemade nut butter–based dressings. This increased the caloric density while allowing him to eat his favorite meal for disease prevention. The next adjustment was to increase his serving sizes for grains and beans and make space for snacks and smoothies. At first, Nathan was apprehensive about weight gain, but he soon realized the benefit of properly fueling his workouts and committing to a well-rounded dietary approach.

– Matt

Meeting energy needs is the first—yet often neglected—nutritional priority for all athletes. However, discussions about meeting energy needs are usually not a priority unless the athlete needs to lose or gain weight or is vegetarian. Although I sometimes find the latter amusing, I usually find it frustrating. During my years of practice, I have found that certain athletes—vegetarian or not—have trouble meeting energy needs. Typically, the athletes who struggle to meet energy needs have excessively high energy expenditures and make food choices that are bulky or too high in fiber. Many also have hectic schedules that do not allow enough time to cook or eat. A vegetarian diet low in energy-dense foods can contribute to the problem. Therefore, this chapter focuses on enhancing your understanding of your own energy needs, why neglecting these needs over the long run may be a recipe for disaster, and how you can meet these needs on a plant-based diet.

Energy, Calories, and Joules

In the United States, the term calorie and energy are often used interchangeably. Elsewhere, the joule is used in place of the calorie. Calories and joules are simply terms used to quantify energy (see box 2.1). Skipping the hardcore thermodynamics lecture, the body releases the energy stored within the chemical bonds of certain foodstuffs we know as carbohydrate, fat, protein, and alcohol, and temporarily traps this released energy within the chemical bonds of molecules called adenosine triphosphate (ATP) and creatine phosphate (PCr) (Some heat is released at the same time.). The energy stored within ATP and PCr is used to fuel muscle and other energy-generating activities in the body, ultimately releasing heat energy. The overall process is similar to using wood to fuel a fire and generate heat, except that instead of using the energy

---

Box 2.1

Calories and Joules

The calorie we refer to when we discuss the energy content of food is really a big calorie, or a kilocalorie.

A kilocalorie is the amount of heat required to raise 1 liter of water 1 degree centigrade from 14.5 to 15.5 degrees Celsius. The joule is the international unit of work or energy. It is the work done by a force equal to 1 Newton acting over a distance of 1 meter. The kilocalorie is equivalent to 4.2 kilojoules.

Obtain weight in kilograms (weight in pounds divided by 2.2). Estimate daily energy expenditure (DEE) by multiplying body weight in kilograms by the approximate energy expenditure factor from table 2.1 (kcal/kg/day). The factors vary for men and women and by perceived overall activity level: moderate, heavy, or exceptional. For example, a 52-kilogram female athlete who trains moderately has an estimated DEE of 1,924 kcal/day, whereas the same female athlete would have an estimated DEE of 2,652 kcal/day if she were undergoing an exceptional training regimen.

immediately, the body temporarily stores food energy as ATP. Thus, the body is able to break down the energy stored within the chemical bonds of carbohydrate, protein, fat, and alcohol in food and provide 4, 4, 9, and 7 calories per gram respectively. Vitamins and other organic matter do not provide energy to the body because their chemical bonds cannot be broken down and used as fuel. That said, a calorie and a joule are both simply units of energy similar to how inches and centimeters are units of length.

Energy Needs of Vegetarian Athletes

Daily energy needs vary considerably among individual athletes and depend on many factors. These factors include your sex, body size, body composition, training regimen, and nontraining activity patterns. If you are a growing child or teen athlete, additional energy is needed to support growth and maturation.

Over the past 20 or so years, researchers have learned a lot about the energy needs of athletes, thanks to the development of a technique called doubly labeled water.[1] This technique has allowed scientists to measure—outside the laboratory—free-living energy expenditure in athletes as they carry out their habitual training and daily activities. Using this technique, the energy needs of athletes have been shown to vary from approximately 2,600 calories per day in female swimmers[1] to nearly 8,500 calories per day[2] in men participating in the Tour de France bicycle race. In comparison, the energy expenditure of elite female runners and elite synchronized swimmers has been estimated to average approximately 2,800 calories per day[1,3] and that of elite lightweight female rowers,[4] English Premier League soccer players,[5] and elite male table tennis athletes[6] to average between 3,500 and 4,200 calories per day. The energy needs of a male ultramarathoner who ran around the coast of Australia averaged 6,320 calories per day.[7] While the energy expenditures of less-competitive, less-active, or smaller athletes are likely to be less than these examples, they are most certainly greater than the 2,000 calories for women and 2,500 calories for men used as reference intakes on food labels in the United States.

Vegetarianism does not necessarily affect energy needs. Nonetheless, several groups of researchers have found that energy needs at rest (termed resting energy expenditure, or REE) were 11 percent[8] to 21 percent[9] higher among vegetarians than their matched meat-eating counterparts. Although the researchers were not sure why the vegetarians had a slightly higher REE, they speculated that it was the result of the habitual high-carbohydrate composition,[8] which may have increased the activity of the sympathetic nervous system (SNS), or the higher polyunsaturated fat composition of the vegetarian diet.[9] Other researchers have hypothesized that long-term consumption of high-carbohydrate diets stimulates SNS activity, which is a known stimulator of REE, whereas diets higher in polyunsaturated fat may result in "leakier" cell membranes, which may be beneficial for obesity prevention.

Vegan View: Is a Whole-Food Plant-Based (WFPB) Diet Best for Athletes?

The WFPB diet focuses on eating whole plant foods while avoiding oil, refined grains, sugars, and drinking calories in the forms of smoothies and juices. This eating pattern is associated with a strong reduction in chronic diseases, especially heart disease and type 2 diabetes, and has been extremely successful for weight loss.

But is it ideal for athletes? We know that eating more whole plant foods has advantages, as documented throughout this book, but there is no research on whether strictly following WFPB is better than eating mostly whole foods. The WFPB diet works for weight loss because it is high in volume and low in calories, but for athletes who need 5,000 to 10,000 calories a day, consuming enough while following WFPB may be a challenge. Limited stomach capacity and an extremely high fiber intake could cause problems for some athletes, and fueling with only whole foods while training can be logistically complicated. You can carry only so many bananas and dates!

To combine WFPB with sports nutrition, consider using smoothies to consume more calories quicker, and trade out some whole grains for refined versions. Nuts, nut butters, seeds, and dressings or sauces made from these ingredients can boost calorie content. This way, fruit and vegetable intake remains high while freeing up stomach space to meet energy needs.

Estimating Your Energy Needs

Having a little knowledge of how much energy you need daily to function in your everyday activities as well as train in your given sport should help you meet your energy needs and consume a healthy, well-balanced training diet. Unfortunately, the doubly labeled water technique for measuring energy expenditure is not available to most athletes, unless you are lucky enough to live near a university or research institution that studies the energy needs of active people. Nevertheless, your daily energy expenditure (DEE) can be approximated in several ways. Before we begin, however, let's look at the components that make up DEE and define your daily energy needs.

In adults, the daily energy requirements are made up of various components, including the energy needed to maintain normal body functions, digest food, support training and nontraining activities, and handle the aftermath of exercise. Specifically, resting energy expenditure, or REE, is the energy required to maintain normal body functions such as breathing, heart beating, and brain function. The thermic effect of food (TEF) refers to the energy required to digest, absorb, and metabolize food. Although somewhat self-explanatory, the energy expenditure during training, or TEE, represents the energy expended during scheduled training, practice, and competition sessions that are specifically related to the athlete's sport, whereas the energy expenditure during

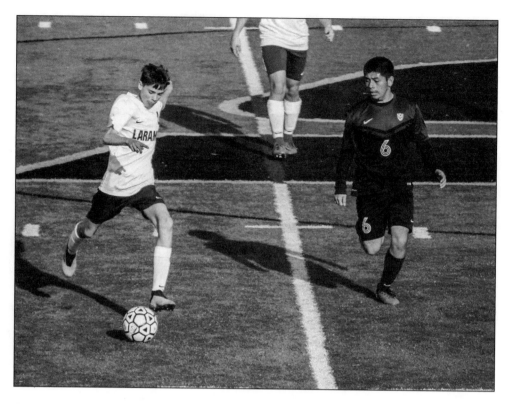

Teen athletes have higher energy needs due to growth as well as the energy demands of their sport.
Courtesy of Laura Tangeman.

nontraining activities, or NTEE, is the amount of energy needed to perform all physical activities that are not related to training. These activities include those associated with food preparation, health and hygiene, work, and leisure. Finally, the temporary increase in REE that occurs after a bout of exercise, termed the excess postexercise oxygen consumption, or EPOC, is partially caused by the increase in body temperature, which remains elevated for a time after exercise, as well as the additional energy required to remove lactate and resynthesize ATP and PCr.[10]

Just how much these components contribute to your daily energy expenditure depends on your activity level. In nonathletes, REE typically makes up about 65 percent of DEE, but it may contribute less than 50 percent of the total needs in athletes who are training heavily. Similarly, the contribution of TEE and NTEE varies with each athlete and depends somewhat on the athlete's nontraining occupation. For example, the NTEE of an athlete whose occupation requires little physical activity (e.g., student, bank associate, computer programmer) will make up a much smaller part of his or her DEE than the NTEE of an athlete whose occupation requires more physical activity throughout the day (e.g., construction worker, waitress, mail carrier delivering mail on foot).

An athlete's TEF and EPOC typically comprise much less of his or her DEE than the other components and, in fact, are often ignored in most methods of prediction because they are typically within the margin of error associated with the estimate. Nonetheless, research has suggested that an estimated 6 to 10 percent of the total energy consumed is required to digest and metabolize food (or 60-100 calories following the consumption of a 1,000-calorie meal), whereas an additional 6 to 15 percent of the total energy cost of a long, more vigorous training session (or 60-150 additional calories following a 1,000-calorie workout) may be needed as a result of EPOC.[10]

Although most of the components of energy expenditure need to be measured in a laboratory, a variety of prediction equations derived from laboratory data can be used to estimate DEE or the various components of TEE. Athletes can either directly estimate DEE or estimate DEE from the sum of its components. The easiest method is to directly estimate DEE by multiplying your body weight in kilograms by an activity factor that best describes your physical activity patterns (see box 2.2). By the direct method, your physical activity pattern lumps your training and nontraining activity levels into one package. For active and athletic people, the activity factors are classified as moderate, heavy, or exceptional. The activity level of ultraendurance athletes or Ironman triathletes is not categorized in this quick method. Nevertheless, this method can at least give you an approximate idea of your energy needs.

The second method for estimating your daily energy needs is to estimate each of the major components of DEE, and then add them together. Although

---

Box 2.2

Quick Calculation for Estimating Daily Energy Needs

Category	ENERGY EXPENDITURE (KCAL/KG/DAY)	
	Men	Women
Moderate: the activity level of a fitness enthusiast who works out for approximately 30 minutes, three or four times per week		
kcal/kg/day	41	37
Heavy: the activity level of an athlete who trains for 45 to 60 minutes, five or six times per week		
kcal/kg/day	50	44
Exceptional: the activity level of an athlete who trains one to two hours, six days per week		
kcal/kg/day	58	51

Data from M. Manore and J. Thompson, *Sport Nutrition for Health and Performance* (Champaign, IL: Human Kinetics, 2000), 473.

somewhat cumbersome, estimating DEE from its components accommodates more variation in activity patterns and is the method I have used for years to help educate athletes about their energy needs (see table 2.1). I have found that working through the calculations with athletes helps them realize why energy needs are so high—or why they are not as high as they think—and how changes in their training during the preseason or off-season should influence their energy intake. The activity also helps athletes realize how their activities

TABLE 2.1 Calculation of Daily Energy Needs

Energy expenditure component	Formula	Example: Female college soccer player who practices for 90 min and lifts weights for 30 min. Weight = 66 kg; body fat = 21% (lean body weight = 52 kg)	Example: Male cyclist who works as a musician and averages 150 miles (241 km) per week (average of 25 miles/day at 20 mph [32 km/h] for 75 min). Weight = 86 kg; body fat = 16% (lean body weight = 72.2 kg)
Resting energy expenditure (REE)*	REE = 500 + (22 × fat-free mass in kg)	500 + (22 × 52) = 1,644 kcal	500 + (22 × 72.2) = 2,088 kcal
Energy expenditure during nontraining physical activities (NTEE)	Light activity (student, bank associate, secretary) = 0.3 × REE	Assume light occupational activity (student): 0.3 × 1,644 kcal = 493 kcal	Assume moderate occupational activity (stands, moves, loads, and unloads equipment regularly, some sitting): 0.5 × 2,088 kcal = 1,044 kcal
	Moderate activity (sales clerk, fast-food worker, electrician, surgeon) = 0.5 × REE		
	Heavy activity (construction worker, waitress, mail carrier delivering mail on foot) = 0.7 × REE		
Energy expenditure during training (TEE)	Refer to physical activities charts (found in many nutrition or exercise physiology texts)	A 66 kg athlete uses ~7.2 kcal/min for soccer practice and 6.1 kcal/min for weight training: 7.2 kcal/min × 90 min = 648 kcal; 6.1 kcal/min × 30 min = 183 kcal	An 86 kg athlete uses ~18.4 kcal/min when cycling at a steady 20 mph (32 km/h) pace (hills and wind ignored): 18.4 kcal/min × 75 min = 1,380 kcal
Total daily energy expenditure (DEE)	REE + NTEE + TEE = DEE	1,644 + 493 + 648 + 183 = 2,968 kcal/day	2,088 + 1,044 + 1,380 = 4,512 kcal/day

*The Cunningham equation for estimating REE[13] has been shown to more closely estimate the actual REE of endurance-trained men and women[14] than other available equations. Calculation of total daily energy expenditure ignores increases in REE that may be the result of following a vegetarian diet (which may raise REE by approximately 11%), the thermic effect of food (which may increase DEE by 6-10% of energy intake), and excess postexercise oxygen consumption (which may add an additional 6-15% of the total cost of exercise) on days the training is vigorous. If you do not know your percentage of body fat, use a range of 5 to 15 percent for a man and 17 to 25 percent for a woman. Values for energy expenditure are for energy needs above resting and were estimated using values from appendix A by subtracting calorie expenditure per minute for lying quietly (top of table) from calorie expenditure per minute for the given activity.

of daily living, including sitting at a desk or with their feet propped up watching television, influence their daily energy needs.

Dangers of Inadequate Energy Intake

To perform optimally and maintain good health, all athletes need to strive for what scientists call a neutral energy balance. A neutral energy balance is simply a condition in which the sum of energy consumed from food, fluids, and supplements equals the energy expended during rest, daily living, and sport-related activity. Although some athletes may need to tilt the energy balance to gain or lose body mass, which is discussed in chapter 13, it is important for athletes to maintain this energy balance, particularly during the season and during times of high-volume aerobic or strength training.

Sufficient energy consumption is important for maximizing the effect of training, promoting adequate tissue repair, maintaining or promoting lean body mass, and meeting your overall nutrient needs. Many athletes do not realize that training, hard racing, and competition are catabolic (i.e., wasting) events, and that the nonexercise, or recovery period is when anabolic events such as tissue repair, remodeling, and growth occur. Inadequate energy intake during the recovery period can result in loss of, or failure to, gain skeletal muscle and bone mass and can increase the risk of injury, illness, and fatigue.[12] It may also lead to lower circulating concentrations of male and female hormones, particularly testosterone and estrogen, and result in menstrual cycle dysfunction in female athletes (Avoiding Pitfalls of Low Energy Consumption on page 27). Information concerning testosterone will be discussed in chapter 13.

Getting Adequate Calories From Plant Sources

Most athletes naturally consume enough calories while eating a vegetarian diet. You work out, you are starving, you eat. End of the story. For some athletes, however, it is not this easy and may even pose a constant struggle. You train, you are not in the least bit hungry, you grab a granola bar or banana, you rush to class or work, and suddenly—an hour later—you are ravenous. But, you have no food. Or, you exercise, you eat, you get full, you rush to work, and suddenly a few hours later you are hungry, and again you have no option to easily obtain food.

You can remedy this situation with a little knowledge and some planning. First, if you have not already done so, estimate your energy needs using one of the methods outlined in box 2.2 or table 2.1 and divide your requirements by three to estimate how much you would need to eat if you ate only three meals a day. If you were the female soccer player in the example in table 2.1, you would have to eat approximately 989 calories at each meal. If you were the male cyclist in the example, you would have to eat about 1,504 calories at each meal. Is this even possible? Probably yes if you stop at a fast food burger joint. Probably not on a high-carbohydrate, mostly whole-foods, plant-based diet! In working with athletes over the years, I have found that most people with high energy needs or hectic schedules or both do better if they "graze," or strive to eat five to eight small meals or snacks throughout the day.

Next take your estimated daily energy requirement and subtract either 750 calories (if your daily needs are fewer than 4,000 calories) or 1,500 calories (if they are more than 4,000 calories). Now divide the remainder by three. The 750 or 1,500 calories was subtracted to account for three 250- or 500-calorie snacks. Again, if you were the female soccer player, you would need to eat approximately 740 calories at each of three meals and consume three 250-calorie snacks (see box 2.3 for snacks that contain approximately 250 calories). If you were the male cyclist, you would need to eat approximately 1,004 calories at each of three meals and consume three 500-calorie between-meal snacks. There is no magic to the 250- or 500-calorie snack, however. You can play around with this to help determine a pattern that works for you. Athletes with early-morning or midafternoon training sessions might also try a plan consisting of four meals plus a snack, which allows an extra meal before or after the workout.

Second, assess your food supply. Do you have food on hand when you are hungry? If not, make it a priority to stock your pantry, desk drawer, workout bag, or car with healthy nonperishable snacks, such as dried fruit, nuts, crackers, and granola bars. If you have regular access to a refrigerator or freezer, stock it also. In working with college athletes, I noticed that most fail to eat enough fruit—even the vegetarians. I often suggest they go to the grocery store once a week and buy a combination of 21 pieces of fruit, three pieces for each day of the week. Each piece has approximately 100 calories and is full of vitamins, some minerals, and many antioxidants. You can also keep a bag of trail mix handy, or make your own by mixing different types of nuts and dried fruit. A nut butter and fruit preserve sandwich is also a quick fallback.

Third, if you eat regularly but feel you get full prematurely, assess your food choices. If your diet mimics the WFPB diet and your energy needs are high, you may need to select breads, cereals, and grains that are more refined about a third to half of the time, and also substitute fruit juice for some of your servings of fruits and vegetables. Although fiber is important, it is common for vegetarian athletes to consume two to three times more than the daily recommended intake of 20 to 38 grams. Diets with excess fiber are not harmful but are bulkier than more-refined diets and may prohibit the intake of high volumes of food and energy. Cyclists, for example, participating in a laboratory-simulated Tour de France had difficulty meeting their daily energy needs of 8,000 to 10,000 calories when they selected whole-grain and high-fiber foods.[15] Some scientists also question whether diets too high in fiber interfere with mineral absorption and the normal metabolism of various steroid hormones, including estrogen and testosterone.

Box 2.3

Grazing Foods That Provide Approximately 250 Calories

Granola bar

Two large or four small pieces of fruit

One large apple or banana with 1-1/2 tablespoons (24 g) of peanut butter

1/2 ounce (14 g) of nuts mixed with 1/2 ounce (14 g) of dried fruit (approximately 1/4 cup [37 g] mixture)

1-1/2 ounces (42 g) of raisins or other dried fruit

One peanut butter and jelly sandwich

2 ounces (57 g) of pretzels (regular or whole wheat)

One large bagel plus 1 tablespoon (15 g) of nut butter

1 cup (245 g) of nonfat yogurt, sweetened and with fruit

1 slice of vegan cheese and 1 ounce (28 g) of regular or whole-grain crackers

Two 2-1/2-inch (6.3 cm) oatmeal or raisin cookies and 1 cup (236 ml) of soy milk

1 ounce (28 g) toasted walnuts and 1/2 cup (102 g) sliced apple

8 ounces (236 ml) of chocolate almond milk, Ensure, or Boost, or other liquid supplement (Note: Boost has slightly fewer calories)

One healthy smoothie (recipe in table 14.5 on page 262, contains approximately 300 calories depending on ingredients selected)

Use the food label and the information available at the USDA Food Composition Databases site (https://ndb.nal.usda.gov/ndb) to estimate the energy content of your favorite snack foods.

Avoiding Pitfalls of Inadequate Energy Consumption

Many athletes—including vegetarian athletes—who are driven to either excel in their sport or improve their body image may consume energy inadequate to support the range of body functions necessary for optimal health and performance.[16] Insufficient energy intake reduces the amount of energy available for optimal body functions and may result in a variety of both physical and psychological complications. Relative energy deficiency in sport (RED-S) was recently coined by a special medical group of the International Olympic Committee and defines the cluster of complications that are observed in both female and male athletes.[12] These consequences may include (but are not limited to) menstrual disturbances, endocrine dysfunction, disordered eating, low bone density and other factors, including GI, renal, neuropsychological, musculoskeletal, and cardiovascular dysfunction.

Endocrine Dysfunction and Amenorrhea

Amenorrhea (or lack of regularly occurring menstrual cycles) may be experienced by any active woman but may be more common in athletes participating in endurance and aesthetic sports, including dance and gymnastics. Male athletes may also experience low testosterone and reduced libido, but these complications are less well studied. The mechanism responsible for disrupting normal menstrual function (and presumably lowering testosterone in men) is not well understood, but accumulating scientific evidence suggests that the disruption may be caused by low energy intake or a constant energy drain.[17] The hormone leptin, which is made by our fat cells, is thought to be one of the key signals that the body is not getting adequate energy.[18] Several studies in the 1980s, predominately in endurance runners, found that amenorrheic athletes report reduced intake of total energy, protein, and fat and higher intakes of dietary fiber than their normally menstruating teammates.[19-21] Although there is indication that menstrual-cycle disturbances may be higher in vegetarians[22] and vegetarian athletes,[20,23] these findings are not consistently reported[22,24] and can be explained by recruitment bias and study-design issues. For example, studies commonly define vegetarians as people who eat small quantities of meat and not necessarily a vegetarian diet.[25] Studies may also attract a biased sample of vegetarians because women with menstrual-cycle disturbances may be more likely to volunteer for a study on menstrual-cycle disturbances.[22]

Disordered Eating

Disordered eating is common among athletes who perceive that they can succeed by achieving or maintaining an unrealistically low body weight through excessive energy restriction or excess exercise or both. While disordered eating is more common in female athletes, male athletes can also develop disordered eating patterns.[12] Several studies have noted that disordered eating behaviors tend to be more prevalent among vegetarians.[26-29] Most experts believe this is because vegetarianism is seen as a socially acceptable way to reduce energy intake and *not* because being vegetarian causes eating disorders.[30,31] Study design issues may also play a role.[25,31]

Low Bone Density and Osteoporosis

Low circulating estrogen levels in female athletes associated with loss of monthly cycles combined with reduced energy and nutrient intake can predispose athletes to reduced bone density, premature osteoporosis, and increased risk of stress fractures or other overuse injuries.[12,16] A recent study of 175 young female athletes, for example, showed that those with menstrual dysfunction were at increased risk for stress fractures.[32] Low bone mineral density is also thought to be common in male athletes with low energy intake, but this issue is less well-studied.

Other Health and Performance Consequences

RED-S can have other serious nutrition and health consequences beyond disrupting reproductive function and bone health. Athletes with low energy intake and availability may develop nutrient deficiencies (including anemia), chronic fatigue, and reduced muscle gains with training and are also at increased risk of infection and illness. Additional information on meeting vitamin and mineral requirements is found in chapters 5 through 8. Athletes should also be aware that physiological and medical complications involving the heart, gut, kidney, and skeletal muscle may result from low energy availability. While their long-term consequences are not yet known, such imbalances in energy intake and expenditure compromise both optimal health and performance.

Evaluation and Treatment

Athletes experiencing any of the signs and symptoms of RED-S should talk to their personal or team physician. Loss of the menstrual cycle is unhealthy and is not a normal part of training. In many cases, the unintended consequences of RED-S, including reproductive function, can be restored by increasing energy intake.

If you are new to a plant-based way of eating, are striving to improve your eating pattern, or are simply overwhelmed, chapter 12 provides guidelines for customizing a meal plan to meet your energy and nutrient needs. The next three chapters offer information on fine-tuning your energy intake to ensure a balance between carbohydrate, fat, and protein fuel—which ultimately influences your performance and even your health. Read on!

3 Finding the Right Carbohydrate Mix

A first-year student on the women's soccer team came to see me a week after the first Friday–Sunday match of the season. She had been one of the coach's top recruits and had a good scoring record playing on the boys' (not girls') team in high school. Given her athletic history, she was thrown into college play early in the season alongside her more-experienced junior and senior teammates. "Ever since Friday it has been an effort to run," she told me. She went on to explain that she had been experiencing tiredness and fatigue all week that was isolated to her quads and was particularly noticeable after climbing stairs or running during practice. She denied any association with muscle soreness or tenderness and then added, "I don't know what is wrong. I felt great during preseason."

I inquired further and learned that the coach had kept her on the field for most of the match on both Friday and Sunday. I took a detailed diet history and was not surprised to find that her carbohydrate intake over the last few weeks had been low. Overall she made good food choices and had eaten adequately during preseason (as I had also observed during my close interaction with the team), but she had unconsciously cut back on her carbohydrate intake, particularly fruit, after classes had started. I estimated that she needed 411 to 462 grams of carbohydrate per day (8-9 g/kg body weight) to support her prolonged practices and nearly 90-minutes of playing time during games, but over the last week she appeared to be averaging only approximately 340 (6.6 g/kg body weight). I suspected that she was experiencing a classic bout of glycogen depletion, initiated by the weekend matches that she had not been able to remedy during the week. I sent her home with a prescription to eat a high-carbohydrate meal that night and gave her ideas for keeping her carbohydrate intake within the recommended range during the season. I never saw her in my office again, but the word from her coach was that she was playing and feeling well.

– Enette

As an athlete, you should consume a diet made up mostly of carbohydrate. Carbohydrate—in the right mix—is needed to properly fuel your muscles and brain and to optimize your training, performance, and health. Getting the right amount of carbohydrate fuel from a vegetarian diet is easy because it is naturally carbohydrate packed, and it can also provide the right mix at the right time. That said, however, vegetarian athletes are not immune to bad training days, most noted by fatigue, reduced precision, lack of power, and "dead" muscles. Bad training days may occur regularly if you don't understand the importance of carbohydrate fuel or know how much is required during each stage of your training. They may occur because you are not yet armed with the adequate carbohydrate know-how, even if you are already on a vegetarian diet. Thus, this chapter reviews how to make sure you get enough carbohydrate fuel for each stage of training and in the right mix. It will also discuss why you should not be fooled by the current low-carbohydrate craze, which can result in detrimental effects to your training and performance.

Why Athletes Need Carbohydrate

In chapter 2, we briefly discussed how your body gets energy from foodstuff and that it is the energy released from within the chemical bonds of carbohydrate, fat, and even protein that allows you to live. Although carbohydrate, fat, and, to a lesser extent, protein are used to fuel physical effort, carbohydrate is the only fuel that can sustain the moderate- to high-level effort that is required in most sports and athletic endeavors. Carbohydrate is also the preferred fuel for the brain and central nervous system and the only fuel these systems can use without weeks of adaptation that allows the brain to use products of fat metabolism, called ketones or ketone bodies.

As most athletes know, carbohydrate can be stored in skeletal muscle and liver in a starchlike form called glycogen. The body's glycogen stores, however, are limited. Glycogen can become depleted during continuous steady-state exercise lasting at least 60 minutes and during intense intermittent activities that include stop-and-go running, intense court play, and brisk hiking on difficult terrain. In fact, glycogen levels are likely depleted at the end of an intense soccer, basketball, or hockey game in team members who play the majority of the game.

Research has shown time and time again that muscle and whole-body fatigue develop at about the same time that glycogen stores become low. The reasons are relatively simple. First, active muscles that have been exhausted of their carbohydrate stores are forced to rely primarily on fat for fuel. Fat cannot be "burned" as rapidly or efficiently as carbohydrate, so you are forced to slow your pace and eventually stop exercising. What this means for you is that you produce less adenosine triphosphate (ATP) energy for a given amount of oxygen consumed when fat instead of carbohydrate is used as fuel. Second, the liver—exhausted of its carbohydrate stores—is now unable to serve as a storage reservoir for blood sugar and must struggle to maintain blood sugar level by converting protein (amino acid) sources to blood sugar. This process, termed *gluconeogenesis,* which means new-sugar formation, is slow and typically cannot keep pace with the rate at which the exercising muscle takes up sugar. The result is often low blood sugar, which is characteristically accompanied by lightheadedness, lethargy, and overall fatigue.

Although the body's enzymes—machinery for making blood sugar from amino acids—are typically regulated through training, athletes at any level can experience low blood sugar. Most likely you have experienced this feeling yourself—at least once—which in some athletic circles is called *bonking* or *hitting the wall.*

Carbohydrate for Optimal Performance

Diets high in carbohydrate are important in most sports because they maintain glycogen stores in muscles and the liver and also affect the ability to adapt to training.[1] Extensive research conducted in this area has found that high-carbohydrate diets prolong exercise time before fatigue and help maintain power output during both continuous and highly intense intermittent exercise,[2] including the intermittent variable-speed running common in many team sports.[3] Overall, diets rich in carbohydrate increase your capacity to exercise longer before exhaustion and maintain your ability to sprint toward the end of exercise. For endurance athletes, this means you will be able to maintain a faster pace for longer and better preserve your sprinting potential at the end of long training runs or races. A recent study highlighted this performance benefit in male adolescent runners asked to complete a 10K race after consuming a high- (7.1 g carbohydrate/kg body weight), moderate- (5.5 g/kg) or low-carbohydrate (2.5 g/kg) diet for two days before.[4] The high-carbohydrate diet allowed for higher running speed in the final 400 meters of the 10K race, and produced better overall performance than did the lower carbohydrate diet.

For athletes involved in stop-and-go sports such as soccer, football, rugby, volleyball, basketball, tennis, and hockey, this means you will be able to play (or practice) longer before feeling fatigued and also maintain your ability to sprint, jump, slam, or tackle at the end of a game. Fewer studies, however, have attempted to evaluate the benefit of an overall high-carbohydrate diet on performance during stop-and-go team sport. Most of those studies have been in soccer (known as football outside the United States). For instance, a study conducted at the Karolinska Institutet in Stockholm, Sweden, in the late 1990s found that male soccer players performed approximately 33 percent more high-intensity exercise movements during a 90-minute soccer game with four players to a side when they consumed a high- compared to a low-carbohydrate diet.[5] A similar, more recent study found that male professional soccer players covered more distance at all speeds (from jogging to all-out sprinting) during a typical 11-to-a-side soccer match when they followed a high-carbohydrate diet that provided 8 g carbohydrate/kg body weight, compared to when they followed a low-carbohydrate diet that provided only 3 g carbohydrate/kg body weight.[6]

Also of interest to athletes is the fact that carbohydrate can maintain an optimal bioenergetic state, the balance between high-energy creatine phosphate (PCr) and its breakdown products, in exercising muscles longer than fat can.[7] This could ultimately affect regeneration of ATP for the ATP–PCr system. As discussed in chapter 2, this energy system is used primarily for power and

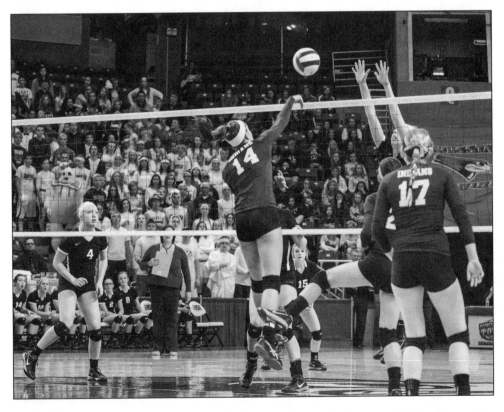

A vegetarian diet rich in a variety of carbohydrate sources can help prevent fatigue toward the end of a game.

speed activities that last less than 10 seconds, such as sprinting, jumping, serving, spiking, blocking, tackling, digging, and batting.

In a study conducted early in my career, my colleagues and I had active men and women follow a vegetarian diet that was either rich in carbohydrate (7.5 g carbohydrate/kg body weight) or low in carbohydrate (1.5 g carbohydrate/kg body weight) for five days.[7] Both diets met the subjects' energy requirements and were randomly assigned based on a coin toss. The subjects exercised their quadriceps muscles on a device similar to a knee-extension machine, and the exercise got progressively more difficult every two minutes. While the participants were exercising, we measured the bioenergetic state of their muscle using a magnetic resonance imaging (MRI) machine. This technique, called magnetic resonance spectroscopy, allowed us to study muscle metabolism without taking a muscle biopsy. The participants were able to exercise an average of 5 minutes, 40 seconds when they followed the carbohydrate-rich diet and an average of 5 minutes, 10 seconds when they followed the carbohydrate-poor diet. Most notably, we found that the PCr concentrations in the working muscles were preserved for longer on the carbohydrate-rich diet. Had this been an athletic competition, the high-carbohydrate diet may have allowed the competitors to get in an extra jump, punch, jab, or dig. Who knows how it would have helped in double overtime.

Determining Carbohydrate Needs

Optimal carbohydrate intake depends on several factors, including your body size, the fuel demands of the sport (or sports) you participate in, and your training adaptation and body composition goals.[1,8] Determining exactly how much you need involves trial and error and is likely to vary according to your training and competitive season.

Under the umbrella of the most recent recommendations, it is suggested that athletes periodize their intake over the week and according to training cycles of the seasonal calendar. As outlined in table 3.1, athletes should strive for higher carbohydrate intakes of 6 to 10 grams per kilogram of body mass per day and at least 12 grams per kilogram during times of higher training volume and intensity. They may have lower demands of only 3 to 5 grams per kilogram of body mass per day when performing low-intensity or skill-based training. In addition, at times during training, lower carbohydrate intake may enhance training adaptation or weight loss over the short term. Additionally, whether you aim for the upper or lower end of the range will also vary among athletes and depends somewhat on your total energy requirements; some athletes simply burn more carbohydrate and thus have higher demands (even when they are off the court) than other athletes have. Refer to table 3.1 to estimate your daily carbohydrate requirements.

TABLE 3.1 Estimating Daily Carbohydrate Needs

Enter your body mass (weight) in kilograms (weight in pounds divided by 2.2).	_____ kg *(line a)*
Enter estimated range of carbohydrate needed to support your current level of training and performance (see bullet points). <ul><li>Light-intensity or skill-based training: 3-5 g carbohydrate/kg</li><li>Moderate exercise program (e.g., ~1 hr/day): 5-7 g carbohydrate/kg</li><li>Endurance program (e.g., 1-3 hr/day of moderate to high-intensity exercise): 6-10 g carbohydrate/kg</li><li>Extreme exercise commitment (e.g., >5 hr/day of moderate to high-intensity exercise): 8-12 g carbohydrate/kg</li></ul>	_____ to _____ g/kg *(line b1) (line b2)*
Multiply *line a* by *line b1* to get the estimated lower range.	_____ g carbohydrate/day
Multiply *line a* by *line b2* to get the estimated upper range.	_____ g carbohydrate/day
You may need to meet or exceed your estimated upper range on the day before or after (or both) a particularly vigorous or long training session or competition.	

Adapted from L.M. Burke, A. Hawley, S.H.S. Wong, and A.E. Jeukendrup, "Carbohydrates for Training and Competition," *Journal of Sports Sciences* 29, suppl. 1 (2011): S17-S27.

Estimating Carbohydrate Intake

Every athlete should count carbohydrates at least once. This exercise helps you determine whether you are meeting your estimated needs and forces even vegetarians to learn a little more about which foods are the richest sources of carbohydrate. Knowing carbohydrate sources is also useful in assuring that you consume adequate carbohydrate before, during, and after exercise, which is discussed in chapter 9.

To give carbohydrate counting a try, simply pick a day or two that is representative of your intake and keep a running tally of the carbohydrate-containing foods and beverages you eat and drink. All foods except cheese, oils, and meat contain countable amounts of carbohydrate. Remember to include sport drinks and supplements consumed during your workout. The carbohydrate content of selected vegetarian foods is listed in table 3.2. Serving sizes are listed according to the recommendations in United States Department of Agriculture's (USDA) MyPlate (see appendix B or www.choosemyplate.gov). This information, along with the food label (which in the United States and other countries lists the carbohydrate content of most foods in grams per serving), should give you an idea of whether your intake is close to your recommendations. An example of a carbohydrate-counting log is shown in table 3.3.

Once you have tallied your daily needs, compare it to your estimated needs (table 3.1). If you are meeting your needs and are feeling strong, congratulations! If you are falling short, try to add carbohydrate foods for a week or two and see how you feel. If you notice no difference, your diet may be just fine. The

TABLE 3.2 Approximate Carbohydrate Content of Various Foods and Beverages

Food	Portion	Carbohydrate (g)
GRAIN EQUIVALENTS		
Bagel	Mini bagel	15
Bagel	Large (3-4 oz)	45-60
Biscuit	Small (2 in. diameter)	15
Bread, sliced	1 slice	15
Cornbread	1 (2 in. cube)	15
Crackers, whole wheat	5 crackers	15
Crackers, rounds or squares	6 to 8 crackers	15-20
English muffin (or bun)	1/2 or 1 side	15
Grains (most) including barley, bulgur, couscous, farrow, polenta, quinoa	1/3 to 1/2 cup	15
Muffin	Small (2-1/2 in. diameter)	15-20
Oatmeal	1/2 cup (1 packet of instant)	15
Pancake	4-1/2 to 5 in.	15
Pasta	1/3 cup cooked (1 oz dry)	15
Popcorn	3 cups, popped	15
Ready-to-eat cereal	1/3 to 1-1/4 cup (varies)	15-20
Rice	1/3 cup cooked	15
Tortilla, corn or flour	1 small (6 in.)	15
Wild rice	1/2 cup cooked	15
VEGETABLES		
Broccoli	1 cup cooked	5-10
Greens (collards, mustard, turnip, kale, spinach)	1 cup cooked	5-10
Salad greens (lettuce, spinach, and so on)	2 cups raw	5-10
Carrots, winter squash, pumpkin	1 cup	15
Sweet potato	1 cup	30
Beans, peas, lentils	1 cup	30-45
Corn	1 cup	30
Potato, baked or mashed	1 medium or 1 cup	30
Other vegetables (cucumber, asparagus, green beans, mushrooms, onions, tomatoes)	1 cup raw or cooked	5-10

Food	Portion	Carbohydrate (g)
FRUITS		
Fruit, all	1 cup	15
Orange, peach, pear	Medium	15
Apple, banana	Large	30
Fruit, dried	1/3 to 1/2 cup	60
Fruit juice, lemonade	1 cup	30-45
MILK AND YOGURT		
Milk, plain yogurt	1 cup	12
Yogurt, sweetened and flavored	1 cup	40-45
SPORT AND DISCRETIONARY FOODS		
Fluid-replacement beverage	1 cup	15-19
Soda	12 oz	40-45
Sport bar	1 bar	40-60
Sport bar, high protein	1 bar	2-30
Sugar	1 tbsp	15
Jelly, jam, honey, preserves	1 tbsp	15

Note: Developed based on MyPlate serving equivalents for grains, vegetables, fruits, milk and discretionary calorie; carbohydrate content approximated according to the Dietetic Exchange List for Meal Planning, 2003, and selected food labels. Refer to appendix F for guidance on converting English units to metric.

volleyball player whose carbohydrate log is presented in table 3.3 was asked to add a few more servings of carbohydrate at dinner after it was determined that her log accurately reported what she ate and her portion sizes. Finally, if you are falling short and feeling tired, fatigued, or dead legged, by all means start counting carbohydrate daily until eating a higher-carbohydrate diet becomes second nature.

Carbohydrate counting is also particularly helpful when you are bumping up the volume or intensity of your training, or are entering an intense competitive season. For best results, counting carbohydrate during these times should be combined with the use of a training log or performance feedback from a coach or training partner. You may, for example, note that low carbohydrate intake on a particular day was followed by poor running, lightheadedness, or excessive moodiness during or after a training session. Occasional carbohydrate counting may also be useful to athletes prone to weight gain because consuming excessive calories—even in the form of carbohydrate—can result in weight gain.

TABLE 3.3 Sample Log for Counting Carbohydrate

Food	Carbohydrate (g)
1-1/2 cups cornflakes (3/4 cup = 1 oz serving)	44
1 cup 1% milk	12
12 oz (1-1/2 cups) orange juice	45
White bread, 2 slices	30
2 tbsp peanut butter	—
1 can (~2 cups) fruit cocktail in light syrup	60
1 large handful (~1 cup) grapes	30
Jelly beans (~2 oz)	54
1/3 cup granola	15
1/4 cup almonds	—
2 cups vegetarian chili (contains ~1 cup beans topped with 1 cup onion, green peppers, and tomato sauce combined)	30-45 5
~2 oz cheddar cheese	—
15 saltine crackers	30
Total	355-370

Note: Reported daily carbohydrate intake for a 141-pound (64 kg) female volleyball player involved in off-season training. Her carbohydrate goal range was 384 to 448 grams of carbohydrate per day (6-7 g carbohydrate/kg body mass). Carbohydrate counting is most accurate if portion sizes are accurately measured and food labels are used to supplement the information presented in table 3.2. Refer to appendix F for guidance on converting English units to metric.

A study conducted at the University of Birmingham in the United Kingdom illustrates how the carbohydrate level of your diet might affect your training and mood, which, in addition to your teammates or training partner, may even be detected by your significant other, children, or coworkers.[9] Researchers asked seven trained male runners to perform two 11-day training periods in which training was intensified over the last 7 days of the 11-day session. During one period, the runners consumed a moderate-carbohydrate diet that provided 5.4 grams of carbohydrate per kilogram per day. During the other period, they consumed a high-carbohydrate diet (8.5 g carbohydrate/kg/day). The order of the diets was randomly assigned. The researchers found that although some aspects of the athletes' mood and performance were negatively affected by the intensified training, the high-carbohydrate diet better maintained the athletes' mood and endurance performance (measured during a 10-mile [16 km] outdoor race) over the course of the 11-day training period. They concluded that a carbohydrate diet may be particularly important during periods of intensified training to reduce the symptoms of overreaching. *Overreaching* is the preferred term for short-term overtraining.

Components of the Carbohydrate Mix

Finding the right carbohydrate mix is a bit more difficult than ensuring that you are getting enough carbohydrate. This is because the right mix is likely to be different from person to person and to vary somewhat across your training and competitive year. To help you find the right mix, this next section reviews the various components of the mix along with the definitions of carbohydrate— simple, complex, high glycemic index, and low glycemic index—gluten, and FODMAPs (fermentable oligosaccharides, disaccharides, monosaccharides, and polyols). Although it is generally more important to incorporate a variety of mostly whole grains, colorful fruits and vegetables, and, to a certain extent, sport products into your mix than to focus on only complex carbohydrate or foods with a low glycemic index (GI), emerging evidence reveals that avoidance of certain carbohydrate foods may be beneficial for athletes with a history of gastrointestinal or other issues. Table 3.6 on page 48 can help you determine whether you might benefit from altering your carbohydrate mix to improve your health and performance.

Important Considerations

Your daily choices of the foods presented in table 3.2—including grains, fruits and vegetables, milk, sport products, and desserts—are what make up your carbohydrate mix. Balancing these carbohydrate-containing foods in your diet is necessary for ensuring that you consume adequate nutrients and obtain a variety of disease-preventing and possibly recovery-enhancing phytochemicals. Achieving this mix requires that you have knowledge of the other food categories, or food groups, which we address again in chapter 12. For now, however, let's think carbohydrate.

Grains vs. Fruits vs. Vegetables vs. Dairy

If you look at the various food guidance models available in the United States and other countries, including USDA's MyPlate, Great Britain's Eatwell Guide, Canada's New Food Plate and Japan's spinning top, among others (see appendix B), the consensus is that the bulk of your carbohydrate should come from grains supplemented with carbohydrate from vegetables, fruits, milk, and, if desired, other discretionary foods. The MyPlate recommendation for a 2,400- to 3,000-calorie diet is 8 to 10 servings of grains. The grains are a staple because, in addition to carbohydrate, they also provide protein, B vitamins, and iron and, if not overly processed, are a more satiating source of carbohydrate than many fruits and vegetables. Whole grains, in addition, provide fiber, zinc, magnesium, and selenium.

Fruits, on the other hand, provide fiber, potassium, folate, and vitamin C. Dark-green and orange-red fruits also provide carotenoids, some of which may be converted to vitamin A. Although they provide about the same amount of carbohydrate per cup, fruits are higher in natural sugar and water and are typically lower in complex carbohydrate. This may make them appealing after a workout but less likely to satisfy an hour or so after consumption. It is not understood why fruits tend to be less satiating than grains, but it may be related to their negligible protein content. However, the carbohydrate in many fruits—including cherries, plums, peaches, and apples—is absorbed slowly, yielding a rather low glycemic index. This may be helpful for some people (described later in this chapter), but they may need to be avoided before exercise by people who experience gastrointestinal distress or irritable bowel syndrome. Both factors will be discussed later in this chapter. Fruits overall should not be limited because of their high sugar content and, contrary to popular belief, do not cause spikes and subsequent falls in blood sugar.

In contrast to grains and fruits, vegetables come in starchy and nonstarchy varieties. Starchy vegetables—including root vegetables and legumes—are carbohydrate packed (a half cup [90 g] cooked contains 15 grams of carbohydrate), whereas nonstarchy vegetables—such as asparagus, broccoli, cauliflower, snap peas, and leafy greens—contain little carbohydrate (a half cup [90 g] contains 5 grams or less of carbohydrate). Like fruit, vegetables are a source of fiber, potassium, folate, vitamin C, and carotenoids but also contain protein, iron, calcium, and other minerals. Although all vegetables are good for you, vegetarian athletes may need to alter the mix of these vegetables according to their training regimens. For example, when energy needs are high, eating a large helping of nonstarchy vegetables can literally fill you up, at least temporarily, before you are able to consume an adequate supply of carbohydrate. When you are injured, redshirted, or unable to compete for a prolonged period, however, eating this same serving of nonstarchy vegetables may help you feel full and prevent unwanted weight gain. Some vegetables, like certain fruits, may also trigger gastrointestinal symptoms in certain athletes, so you may need to try different vegetables to see what works best for you.

Finally, some dairy products, particularly milk and yogurt, are also sources of carbohydrate (12 grams per cup [236 ml]) as well as protein and calcium. Nearly 100 percent of the carbohydrate in milk is in the form of lactose (or milk sugar), which many adults cannot easily digest. The lactose content of yogurt is also high but is much lower than that of milk and apparently decreases daily (even as it sits in the refrigerator) because its natural bacteria breaks down lactose to glucose and galactose. Glucose, sucrose, and even high-fructose corn syrup provide additional carbohydrate in fruit-containing and flavored yogurt. It is not necessary to include carbohydrate from dairy in your mix, but it does provide additional carbohydrate for vegetarian athletes who are able to digest lactose. Athletes who experience abdominal discomfort, bloating, or gas after consuming milk or yogurt may be lactose-intolerant and may want to cut back on or eliminate these foods from their diets (see chapter 6 for information on getting adequate calcium without consuming dairy products). Lactose-intolerant adults who want to continue consuming dairy products can buy low-lactose versions or take tablets that contain the enzyme lactase, which aids in the digestion of milk sugar.

Although most food guidance systems were not designed with athletes in mind, the recommendation to obtain the bulk of carbohydrate from grains is appropriate for athletes. My own eating habits follow this trend. I have found over the years that if I don't eat enough rice and grains over the course of several days, I don't feel satisfied and end up with uncontrollable cravings for any and all grain products. The summer I participated in RAGBRAI (Register's Annual Great Bicycle Ride Across Iowa), I spent the week eating mostly fresh fruit, higher-fat pastries, and cheese pizza because vegetarian options were hard to come by. About five days into the weeklong ride, I was craving bread so much that I stopped at a small store, bought a loaf and devoured nearly the whole thing. That said, however, I have also encountered a few vegetarian athletes who feel the food guidance models, including MyPlate, are too heavy on the grains. These athletes claim they do fine eating mostly fruits, vegetables, legumes, and nuts and fewer grains. Learn to listen to your intuition on this one.

Color

Several national nutrition campaigns in the United States, including MyPlate and the Produce for Better Health (PBH) Foundation's More Matters, have taken the message of increasing consumption of fruits and vegetables one step further and placed a public health emphasis on color. Why? Because colorful fruits and vegetables provide the range of vitamins, minerals, and phytochemicals the body needs to maintain good health. The message from MyPlate is to include dark-green vegetables, orange vegetables, legumes, starchy vegetables, and other vegetables in your diet regularly. The message from PBH is to ensure there is a rainbow on your plate (see https://pbhfoundation.org/pub_sec/edu/cur/rainbow). The spectrum of colors is explained in table 3.4 and consists of five groups: blue and purple, green, white, yellow and orange, and red. As athletes, striving to eat a variety of colorful phytochemical-rich fruits and vegetables provides a source or antioxidants and may not only lower your risk of some chronic diseases, such as cancer and heart disease, but may also optimize your ability to recover from strenuous exercise. More information on phytochemicals will be discussed in chapter 11.

Whole vs. Processed

During a meeting of the American College of Sports Medicine many years ago, I attended a session that focused on the nutritional needs of male athletes training for and competing in distance stage bicycle races such as the Tour de France.[10] During this session, it was emphasized that focusing on whole grains was not a good idea for these athletes because the low energy density of whole compared to processed grains and other whole foods made it more difficult for these athletes to meet their extreme energy and carbohydrate

TABLE 3.4 Phytochemical Color Guide for Fruit, Vegetables, and Herbs

Phytochemical	Color (and specific flavonoid)	Found in (examples)
Flavonoids	Blue and purple (anthocyanidins, flavonols, flavan-3-ols, proanthocyanidins)	Blueberries, blackberries, plums, grapes, red wine, dark chocolate, grape juice, grape skin
	Green (flavones, flavanones, flavonols)	Parsley, spinach, grapes, celery, lettuce, thyme
	White (flavanones, flavonols)	Onions, apples
	Yellow and orange (flavanones, flavonols)	Citrus fruits and juices
	Red (anthocyanidins, flavonols, flavones, flavan-3-ols, flavanones, proanthocyanidins)	Cranberries, raspberries, red onions, red potatoes, red radishes, strawberries, grapes, beets, red peppers
Carotenoids	Green (beta-carotene, lutein, zeaxanthin)	Spinach, collard greens, kale, broccoli, brussels sprouts, artichokes
	Yellow and orange (alpha-carotene, beta-carotene, beta-cryptoxanthin, zeaxanthin)	Pumpkin, sweet potato, carrots, winter squash, apricots, tangerines, oranges, papayas, peaches, nectarines
	Red (leutine)	Tomatoes and cooked tomato products, watermelon, pink grapefruit, red peppers
Other phytochemicals	Blue and purple (ellagic acid, resveratrol)	Blueberries, blackberries
	Green (indols, isothiocyanates, organosulfur compounds)	Broccoli, brussels sprouts, cabbage, kale, leeks, chives
	White (indols, isothiocyanates, organosulfur compounds)	Cauliflower, leeks, garlic, onions, shallots
	Red (ellagic acid, resveratrol)	Raspberries, strawberries, red grapes, grape juice, grape skin, red wine

Adapted from "Phytochemical List," Produce for Better Health Foundation, accessed January 17, 2019, https://pbh-foundation.org/about/res/pic/phytolist/.

needs. The point hit home. I had experienced trouble with the same thing several years earlier (although I was not training for the Tour). At the time I had been a vegetarian for about a year and estimate that I was "burning" more than 3,000 calories a day cross-training and riding 100 to 150 miles (160-241 km) a week. I was making spaghetti with whole-wheat pasta, eating brown rice, baking bran muffins, and eating lots of fruit, and I could not eat enough food. My stomach got full, but I still felt hungry—yes, I thought this was physiologically impossible. The solution for both the elite cyclists and me was the same—relax on the whole foods. The right mix for an athlete is one that includes some whole grains and some more-processed versions. Even the USDA's Dietary Guidelines for Americans and MyPlate suggest that we aim for half of our grains to be whole grains.

Sport Products and Desserts

Okay, we all know modern athletes do not live by bread alone. What about other carbohydrate sources like lemonade, sport drinks, sport bars and gels, recovery drinks, and, heavens yes, frozen yogurt, dairy-free frozen dessert (such as Tofutti), and grandma's homemade cherry pie? These are added-sugar foods and beverages in which sugar or syrups have been added during processing or preparation. On MyPlate, they are considered luxuries and make up your discretionary calories. Although they are allowed in a healthy diet, MyPlate suggests that you limit foods that provide discretionary calories. This limit is approximately 50 grams of added sugars for active individuals consuming 2,000 calories per day and 75 to 80 grams for an athlete taking in 3,000 to 3,200 calories per day.

Given these guidelines, let's first address sport products. Although I am a firm believer in whole foods, I find—as I suspect many athletes do—that some products (including sport drinks, gels, and honey packets) can be a convenient necessity. When I competed in my first 100-mile (160 km) bike ride back in the late 1980s, I ate at least six bananas during the ride. I started the ride with two wedged in my sport bra (I was new to the sport and did not yet have a jersey with pockets), and as much as I like bananas, I was pretty sick of them for weeks after the ride. I became a thankful fan when the first sport gel arrived on the market. Although there are no hard-and-fast rules for athletes concerning the use of supplemental sport foods, my rule is to eat meals and snacks made with real foods and use sport foods as supplements if needed during longer training sessions or competitions. Remember that if you follow the recommendation from MyPlate and consume 2,000 to 3,200 calories per day, you could consume 50 to 80 grams of carbohydrate as supplements—if you ate no dessert—which is enough to support one to two and a half hours of training (see chapter 9). This sounds fairly reasonable to me.

Now let's get to dessert. When I am training hard, I am a fan of desserts. In working with athletes over the years, I have found that a daily dessert treat is usually appropriate as long you don't get carried away. Believe me, I have seen resident athletes at the U.S. Olympic Training Center in Colorado Springs attack the poor chef as he emerged from the kitchen with a plate of warm cookies. For vegetarian athletes, a few cookies, a piece of pumpkin cake, a dish of pudding, frozen yogurt, or Tofutti will add extra calories, and if the choices are right, even some nutrition. My rule on dessert is to have homemade if at all possible—that way you can sneak in some whole grains, nuts, and good oils—and to choose ones that are low in saturated fat and contain fruits or vegetables. Dark chocolate is OK too (the higher the percent cocoa the better). Examples of appetizing fruit desserts include frozen yogurt with bananas or berries, fruit cobbler, baked apples, pumpkin muffins, rhubarb bread, and dark-chocolate zucchini cake. Together, dessert and your sport supplements should—as MyPlate suggests—make up only a small portion (10-20%) of your calories.

Less-Important Considerations

If you had even a little background in vegetarian or sports nutrition before reading this book, you may be wondering why I have so far neglected to discuss simple and complex carbohydrate and the glycemic index (GI), which is a method of classifying carbohydrate sources based on their functionality or how quickly they appear in the bloodstream after consumption. This is because I feel strongly, based on the research and my experience, that it is more beneficial to be concerned about eating a variety of wholesome foods—which include fruit and fruit juice—rather than to be concerned about whether a carbohydrate is simple or complex or elicits a certain glycemic response.

Complex vs. Simple Carbohydrate

Vegetarian athletes have several reasons for not being overly concerned—as many still are—about the amount of simple (sugars) compared to complex (starchy) carbohydrate they consume in their diet (see table 3.5). The first is that simple carbohydrate, including fruit, fruit juice, and milk are not necessarily less healthful than more-complex carbohydrate, which includes whole-wheat bread, potatoes, and cereal. Rather, it is that these foods should be consumed in the right mix, limiting the more-processed versions because these foods tend to be lower in nutrients, phytochemicals, and fiber. Second, from a performance standpoint, there is no evidence that complex carbohydrate or simple carbohydrate is more advantageous for athletes during training. In fact, researchers have known for quite some time that diets either high in complex carbohydrate or high in simple carbohydrate are equally effective at improving endurance (compared to a low-carbohydrate diet)[11] and in restoring glycogen in the 24-hour period after exercise.[12] One benefit of a diet higher in more-complex carbohydrate, however, is that it tends to result in slightly higher muscle glycogen stores over a 48-hour period when athletes rest and do not train.[12]

TABLE 3.5 Classification of Carbohydrate Sources

Type	Example
Simple: Monosaccharides (one sugar unit)	Glucose or blood sugar Fructose or fruit sugar Galactose
Simple: Disaccharides (two sugar units)	Sucrose or table sugar (glucose + fructose) Lactose or milk sugar (glucose + fructose) Maltose (glucose + glucose)
Slightly complex: Oligosaccharides (short-chain carbohydrate containing a "few" sugar units)	Glacto-oligosaccharides and fructo-oligosaccharides, including inulin
Complex: Polysaccharides (many sugar units)	Maltodextrin (short straight chain) Amylose starch (straight chain of glucose) Amylopectin starch (branched chain of glucose) Polycose (commercial product of glucose units)
Polyols (sugar alcohols)	Mannitol, sorbitol, xylitol

Vegan View: Is Sugar Vegan?

Those who are new to veganism are often surprised to learn that some sugar is refined through processing with animal bones. As archaic as it might sound, part of the refining and whitening of cane sugar is done with bone char. Therefore, some vegans avoid refined sugar. Fortunately, the use of bone char is being phased out, and beet sugar, which never uses bone char, is now more common than cane sugar.

If you want to avoid bone-char-refined sugar, you can choose beet instead of cane, choose organic versions, which never uses bone char, or select a less-refined sugar like Sugar In The Raw or Sucanat brands. Another option is to switch to a liquid like agave or maple syrup, if your recipe and use allows.

The inevitable question then is how strict should you be when eating out or reading package labels? That answer varies among vegans and in the end is up to you. Some sugar-containing products may be certified vegan and a simple Internet search will tell you what others have found. Another option is to not worry too much about minute ingredients away from home. Even if a sugar is refined with bone char, the end product is still free of animal products. Additionally, the sugar issue can cause confusion at food establishments. For example, my local ice cream shop carries four popular vegan flavors every day and nearly stopped providing them because a vegan was irate over the unknown sugar source. In this scenario, the big picture—having delicious vegan options next to traditional ice cream—trumps the limited impact of choosing one sugar over another.

Low-Glycemic vs. High-Glycemic Index

Vegan athletes also have several reasons they should not be overly concerned about the GI of the foods that make up their carbohydrate mix. The first is that the GI, which is a measure of how quickly the carbohydrate in an individual food appears in the bloodstream after consuming a standard 50- or 100-gram portion, is quite controversial. Although low glycemic–index diets offer some promise for weight loss, blood sugar control, and improved overall health,[13] the evidence from scientific studies is not particularly compelling and can be confusing.[14] Furthermore, because the GI is measured in individual foods, its application to mixed meals and the overall diet has been criticized. Indeed, the GI of a food, such as a banana, can change quickly with ripening, cutting, or smearing with a little nut butter. With respect to its benefit to athletes, a food's GI is likely to be an important consideration only during exercise or in the preexercise and postexercise meal (as will be discussed in chapter 9), but no research suggests that athletes—particularly vegetarian athletes—will be faster, leaner, or healthier if they consume a low glycemic index training diet.

Considerations of Emerging Importance

If you discuss food with your training partners, relatives, or nonathletic friends, chances are you know someone who avoids gluten or has been following a low-FODMAP diet. These two diets have become increasingly popular among the general U.S. population and are even being considered by athletes. While both diets are appropriate for certain athletes, they do not improve performance and are not for everyone.

Gluten-Free Diets

Gluten-free diets have become quite the rage in the last 10 years, so much so that I have had perfectly healthy athletes walk into my office feeling pressured to eliminate the evil gluten. The unfortunate truth is that many don't even know what gluten is or why someone should eliminate it. Gluten is a protein found in grains such as wheat, rye, and barley that gives certain breads their characteristic chewiness. It is discussed here because its elimination can leave some athletes struggling to meet their carbohydrate needs.

While a gluten-free diet is essential for the treatment of people with celiac disease—a digestive and autoimmune disorder that results in damage to the lining of the small intestine when foods with gluten are eaten—and nonceliac gluten sensitivity, there is no evidence that gluten promotes weight gain, zaps energy level, or is responsible for chronic disease. Eliminating gluten can also alter fiber and nutrient intake and results in unnecessary food restriction. In a recent study, 13 nonceliac endurance cyclists followed a gluten-free or a gluten-containing diet in a randomly assigned order for 7 days, which was separated by a 10-day washout period.[15] The gluten-free diet did not result in improvement to performance, gastrointestinal function, or well-being.

A recent randomly assigned clinical rechallenge study in 37 nonathletes found compelling evidence to suggest that many of the effects perceived to be caused by gluten may be related instead to FODMAPs, and therefore caused by components of wheat besides gluten.[16] Visit your doctor if you feel you have gastrointestinal or other problems related to intake of wheat-containing foods. Unless you have a medical reason for eliminating gluten, however, there is no reason to do it. Eliminating foods with gluten can limit variety and ultimately impair both health and performance.

Low-FODMAP Diet

FODMAP is an acronym for fermentable oligosaccharides, disaccharides, mono-saccharides, and polyols, which are carbohydrate-based molecules found in food (see table 3.5). This diet is based on the principle that FODMAPs—found in many familiar foods in the diet (see appendix C)—are more difficult to digest and absorb and many are rapidly fermented by the bacteria in the gut. This can lead to gas, bloating, and diarrhea in susceptible individuals. Diets that are low in FODMAPs are becoming fundamental therapy in the management of irritable bowel syndrome.[17,18]

While no evidence to date suggests that healthy individuals without irritable bowel syndrome (IBS) would benefit from low-FODMAP diets, preliminary research in athletic populations has suggested that athletes with recurring exercise-associated gastrointestinal distress may benefit from short-term FODMAP reduction to minimize symptoms including bloating, abdominal cramping, flatulence, and diarrhea during exercise and major competitions.[19,20]

Carbohydrate Wrap-Up

As discussed in this chapter, evaluating your carbohydrate mix is somewhat involved because it includes honestly assessing many aspects of your current eating. Some of these aspects are important for performance only, and others influence only health. Although the information in table 3.6 is helpful, keep in mind that the right mix might change as you progress through your yearly season. For example, it is probably prudent to routinely increase the variety in the color of your food, but you could also find that you need to change your discretionary calories or amount of whole vs. processed foods or starchy vs. nonstarchy vegetables according to your energy requirements and training level. You might also find that avoiding FODMAPs might be beneficial before major competitions if you previously developed gastrointestinal symptoms on race day. During the off-season or when you are training less, eliminate your dependence on sport drinks and focus on eating more whole foods. When you are in the heart of your season, enjoy the convenience of these products.

Also keep in mind that the carbohydrate mix that works for you might not be the one preferred by your training partner or suggested by MyPlate. Rather, what is important is that you meet your carbohydrate and nutrient needs by consuming a variety of grains, colorful fruits and vegetables, and, if desired, sport supplements in a mix that works for you. This will inevitably affect your health and your performance. Stay tuned, now, as we move on to fat.

TABLE 3.6 Are You Getting the Right Carbohydrate Mix?

Evaluation question	Suggestion for change
Do you find it a struggle to maintain your weight?	No. No reason to change.
	Yes, I struggle to keep weight on. Replace some of your whole-grain and whole foods with more-processed versions. Eat regular pasta, white bread, and fruit and vegetable juices in place of some whole-grain and whole-fruit versions.
	Yes, I am a few pounds overweight. Eat more whole-grain and whole foods. Substitute regular pasta, breakfast cereal, and fruit juice with whole-wheat pasta, cooked grains such as oatmeal and barley, and whole fruit. This will increase the fiber content of your diet and may reduce hunger by making you feel more full or satisfied.
Do you eat a variety of carbohydrate sources from the grain, vegetable, and fruit groups?	No. Assess what you lack and add these to your diet. The guidelines presented in MyPlate or other researched food models are a great place to start.
	Yes. Good job.
Do you eat a selection of colorful fruits and vegetables?	No. Incorporate more of the fruits and vegetables listed in table 3.4. This will help you reduce your risk of cancer and other chronic diseases and may improve your ability to recover from strenuous exercise.
	Yes. Keep up the good work. You have taken a step toward reducing your risk of cancer and other chronic diseases and may even be improving your ability to recover after strenuous exercise.
Do you regularly experience symptoms associated with IBS, including abdominal pain, gas, constipation, diarrhea, or persistent exercise-associated gastrointestinal dysfunction?	No. It is important to remember that FODMAPs are important dietary constituents that favor growth of beneficial bacteria, increase stool bulk, and even enhance gut health and immune function. Most people are not sensitive to FODMAPs, and their unnecessary restriction limits food variety on a vegetarian diet.
	Yes. A low-FODMAP diet shows promise as an effective dietary treatment for most people suffering from IBS.[17] Preliminary research suggests that the short-term low-FODMAP diet may be efficacious in the management of daily gastrointestinal symptoms in athletes.[20] Consulting a registered dietitian who is knowledgeable about FODMAPs and sport nutrition is highly recommended.
Do you experience gastrointestinal or other symptoms that may be associated with the consumption of wheat products?	No. Evidence does not indicate that gluten-free diets influence elements of health or exercise performance among nonceliac athletes.[15] Bread and other wheat products are an important source of the B vitamins, iron, magnesium, and fiber. The unnecessary restriction of these products is not recommended in a vegetarian diet.
	Yes. See your physician if you think you may have celiac disease or gluten sensitivity. Both conditions are rare. Consultation with a registered dietitian is important for ensuring adequate nutrient intake on a gluten-free, vegetarian diet for athletes.

Evaluation question	Suggestion for change
Do you use sport supplements?	No. There is no reason to use these items. However, fluid-replacement beverages and carbohydrate bars and gels are convenient products that help athletes in heavy training meet their carbohydrate needs.
	Yes. Fluid-replacement beverages and carbohydrate bars and gels are convenient products that help athletes in heavy training meet their carbohydrate needs. These items, however, should not replace real food. Cut back on their use if they make up more than 20% of your total calories or have become your regular lunch or dinner.
Have you been trying to follow a diet that has a low-glycemic index or that avoids sugar?	No. Because these factors don't seem to matter in the big picture, you are right on target.
	Yes. Focus instead on getting a variety of grains, whole grains, fruits and vegetables, and legumes. Glycemic index and sugar don't seem to matter in the big picture. Even if you have diabetes or prediabetes, the total carbohydrate content of the food and its nutrient content are more important. Remember also that sugar is found naturally in many foods including fruit and milk.
Do you eat sweets or dessert regularly?	No. Great. But allow yourself to splurge if you want to every once in a while.
	Yes. Enjoy yourself. Strive, however, for choices that are low in saturated fat and trans fat and provide nutrients. Good choices include frozen yogurt (or tofu) topped with fruit, fruit cobbler, baked apples, and whole-wheat versions of banana or pumpkin breads and oatmeal chocolate chip cookies with pecans.

4 | Choosing Smart Fat Over No Fat

My training group had just ridden the century
(160-kilometer bike ride) from hell. We were starved!
One of my training partners, however, just sat there
sipping her sport drink while the rest of us devoured
a special Cajun stew (no sausage) prepared by
the famous New Orleans chef Paul Prudhomme.
It wasn't that she didn't like Cajun food; she just
knew that the dish contained too much fat. She
looked miserable. We had specifically traveled to
this small-town Cajun festival to participate in the
athletic events (it hosted a 5K run on Saturday morning followed by a century bicycle ride on Sunday) and
enjoy the food and festivities. The weather in early
June had been hotter and more humid than we had
planned. Between that, a few wrong turns, and a
flat tire, it had taken us a little longer than normal to
finish the century. Now that the work was over, we
had the afternoon to relax (before our drive home)
and enjoy some local fare. I felt bad, however, that
my training partner was unable to enjoy herself.
Despite riding more than 100 miles (160 km) and
competing in a 5K run the day before, she was afraid
to eat a single gram of fat. On the way out of town,
she made a beeline for the Wendy's drive-through
and ordered two plain baked potatoes with broccoli.

– Enette

When I wrote the first edition of this book in the mid-2000s,
dietary fat was out. We were on the heels of recovery from
the 1980s dietary guidelines, which identified a reduction in
dietary fat as the single most important change needed to
improve health and prevent disease, mainly heart disease.[1]

The real reason was to target reduction of saturated fat but that message was thought to be too complex for the U.S. public, so total fat was targeted instead. With this revision of the book, it is both fortunate and unfortunate that fat is now in. In fact, fat and protein are considered the "cool kids" and carbohydrate seems to not "fit in." The truth of the matter is that while fat is important for athletes—to aid in the absorption of fat-soluble nutrients, synthesize hormone regulators, serve as a dense source of fuel, and enhance the flavor of our foods—consuming too much of it is not good either. Too much dietary fat can displace valuable carbohydrate calories and, if it is saturated, can elevate "bad" low-density lipoprotein (LDL) cholesterol levels and increase even an athlete's risk for heart and other vascular diseases. This chapter directs you toward choosing smart fat over no fat or high fat. It reviews the importance of fat—but not too much fat—in an athlete's diet, provides information on the types of fat most associated with health, and provides tips for getting the healthy fat sources into and the not-so-good fat sources out of your diet.

Why Athletes Need Fat

Fat is a necessary component of the diet. It provides essential fatty acids and associated nutrients such as vitamins E, A, and D, and aids in the absorption and transport of not only these nutrients but also other fat-soluble phytochemicals found in plant foods. The essential fatty acids—alpha-linolenic acid and linoleic acid—are the precursors for many regulatory compounds within the body and include the major regulators of the inflammatory process (discussed further in chapter 11). The fat-soluble vitamins and phytonutrients—carotenoids and lycopene to name a few—serve as antioxidants and are associated with a reduced risk of chronic diseases including certain cancers. In addition, dietary fat is a component of the cell's protective membrane barrier and thereby helps the skin and other tissues remain soft and pliable.

Fat also serves as a source of energy. As discussed in chapter 3, fat and carbohydrate are the main energy fuels used during exercise. In the sport nutrition world, a greater emphasis is typically placed on dietary carbohydrate both because carbohydrate stores in the body are limited and because carbohydrate is the only fuel that can support intense bouts of exercise. *Period.* This does not mean, however, that fat is unimportant. Fat serves as a constant fuel source during exercise and could theoretically supply most of the fuel needed during light to moderate efforts. Carbohydrate fuel is simply needed for more-intense efforts. This is because fat cannot be metabolized (or broken down) rapidly enough to support the rapid energy demands of more-intense efforts. Increasing the muscles' ability to use fat as a fuel through endurance training is thought to preserve or spare carbohydrate for use during quick or intense physical effort, which is required during most training and competitive efforts. It is well established, in fact, that the maximal fat oxidation rate is reached during moderate-intensity exercise, corresponding to 59 to 64 percent of $\dot{V}O_2$max (an estimate of the body's maximal aerobic capacity) in endurance-trained athletes and 47 to 52 percent in those less trained. This is the intensity of a light jog for a trained athlete.

The source of fat used to fuel exercising muscle comes predominantly from fat stored in both body fat (termed adipose tissue) and in skeletal muscle itself. The small amount of fat that circulates in blood as triglycerides (serum triglycerides) is another possible source but contributes only a negligible amount even after a high-fat meal. The fat stored within the muscle as droplets (see figure 4.1) is the ideal source during exercise because it provides a direct source of fat to the mitochondria, the cell's ATP-generating powerhouse. In fact, the fat droplets often appear to be completely encircled by the mitochondria in the well-trained athlete, as can be seen in figure 4.1.

Fat stored in adipose tissue as triglycerides, on the other hand, has to travel a lot. It must first be broken down to fatty acids (the chemical form used for energy), be released from the adipose tissue, travel in the blood bound to an escort protein called albumin, and then pass through the muscle cell and mitochondria membranes escorted by other carriers (a transmembrane carrier and carnitine, respectively). And you thought your workout was tough! Although the amount of energy stored in adipose depots is large compared to that in other storage sites, the energy content of the fat stored within the muscle cell is also noteworthy and has been estimated to be 60 to 70 percent more than energy stored as glycogen (see table 4.1).

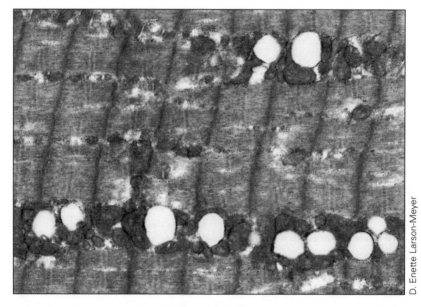

D. Enette Larson-Meyer

FIGURE 4.1   Electron microscopy of the muscle cell obtained from the thigh (vastus lateralis) of a male runner. The fat droplets (bright white circles) are in close contact with mitochondria (darker structures), which are the structures responsible for producing ATP from fat and carbohydrate fuel.

TABLE 4.1   Estimated Energy Stores of Fat and Carbohydrate in a 165-Pound (75 kg) Male Athlete With 15 Percent Body Fat

Energy fuel stores	Components	Energy (kcal)
Fat	Blood fat (free fatty acids and triglyceride)	40
	Adipose tissue	99,000+
	Muscle lipid droplets (intramuscular fat)	2,600
	Estimated total	101,640
Carbohydrate	Blood glucose	80
	Liver glycogen	380
	Muscle glycogen	1,500-1,600
	Estimated total	1,960-2,060

Whether your exercising muscles decide to use fat from adipose tissue or fat stored directly in muscle is influenced by many factors including the intensity and duration of your exercise, your fitness level, sex, genetics, and also your diet. These are the same factors that influence whether your muscles select fat or carbohydrate as the preferred fuel. Although fat stored in muscle as lipid droplets (or intramuscular fat) is still somewhat of a mystery, the last decade has slowly revealed more about the importance of this fuel. This is in part because measuring muscle-fat stores and determining how much of it is "burned" as fuel during exercise is technically difficult. Nonetheless, a variety of state-of-the-art techniques used over the past two decades have helped us understand that muscle fat stores can serve as an important source of fat fuel during moderate exercise (65% $\dot{V}O_2$max) but that it can still be used along with glycogen as a fuel during more-intense efforts (85% $\dot{V}O_2$max) (see figures 4.2 and 4.3). Fat from adipose tissue, in contrast, is used to the greatest extent to fuel light exercise (25% $\dot{V}O_2$max), although limited amounts are used during moderate and more-intense exercise (see figure 4.2).[2,3] This makes sense considering how far fat stored in adipose tissue needs to travel to reach exercising muscle; it simply can't get to the muscle mitochondria fast enough to fuel intense exercise efforts.

Use of muscle fat is also known to increase with exercise duration (i.e., it is a more important fuel source the longer you exercise beyond an hour or two) and depends somewhat on the amount in storage. Aerobically trained athletes store more fat in the muscle fiber and in a more convenient location close to the mitochondria (see figure 4.1) as lipid droplets in a form called intramuscular fat, but this may be dependent on diet. Research from my lab[4,5] and others[6] found that the amount of fat stored in exercised muscles is increased by eating more fat in the diet. In our studies, male[5] and female[4,5] runners completed a two-hour run at 65 percent of $\dot{V}O_2$max and were then fed low-fat (10% fat) and

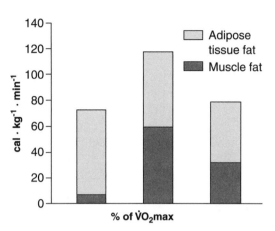

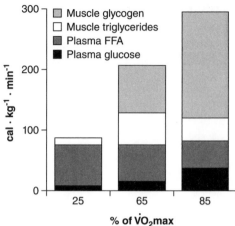

FIGURE 4.2   Contribution of fat from muscle-fat stores, as droplets within the muscle cell, and adipose tissue breakdown, from delivery in blood as free fatty acids, to energy expenditure after 30 minutes of exercise at 25 percent equivalent of walking, 65 percent equivalent of running moderately, and 85 percent equivalent of running intensely of maximal oxygen uptake ($\dot{V}O_2$max).

Adapted by permission from E.F. Coyle, "Fat Metabolism During Exercise," *Sports Science Exchange* 59, vol. 8, no. 6 (1995).

FIGURE 4.3   Proportion of carbohydrate and fat use during exercise.

Reprinted by permission from J.A. Romijn, E.F. Coyle, L.S. Sidossis, A. Gastaldelli, J.F. Horowitz, E. Endert, and R.R. Wolfe, "Regulation of Endogenous Fat and Carbohydrate Metabolism in Relation to Exercise Intensity and Duration," *American Journal of Physiology* 265, no. 3, part 1 (1993): E380-E391.

moderate-fat (35% fat) vegetarian diets for three days in a randomly assigned order on two different occasions. We found that intramuscular fat stores were reduced by an average of 25 percent following the endurance run[5] and that recovery depended on the fat content of the diet.[4,5] Consuming the moderate-fat diet allowed muscle-fat stores to return to baseline the following morning (22 hr later) and to overshoot baseline values three days later, despite the fact that the runners continued to perform 45-minute training runs. Consuming the low-fat diet, in contrast, did not allow intramuscular fat to be restocked even three days after the run.[5] Although our studies did not find differences between men and women, others have alluded to the fact that women may be better able to store and use intramuscular fat.

Dietary Fat and Exercise Performance

In writing the revised edition of this book, pressing questions have emerged concerning the possible ability of higher-fat diets for athletes to enhance either muscle triglyceride stores or the overall capacity to use fat during exercise. This would theoretically decrease reliance on carbohydrate fuel. While such interest in higher-fat diets is not new, their popularity has soared in the last 10 or so years, right alongside those of the extremely low-fat diet. In a Gallup poll from 2014, for instance, 56 percent of Americans reported that they were actively trying to avoid fat in their diets, whereas 29 percent said they were actively avoiding carbohydrate.[7] This suggests of course that low-fat diets have not gone away despite the increasing popularity of high-fat diets. Let's review what we know about these diets for athletes.

Moderate-Fat Diet to Enhance Muscle Fat and Performance

One lingering question from our earlier discussion on the importance of intramuscular fat is whether higher fat consumption designed to stock the muscle with fat can offer a performance advantage. Studies in my lab[4] and others[8] have found, somewhat disappointingly, that enhancing intramuscular fat stores does not affect performance during running or cycling events lasting between two and three and a half hours. In our study, we asked male and female runners to complete a 10K race after running for 90 minutes at a moderately relaxed pace (65% $\dot{V}O_2$max) under two dietary conditions: 1) four days of a diet containing 10 percent fat and 2) three days of a diet containing 35 percent fat plus one day of a low-fat, high-carbohydrate diet (to ensure similar glycogen stores between treatments). The order of the diets was randomly assigned. Although intramuscular fat stores were approximately 30 percent higher after the diet that was 35 percent fat, runners ran remarkably similar 10K races. The study in cyclists was similar. Performance during a 20K time trial completed after three hours of moderate riding was not notably different despite a 70 percent increase in intramuscular fat stores. Whether this type of muscle-fat loading might be beneficial during longer, multiple-day events is not yet known.

High-Fat Diet for Endurance Performance

A second pressing question is whether extremely high fat diets, 60 to 70 percent fat, might enhance fat use as a fuel during exercise and offer a performance advantage.[9] While this would seem unlikely based on our early discussions of carbohydrate fuel, proponents and researchers have questioned whether following high-fat diets for longer than a few weeks might allow the body to adapt by revving up its fat-burning enzymes. Many thought this would be a good thing because the body could be trained to use its endless supply of body fat and not be dependent on carbohydrate fuel.[10] Studies to date, however, suggest that long-term consumption of high-fat diets only partially deliver. They can drastically increase the body's ability to burn fat during moderate-intensity to moderately high intensity exercise but do not dampen the muscles' need for carbohydrate during high-intensity exercise. A study in fat-adapted, male ultramarathon athletes illustrates this point. These athletes—who had consumed a high-fat (>60% fat) diet for at least six months—had peak fat oxidation rates that were more than double those of their sport mates following higher-carbohydrate diets (1.54 vs. 0.67 g fat/min), but still experienced their peak fat oxidation around 70 percent $\dot{V}O_2$max just like participants consuming higher-carbohydrate diets.[11] This means they still required carbohydrate fuel to exercise at higher intensities. Furthermore, exercise capacity is not shown to increase after fat adaptation. Instead, fat-adapted athletes were less efficient during training (with respect to oxygen cost) and experienced an increased perception of effort and an impairment in their response to training.[9,12] Replacing glycogen on the days leading up to competition does not seem to override these adaptations because the fat-adapted body loses its ability to effectively burn carbohydrate fuel and work at high intensities.[13,14] Arguably, surges in intensity—including uphill climbs, breakaways, and sprints to the finish—are

Vegan View: What About Keto Diets?

The ketogenic diet, often shortened to keto, is an extremely low-carbohydrate, very high-fat diet that originated as a treatment for pediatric epilepsy. Significantly more strict than an Atkins-style low-carbohydrate diet, an adherent to the keto diet consumes fewer than 35 grams of carbohydrate per day. That's only 140 calories, or less than 7 percent of calories, from carbohydrate in a reference 2,000-calorie diet. Unlike other low-carbohydrate diets, it is not high in protein, which is only eaten in moderation.

This way of eating forces the body into ketosis—a metabolic state in which fat, in the form of ketones, is the primary source of fuel. Using stored body fat for energy is normally an inefficient process, but severely restricting carbohydrate forces this physiological change and trains the body to burn fat more productively. Theoretically, this could be advantageous for athletes who want to lose weight and potentially gain an energy advantage.

But the evidence is still limited, and fully adapting to a keto diet is extraordinarily arduous and takes significant discipline. If ketosis isn't reached and maintained, the body does not adapt, and the fat-as-fuel pathway remains unchanged. Often people attempting the keto diet don't reach ketosis because the amount of allowable carbohydrate is prohibitively low. All grains, pastas, breads, beans, sugar and other sweeteners, starchy vegetables and nearly all fruit are eliminated (the exceptions are avocados and small amounts of berries). Meats, full-fat dairy, eggs, leafy green vegetables, and oils are emphasized. Advocates warn of a transition time known as the "keto flu," in which bad breath, dry mouth, increased hunger, and excessive urination are potential side effects. Maintaining a keto diet long term requires test strips to measure for ketones in the urine.

Despite the current interest in keto diets for athletes, a review of the literature in its 2017 position paper on body composition, the International Society of Sports Nutrition concluded that a keto diet may compromise high-intensity training output and has not shown superior effects on body composition compared to nonketo diets where protein and calories are matched [52]. Future studies undoubtedly will be done, but as we await the results, the popularity is not matched by data justifying such a restrictive diet.

Source: A. Aragon, B. Schoenfeld, R. Wildman, et al., "International Society of Sports Nutrition Position Stand: Diets and Body Composition," *Journal of the International Society of Sports Nutrition* 14 (2017).

required in all athletic competitions, making high-fat diets unacceptable even for the ultraendurance competitor.[9]

Some of best evidence to date demonstrating the potential detrimental effects of high-fat diets comes from the Australian Institute of Sport. Researchers assigned one group of elite racewalkers, who were initiating an intensive three-week block of training, to a high-fat diet (65%) and compared their results to their teammates assigned to higher-carbohydrate regimens that were either standardized or personalized. They found that the group assigned to the high-fat diet failed to demonstrate training improvements despite the intense training regimen, whereas the higher-carbohydrate groups experienced the expected improvements. Beyond that, the appeal of these diets to the vegan and vegetarian athlete is worth a quick mention. To achieve 60 to 70 percent of energy from fat requires a diet based heavily on high-fat cuts of meat, low-carbohydrate vegetables, butter, cream, and salad dressing. Even the carbohydrate in legumes might be too much. I don't know about you, but I still prefer some bread with my olive oil.

Very Low-Fat Diet and Performance

A final pressing question is whether overzealous fat restriction can influence exercise capacity or performance. Numerous studies in athletes have found suggestions that low-fat diets, typically defined as providing less than 15 percent fat, are not appropriate either (except when followed for a limited number of

Balancing intake of dietary fat is important for the athlete.

Brenda Whitman

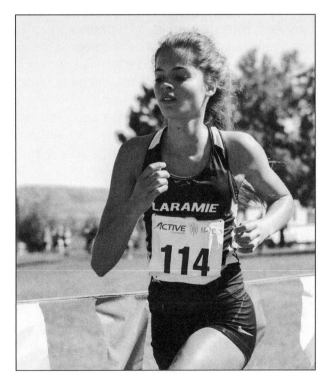

days leading up to a competition). Long-term consumption of low-fat diets are associated with dry flaky skin, compromised immune function,[15] and increased risk for amenorrhea or altered menstrual cycle function.[16-18] Low-fat diets are also known to raise serum triglycerides, even in athletes.[4,5,19] Elevated serum triglyceride concentrations above 150 milligrams per deciliter are thought to be a risk factor for heart disease. Although slightly elevated triglycerides are not a problem for most athletes—who have low triglyceride concentrations to begin with—several healthy runners in my studies have exceeded the 150 milligrams per deciliter mark when placed on a research diet consisting of 10 percent fat. While less is known about performance, a study in runners found that an extremely low fat diet had the potential to impair endurance performance in runners when compared to diets containing slightly more but reasonable amounts of fat,[20] perhaps by reducing triglyceride stores in muscle. Yes, we are back to enjoying a little olive oil or margarine with our bread!

Connection Between Dietary Fat and Body Fat

Before we discuss the fat recommendations for athletes, it is important to review the connection between dietary-fat intake and body fat. Many misconceptions exist on both ends of the fat intake spectrum. Many people, like my training partner in the late 1990s, were afraid to eat even a morsel of fat for fear of weight gain, whereas nowadays people are afraid to eat carbohydrate for the same reason. So what is the evidence? Concerning fat, a handful of studies[21]—including a few of my own[22,23]—have found a positive relationship between dietary-fat intake (as a percentage of calories) and body fat percentage among nonathletes. While this seems to suggest that eating more fat may go right to your hips or your belly, it is important to point out that the reported relationship between dietary fat and body fat is weak (accounting for approximately 10% or less of the variance in body fat), and in one of our studies, it completely disappeared when we accounted for the physical activity level of our participants.[22] In addition, the intake of polyunsaturated fat is shown in some studies to have the opposite effect and is negatively correlated with body fat.[22,24]

On the flipside, a higher carbohydrate intake does increase insulin secretion. The purported problem with insulin is that as an anabolic hormone, it promotes fat deposition in adipose tissue and prevents lipolysis (or fat breakdown) as part of its role in promoting an uptake of glucose into body cells. So if you think we're in trouble, we are not. The problem is the oversimplification of the science. In fact, it goes back to overeating, which is what really makes us put on body fat and gain weight, not simply eating fat or eating protein. Looking back at fat intake, there is a grain of truth to thinking that fat goes right to your hips,[25,26] but it is by promoting unconscious overconsumption of fat-containing foods. Researchers discovered this when they manipulated the fat content of various omnivorous recipes and then allowed sedentary volunteers to eat as much as they wanted.[27] The research volunteers were not privy to the recipe modifications but overate when the higher-fat versions of the same recipes were offered. The researchers speculated this was caused by both the higher energy density of the higher-fat recipes (9 kcal/g for fat vs. 4 kcal/g for carbohydrate) and the enhanced sensory qualities of dietary fats. The participants tended to choose the same volume of food, which resulted in increased energy intake of the high-fat foods because of its higher energy density.

Results from these studies in sedentary subjects, however, should not be taken to mean that plant-based athletes will overeat and increase their body fat stores simply by being a little more liberal with their fat intake at the expense of carbohydrate. Studies in endurance athletes[19,28] have found that body fat is not influenced by following self-selected higher-fat diets that provided up to 50 percent of energy intake for as long as 12 weeks.[19] The other side of the story is that athletes may eat more on an overly processed high-carbohydrate diet perhaps because of the sweeter taste. Manufacturers know this and add sugar to nearly everything. No studies in the literature, however, point to a link between a high-carbohydrate, mostly whole-foods diet and obesity. It is the over-processed carbohydrates that get us. Thus, part of this argument may go back to choosing the right carbohydrate (as discussed in chapter 3) and not overeating. Think, for example, of a person who consumes an entire package of fat-free cookies and still wants the taste of just one or two "real" fat-containing cookies (enhanced with a little whole-grain flour, of course).

Determining Fat Needs

The amount of fat in your overall diet should make up the remainder of energy intake after your carbohydrate and protein needs are met. For many active people and athletes, this will amount to 20 to 35 percent of daily energy intake, which is consistent with the acceptable macronutrient distribution range (AMDR) established by the Institute of Medicine[29] and in agreement with the recommendation of the American College of Sports Medicine, the Academy of Nutrition and Dietetics, and Dietitians of Canada.[30] These recommendations specify that fat intake for athletes be in accordance with public health guidelines, and be individualized based on training and body composition goals. Specifying fat intake as a percentage of daily energy, however, can be complicated because it requires that the athlete know his or her daily energy requirements. Furthermore, the percentage can be misleading because you can consume a higher percentage of energy from fat (and still meet carbohydrate and protein needs). For example, a 165-pound (75 kg) endurance athlete whose energy needs are 4,500 calories per day (as shown in table 4.2), can eat a diet that provides 38 percent of daily energy intake from fat and still meet his or her carbohydrate and protein requirements, which in this example were assumed to be 8 grams of carbohydrate per kilogram of body mass and 1.2 grams of protein per kilogram of body mass. Similarly, a smaller 121 pound (55 kg) athlete

TABLE 4.2   Level of Acceptable Fat Intake for Two Sample Athletes Weighing 75 and 55 kg Respectively, Whose Energy Needs Are 4,500 kcal/day and 2,500 kcal/day

Total daily energy requirements	4,500 kcal/day *(line a)*	2,500 kcal/day *(line a)*
Estimated carbohydrate requirements	Assume 8 g/kg body mass = 600 g/day × 4 kcal/g = 2,400 kcal/day from carbohydrate *(line b)*	Assume 5 g/kg body mass = 275 g/day × 4 kcal/g = 1,100 kcal/day from carbohydrate *(line b)*
Estimated protein requirements (see chapter 5)	1.2 g/kg body mass = 90 g/day × 4 kcal/g = 360 kcal/day from protein *(line c)*	1.2 g/kg body mass = 66 g/day × 4 kcal/g = 264 kcal/day from protein *(line c)*
Estimated fat intake in kcal/day (subtract *lines b* and *c* from *line a*)	4,500 – 2,400 – 360 = 1,740 kcal/day from fat *(line d)*	2,500 – 1,100 – 264 = 1,136 kcal/day from fat *(line d)*
Estimated fat intake in g (divide kcal from fat *[line d]* by 9 kcal/g)	1,740 kcal/day ÷ 9 kcal/g = 193 g fat *(line e)*	1,136 kcal/day ÷ 9 kcal/g = 126 g fat *(line e)*
Estimated percentage of kcal from fat (divide kcal from fat *[line d]* by total kcal *[line a]* and multiply by 100)	1,740 ÷ 4,500 ×100 = 38.7% of daily energy as fat	1,136 ÷ 2,500 × 100 = 45.4% of daily energy as fat

undergoing more skill-based training and requiring 2,500 kilocalories could meet assumed carbohydrate needs of 5 grams per kilogram of body mass and a similar amount of protein on a diet that is more than 40 percent fat. As an interesting exercise, use this table to estimate your own dietary-fat range.

After this discussion, if you are wondering whether dangers are associated with eating too much or too little fat, the answer is still a definite yes—although this may depend somewhat on your sport, training level, and preferences. Diets that are too high in fat, or even protein for that matter, do not provide sufficient carbohydrate to keep glycogen stores stocked, and diets too high in saturated fat are linked to cardiovascular disease. But just because too much dietary fat is not recommended, athletes should also not severely limit fat. This is important to mention again because extremely low-fat vegetarian diets (<10% energy from fat) are recommended by Ornish,[31] Barnard,[32] and others. And while such extremely low-fat diets show promise clinically to improve glycemic control[32,33] and promote regression of coronary atherosclerosis,[31,34,35] they are likely too restrictive for even serious recreational athletes. They may, however, be a consideration for dedicated moderate exercisers or yoga enthusiasts with a history of heart disease or diabetes.

Balancing Good Fat and Bad Fat for Health

In addition to thinking of fat exclusively as an energy source, the specific types of dietary fat needs to be considered in terms of their effect on health, even in vegetarian athletes. Although we have known for a long time that consuming too much saturated fat is "bad" for our health, we really did not appreciate until recently that consuming certain types of fat, at the expense of others, might actually benefit health. Part of this may go back to the oversimplification of our public health message in the United States that too much fat is linked to poor health when, in fact, it is really too much saturated fat. Hence, this section is devoted to reviewing the types of fats and their food sources in an effort to help you adjust your diet as needed. Your overall goal—of course—is to get to know the "good guy" fats and limit contact with the "bad guy" fats. Making smart fat choices should have an impact on your long-term health, but it may also reduce whole-body inflammation and potentially affect your susceptibility to inflammation and injury. This will be discussed more in chapter 11. Results from nearly 150 epidemiological and clinical investigations,[36] including the Nurses' Health Study[37] and our most recent public health guidelines[38-40] support the idea that eating smart fat over no fat may be more effective at preventing coronary heart disease and possibly other chronic diseases.

"Bad Guys"—Saturated Fats and Trans Fats

Unless you have paid little attention to news reports and diet trends, you probably know quite a bit about saturated fats and trans fats (see box 4.1 for a review). Saturated fats are found mostly in animal products and tropical oils and should be limited in your diet because they are linked to increased risk of cardiovascular disease, stroke, and other types of vascular disease. Although not all recommendations expressed in the scientific literature and the media support a focus on saturated fat, hundreds of trials that fed people different fats have shown beyond doubt that saturated fat raises cholesterol, especially the "bad" LDL-cholesterol. The 2015-2020 Dietary Guidelines for Americans,[38] along with the American Diabetes Association (ADA),[39] recommends that saturated fat intake be limited to no more than 10 percent of energy, whereas the American College of Cardiology and the American Heart Association (AHA) place more emphasis on reducing saturated fat intake to less than 5 percent if LDL is elevated[40] (i.e., is more than 100 milligrams per deciliter). Trans fats, on the other hand, are obtained mostly from processed foods in which partially hydrogenated oils are used in their preparation or processing. These fats have been recognized to cause a double whammy by both increasing LDL cholesterol and also decreasing high-density lipoprotein (HDL) cholesterol, or "good" cholesterol. While most health organizations recommend keeping the amount of trans fat in the diet as low as possible, it is hoped these recommendations become a moot point with the 2015 mandate by the Federal Department of Agriculture (FDA) that food manufacturers stop using trans fats by June 2019.[41]

Box 4.1

Classes of Dietary Fats

Dietary fats. Most of the dietary fats in our food supply are found in a chemical structure called *triglycerides.* Triglycerides consist of a backbone molecule called glycerol that holds three fatty acids, thus the name triglycerides. Fatty acids are simply chains of carbon molecules with an acid end that attaches to the glycerol backbone and a stable methyl end. Most of the fatty acids in the diet are long-chains (14-22 carbons), but some foods contain small amounts of short-chain (4-6 carbons) and medium-chain (8-12 carbons) fatty acids.

Saturated fats. Saturated fats include those fatty acids that have all their carbon chains fully saturated with hydrogen atoms. This saturation makes them solid at room temperature. In general, animal fat provides 40 to 60 percent of their fat as saturated fat whereas plants provide only 10 to 20 percent of their fat as saturated fat (see figures 4.4 and 4.5). Commercially available products that were once high in trans fat and sources of partially hydrogenated oils may now be sources of fully hydrogenated, saturated fat.

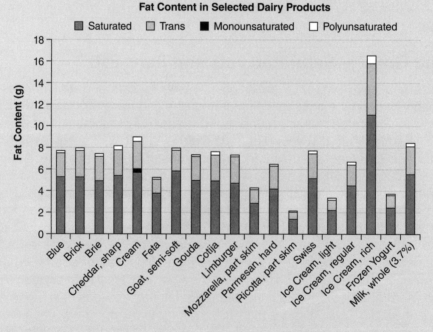

FIGURE 4.4 Amount of saturated, monounsaturated, and polyunsaturated fat in 1 ounce (28 g) of selected cheeses, half a cup (66 g) of ice cream, or 1 cup (236 ml) of whole milk. Note: Most cheese provides 8 grams of fat per serving, with about 5 of these grams coming from saturated fat.

Data from the USDA National Nutrient Database for Standard Reference (Dairy Products and Eggs and Sweets Categories). Available: https://ndb.nal.usda.gov/ndb/.

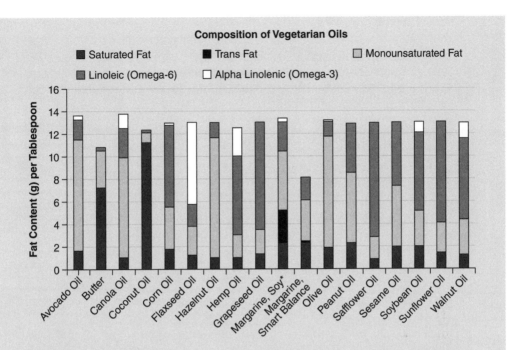

FIGURE 4.5 Amount of saturated, trans, and monounsaturated fats and omega-6 and omega-3 polyunsaturated fats in 1 tablespoon (~ 15 ml) of butter and various vegetable oils.

Data from the USDA National Nutrient Database for Standard Reference (Fats and Oils). Available: https://ndb.nal. usda.gov/ndb. Product information for hemp (seed) oil not contained in the USDA database.

*Varies by brand.

Monounsaturated fats. Monounsaturated fats have one missing pair of hydrogen molecules. They are therefore unsaturated at one location and thus have one double bond. Monounsaturated fats are found in both animal and plant foods, but their richest sources are olive oil, canola oil, most nuts and peanuts, and avocado. A common monounsaturated fat found in the diet is oleic acid.

Polyunsaturated fats. Polyunsaturated fats have two or more missing hydrogen pairs, and thus have two or more double bonds. These fats are further classified by the position of the first double bond from the stable methyl end as omega-6s and omega-3s.

Omega-6 fats. These polyunsaturated fatty acids have the first double bond positioned at carbon number 6. The most common omega-6 in the diet is the essential fatty acid linoleic acid, which is abundant in common plant foods: corn, sunflower, safflower, soybean, and cottonseed oils. Gamma-linolenic acid (found in evening primrose) is also an omega-6 fatty acid. Arachidonic acid is a longer-chain omega-6 found in animal products and is the form used to make the inflammatory eicosanoids. The body can convert linoleic acid to arachidonic acid.

Omega-3 fats. These polyunsaturated fatty acids have the first double bond positioned at carbon number 3. The plant version, alpha-linolenic acid (ALA) is

(continued)

Classes of Dietary Fats *(continued)*

found in specific plant foods, such as flaxseed, flaxseed oil, hemp oil, canola oil, soybean oil, and English (not black) walnuts (see figure 4.5). The longer fatty-acid versions, eicosapentaenoic acid (EPA) and docosahexaenoic acid (DHA) are found mostly in fatty fish, which include salmon, sturgeon, striped bass, and anchovies and in fish oil capsules. Vegan versions derived from microalgae[43] are now available and have been found to be well absorbed and increase both DHA and EPA concentrations in blood.[44] While alpha-linolenic acid has to be elongated in the body to DHA or EPA, which evidence suggests may be a slow or limited process, its conversion is increased when omega-6 concentrations in the diet or blood are low.[45]

Hydrogenated fats and trans fats. Hydrogenation is a process practiced by the food industry in which hydrogen atoms are forced onto vegetable oil molecules under high pressure and temperature. This converts unsaturated fatty acids into saturated ones, thereby converting a liquid oil into a soft solid with improved stability. Partial hydrogenation, in which only some of the oil's unsaturated fatty acids become saturated, produces unusual fatty acids that are called trans-fatty acids. Trans fat has traditionally been found in vegetable shortenings, hard margarines, crackers, cookies, and snack foods. It is hoped it will soon be omitted from our food supply.

Medium-chain triglycerides. Medium-chain triglycerides (MCTs) are saturated fatty acids with a chain of 8 to 12 carbons. Some can be found naturally in milk fat, coconut oil, and palm kernel oil. They are also made commercially as a by-product of margarine production. Medium-chain triglycerides are water soluble and are more easily and rapidly digested, absorbed, and oxidized for fuel than are long-chain triglycerides. MCTs are commonly recommended to people who have problems digesting long-chain fats. Research has not found that MCTs benefit athletes.

The majority of trans fat in Americans' diets comes from processed, packaged foods that are made with margarine or partially hydrogenated oils (cows' milk also contains small amounts). One consideration is what food manufacturers will replace hydrogenated oil with; if it's coconut or palm oil, because both are high in saturated fat, the net gain may be minimal. There is also evidence that palmitic acid, found in palm oil, shortening, and butter may increase risk for a heart condition called atrial fibrillation in susceptible individuals.[42] A quick look at the ingredients of the new Crisco shows palm oil and fully hydrogenated palm oil as key ingredients. Crisco and similar products may be technically free of trans fat (contain less than 0.5 g/tbsp), but they contain 3.5 grams per tablespoon of saturated fat. Healthier? Probably not much. Thus, for now, keep a keen eye out and continue to read the label on processed food products, vegetarian or not.

Being an athlete with a higher energy expenditure than your peers gives you a little more leeway to eat more saturated fat (if you follow the rules of less than 10%), but the unnatural trans fats—in my opinion—should be kept as low as possible, no matter how much energy you expend. While it is great news that as of June 2019, much less trans fat should be found in our food supply because of the FDA mandate, manufacturers may petition to keep trans fat in certain foods. Athletes should therefore still check the food labels and watch for use of fully hydrogenated oils or the return of more saturated fats, including palm and coconut oils. As always, natural fat is still the way to go.

Even though it is prudent for vegetarian athletes to keep saturated fat intake to less than 10 percent of energy, it is probably not necessary to count saturated fat grams unless your LDL level is elevated. Rather, assess your diet for foods and specific brands of food products that may be too high in saturated fat or overly processed fat, and then work toward limiting these foods and replacing them with less-processed sources. For example, replace margarine with olive oil and other flavorful dipping oils and look for recipes using canola and other oils instead of those using the new trans-fat-free Crisco. If you are a cheese-loving vegetarian, strive to limit overconsumption of saturated fat from full-fat dairy. If your LDL cholesterol is elevated, you can estimate your upper limit for saturated fat grams by multiplying your estimated energy needs (from chapter 2) by 5 to 6 percent (the new AHA guidelines)[40] and divide by 9 (9 kcal per gram of fat). For example, if your energy needs are 2,800 kilocalories, your estimated upper range of saturated fat is between 15.6 and 18.7 grams (2,800 $\times$ 0.05 and 0.06 $\div$ 9).

"Good Guys"—Monounsaturated Fat and Omega-3s

Diets that are rich sources of monounsaturated and omega-3 fats (see box 4.1) are advocated for the prevention of heart and other vascular diseases, particularly when they are delivered as part of an overall healthy diet such as the Mediterranean-style diet. [46] Monounsaturated fats, when substituted for saturated fats in the diet, lower LDL cholesterol and favorably influence other cardiovascular risk factors by lowering blood pressure, protecting against LDL oxidation, reducing blood clotting, and protecting the lining of the blood vessels. Omega-3 fatty acids, including both plant and fish forms (described in box 4.1), lower triglycerides, reduce inflammation, and improve immune function. All in all, they appear to reduce the risk for most chronic diseases.

The recommendation to increase the "good guys" is not as straightforward as the recommendation to decrease the "bad guys." While previous guidelines from some public health organizations placed more emphasis on monounsaturated fats, the more recent guidelines emphasize consumption of a dietary pattern that emphasizes intake of vegetables, fruits, and whole grains, and contains low-fat dairy, legumes, fish, poultry, nontropical vegetable oils, and nuts.[40] The ADA[39] suggests that a Mediterranean-style monounsaturated-rich eating pattern may benefit those with type 2 diabetes and that an increase in foods containing long-chain omega-3 fatty acids may be beneficial in prevention of heart disease and also associated with positive health outcomes. The recommendation for omega-3s for the vegetarian athlete also comes with additional considerations. Because the omega-3s and their polyunsaturated counterparts, the omega-6s, both compete to be included as precursors for making a family of hormone-like substances called eicosanoids, it is generally recommended that vegetarians focus more on incorporating omega-3s in the diet[30,47] and less on their omega-6s partners. This is because the eicosanoids are important and potent signal regulators, or mediators, of many biochemical functions such as blood clotting, blood pressure, vascular dilation, immune function, and inflammation. The mediators produced from the omega-3s are thought to be more health promoting than the mediators produced from the omega-6s.

The importance of obtaining higher omega-3s for the vegetarian[47] and the athlete, however, is not well understood.[48] While several recent studies have suggested that omega-3s may be important for inflammatory modulation[49] or reducing exercise-induced muscle damage,[50] the evidence is still preliminary.[48] For now, it may be prudent for vegetarian athletes to ensure somewhat higher intake of omega-3s than the daily recommended intake (DRI),[51] which is 1.1 grams per day for women and 1.6 grams per day for men,[29] while simultaneously limiting intake of linoleic acid.[51] To do this practically, focus on selecting foods that are good sources of monounsaturated and omega-3 fats in place of foods high in saturated fat and omega-6 fats (see figures 4.4 and 4.5). Olive oil is rich in monounsaturated fats, whereas concentrated plant sources of omega-3s include walnuts, flax, chia, camelina, canola, and hemp seeds and their oils. For example, cook using olive, avocado, or canola oils, and bake with canola oil, grapeseed oil, or light olive oil. Also, try incorporating walnuts, ground flaxseed, and other nuts and healthy oils into your meals and snacks (see table 4.3) and at the same time limit intake of corn, safflower, sunflower, and cottonseed oils along with butter, vegetable shortening, and most margarines. If you feel you might benefit from more omega-3s for one reason or another, consider a docosahexaenoic acid (DHA)-rich microalgae supplements along with the consumption of more omega-3-rich plant foods.

Striving for Smart Fat

As with carbohydrate foods, choosing more whole, less-processed fats as part of an overall healthy plant-based diet is important to your health and physical performance. Achieving this "smart fat" approach requires you to do two things. The first is to enjoy eating fat and fat-containing vegetarian foods. Fat sources have wonderful flavors (see table 4.3) and alert your taste buds to the flavors in your grains, vegetables, and fruits. That goes for a sprinkle of roasted nuts or sharp, flavorful cheeses. The second thing you must do is consider the health aspects of fat. Limit the bad guys and focus on incorporating more of the good guys in your diet. By the same token, if you love a food product such as brie cheese, coconut curry, cheesecake, or corn on the cob *with* butter, don't deprive yourself. Just remember to enjoy these foods on occasion. And by all means, get rid of the guilt associated with eating fat.

TABLE 4.3   Characteristics and Recommended Uses for Selected Vegetarian Oils

Oil	Characteristics and recommended uses
Avocado	Made for high heat (when refined); perfect for frying, broiling, or wok cooking; smoke point is 510-520 °F (265-271 °C).
Canola	The ultimate all-purpose oil for cooking and baking, also works well for frying or wok cooking; has a high smoke point in general (400-425 °F [204-218 °C]), but high-heat versions are available.
Flaxseed	Use without direct heat in finished dishes, including salads, grains, and soups or blended into dressings and smoothies. Combines well with tofu, garlic, and onions. Keep refrigerated. Smoke point is 225 °F (107 °C).
Grapeseed	An all-purpose oil with a neutral taste to let other flavors take center stage. Best for short-term, medium-heat cooking, baking, or sautéing. Smoke point is 420-425 °F (204-218 °C).
Hazelnut, toasted	Has the distinctive flavor and aroma of toasted hazelnuts for use in salads and sauces and drizzled in soups. Especially good paired with bitter greens. For best results, use on finished dishes. Smoke point is 430 °F (221°C).
Hemp seed	Provides distinctive nutty flavor and can be added to most recipes. To preserve essential fatty acid content, do not use for frying. Best kept refrigerated. Smoke point is 330 °F (165 °C).
Olive	Suitable for most vegetarian fare, including salads, sautés, and sauces and to dip bread in. Light-flavored olive oil is also good for baking. Smoke point is 320 °F (160 °C) (unrefined), 400-420 °F (204-215 °C) (refined), and 468 °F (242 °C) (light). Do not use unrefined oils for frying at high heats.
Peanut	The unrefined version adds depth and intensity to any sauté or stir-fry. Refined versions are perfect for high-heat applications such as frying or wok cooking. Smoke point is 320 °F (160 °C) (unrefined) and 440 °F (227 °C) (refined).
Pumpkin seed	An opaque oil with the robust flavor of roasted pumpkin. Delicious drizzled over root vegetables (with a little cheese if desired). For best results, use on finished dishes. Smoke point is not available.
Sesame	Great in Asian dishes and salad dressings. Refined versions are acceptable for wok cooking, cooking, or sautéing. Use unrefined and toasted versions for intense flavor, allowing the flavor of the oil into the finished dish. Smoke point is 350 °F (177 °C) (unrefined), and 410-450 °F (210-232 °C) (refined).
Tahini	Use as an ingredient in uncooked or already-cooked dishes, for example in hummus, tabouli, soups, grains, and salads and blended into dressings.
Walnut	Best for short-term, medium-heat cooking, baking, or sautéing. Try it drizzled over vegetables and toasted nuts and in salads or fruit muffins. Allow the flavor of the oil to be part of the finished dish. Smoke point is 320-400 °F (160-204 °C).

Note: The smoke point of the various oils is an approximation and may vary slightly from source to source. Oils should not be heated above the smoke point, which is the temperature at which the oil begins to break down and smoke. Heating above this temperature breaks down essential fatty acids and causes off-flavors. Corn, bean, safflower, and sunflower oils are not reviewed because of their commonality and high levels of omega-6 fatty acids. Many specialty oils are best when stored in cooler temperatures.

That said, you can choose smart fat by being more liberal in your consumption of whole foods containing monounsaturated fats and omega-3-rich alpha-linolenic acid and limiting foods high in linoleic acid (see figure 4.5). You can accomplish this by snacking on nuts, sprinkling ground flaxseed or flaxseed oil in your cereal, smoothie, or salad (it tastes yummy); cooking regularly with olive, grapeseed, or canola oils; and experimenting with different and even new oils. Avocado and coconut are also great additions to recipes. Once you stray from the common refined oils found in grocery stores (corn, sunflower, cottonseed, and safflower), you will discover that individual oils have unique properties and flavors. Some oils, such as canola, are better for baking or cooking at high temperatures, while others, such as olive oil, are perfect for sautéing or dipping and add immense flavor. Some, such as toasted hazelnut or flax, are best simply sprinkled on cooked food or cold salads. Enjoy as we move on to learn more about protein.

5 | Building Muscle Without Meat

She was a recruit for an NCAA DII women's soccer team. Raised vegetarian, the high school senior was concerned about making the transition from eating mostly home-cooked meals to the college cafeteria. She had played mostly club soccer in her younger years and was also on the cross country team her first two years of high school. She tore her anterior cruciate ligament the fall of her junior year playing with a premier-level club she had been excited to make. Looking at her, you could tell she was strong. She had spent the last year and a half strength training and working with a physical therapist to ensure she was ready for college soccer. During our conversation she joked with me about people's typical reaction when they find out she is vegetarian. "The first thing they ask" she said, "is how do you get your protein?" She informed me that she had learned to respond "You don't need to eat meat to get protein," and that her sources were beans, grains, tofu, and eggs. When I did a quick evaluation of her diet, it was clear she easily exceeded the recommended dietary allowance for protein (0.8 g protein/kg) but did not always obtain the higher protein intake recommended for athletes (1.2-2.0 g protein/kg). This often occurred on her low training–volume days but occasionally occurred because she selected lots of fruit, bread, and grains, which she loved. While she did not seem to have performance concerns, we came up with strategies to help her take in more protein both at home and while eating in the college cafeteria.

– Enette

Eating meat to achieve strength and victory has a history in athletics of more than 2,000 years. The diets of athletes in the ancient Olympic era—including the legendary wrestler Milo of Croton who earned five successive Olympic wins from 532 to 516 B.C.—reportedly contained large quantities of meat for "physical strength."[1] And those of laborers and athletes at the turn of the 20th century—including the renowned Harvard and Yale rowing teams—were high in protein because, at the time, protein was considered to be the primary energy source for exercise. In addition, many cultures also believed that consuming the muscle of an animal would result in the transfer of that animal's strength and prowess to the athlete.[2] Certainly, some of these myths still linger as many coaches and athletes continue to believe that large quantities of protein—particularly animal protein—are needed to produce strong and "meaty" athletes. Although protein does play a critical role in an athlete's health and performance, it can be adequately supplied by plant-based diets, including vegan diets. This chapter reviews the role of protein in the diet and discusses how you can easily build muscle strength and mass without meat.

Protein Primer

Dietary protein is necessary for sustaining life. It provides the amino acid building blocks needed to form the structural basis of most of the body's tissue, including skeletal muscle, tendons, hormones, enzymes, red blood cells, and immune cells. Amino acids also serve as a source of energy, and certain amino acids can be converted to blood sugar in a process called *gluconeogenesis,* which is important during both prolonged exercise and starvation. Chemically, each of the 20 different amino acids is structurally distinct, but all contain at least one nitrogen-containing amino group attached to a similar skeleton of carbon, hydrogen, and oxygen.

Our body's requirement for protein is really a requirement for amino acids and nitrogen. As humans, we cannot produce 9 of these amino acids—called the essential amino acids—but are able to make the remaining 11 or so as long as enough nitrogen is consumed in the diet(see table 5.1).[3] Together, the 20 essential and nonessential amino acids are arranged in various combinations to build the many proteins in the body. The arrangement of these amino acid building blocks is unique for each protein in the body as well as in the foods we eat. Closely related species, such as humans and animals, tend to make proteins with a similar spectrum of amino acids, and those of very different species, such as plants compared to mammals, tend to have quite different spectrums. Protein building is initiated after a signal—typically from a hormone or growth factor—to the cell's genetic material (DNA) is communicated to initiate gene transcription and ultimately protein synthesis. In the case of exercise-induced increases in skeletal muscle protein building (or synthesis), a key signal is a molecule called mammalian target of rapamycin (or mTOR),[4] which is stimulated by both resistance exercise and the ingestion of dietary protein.[5]

TABLE 5.1   Essential and Nonessential Amino Acids

Essential amino acids (also called indispensable amino acids) cannot be made by the body and must be obtained through the diet.	Isoleucine* Leucine* Lysine Methionine	Phenylalanine Threonine Tryptophan Valine* Histidine
Conditional amino acids are made by the body but are essential in times of growth because they can't be made at a rate fast enough to support growth.	Arginine Glutamine Proline	Cysteine Glycine Tyrosine
Nonessential amino acids (also called dispensable amino acids) can be made by the body, and thus it is not essential to obtain them through the diet.	Alanine Aspartic acid Serine	Glutamic acid Asparagine

*Branched-chain amino acids

Although the body can make the nonessential amino acids, the essential amino acids must be obtained through the diet. If the mixture of the essential amino acids consumed in the diet does not match that required by the body, the amino acids found in the shortest supply, relative to the amount needed for protein synthesis, are referred to as the *limiting amino acids*. In general, diets based on a protein from a single plant food do not foster optimal growth because the single plant sources do not typically supply enough of all of the needed building blocks for human protein synthesis. For example, maize is low in tryptophan, rice is low in lysine and threonine, wheat is low in lysine, and most legumes, except soy, are low in methionine or tryptophan or both.[6] Diets based on combinations of different plant proteins, [6,7] as well as soy, dairy, fish, poultry, or meat protein, however, can easily supply enough of the right amino acid building blocks for human growth and muscle development.

Determining Protein Needs

As an athlete, your protein needs are most likely—but not necessarily—higher than those of your inactive friends. Whether they are higher, and how much higher, depends on your sport and current training program. For example, if you are a fitness enthusiast or a recreationally active athlete who exercises or plays sports several times a week, your needs are likely met by the recommended dietary allowance (RDA) of 0.8 grams of protein per kilogram of body mass per day. The same may be true if you are taking time off from training or performing light maintenance training during the off-season. This is because the RDA is set two standard deviations above the estimated average requirement for protein of 0.6 grams of protein per kilogram of body weight and is thought to meet the nutrient requirements of 97.5 percent of healthy individuals. If, however, you are training intensely for 8 to 40 hours a week, your protein needs may be about twice the RDA, particularly during the start of the season or a new training regimen, or when muscle mass gain is important.

The consensus of sports nutritionists—which is based on published research on the protein needs of mostly male athletes—suggests that athletes need 1.2 to 2.0 grams of protein per kilogram of body mass per day.[8] While there is some thought that female athletes may require slightly less protein per kilogram of body mass than male athletes,[9] more research is needed before sex-based recommendations can be made. The rationale for the additional protein required during training is based on the additional amino acid building blocks needed to promote muscle protein synthesis, repair exercise-induced microdamage to muscle fibers (endurance athletes know about this) and stimulate synthesis of enzymes and other proteins in our cell's energy-generating powerhouses: the mitochondria. Thus, additional protein is needed for both strength and endurance training. Recent research has also suggested that protein may be needed not only as building blocks but also as a trigger to induce protein synthesis as a result of the signaling molecule mTOR. The amino acid leucine is thought to serve as this key signaling trigger.[10,11]

In addition, inadequate intake of both energy and carbohydrate increases protein needs. During prolonged endurance activity, athletes with low glycogen stores use twice as much protein as those with adequate stores, primarily because amino acids are converted to glucose under these conditions to maintain blood sugar.[12] This, however, can be halted by adequately supplementing

---

Vegan View: "Are You Sure You Are Getting Enough Protein?"

One of the hardest things about being vegan is explaining that yes, you can indeed get enough protein from plant foods. It's frustrating when discussions about plant-based diets are disproportionately spent talking about protein. Some plant-based advocates, including physicians and other health professionals, may even go so far as to state "Protein is a nonissue" or "I have never seen a protein deficiency in a vegetarian" because they are just tired of answering the question. This sentiment is a little troublesome at best and not accurate for everyone because some folks may have protein needs that require extra thought and effort. Even if someone isn't technically deficient in protein intake, he or she might be eating inadequate amounts and exhibiting vague symptoms such as low energy, loss of muscle mass, or simply not feeling satisfied by meals.

Therefore, vegan athletes should first aim to meet protein recommendations—1.2 to 2.0 grams of protein per kilogram body weight—and then adjust from there. Recommendations are based on a range of needs, with actual intake falling along the spectrum. Spending extra time on this chapter to learn about protein sources and needs will help you to meet your own needs and help you explain to inquiring minds that, yes, you do indeed get enough protein!

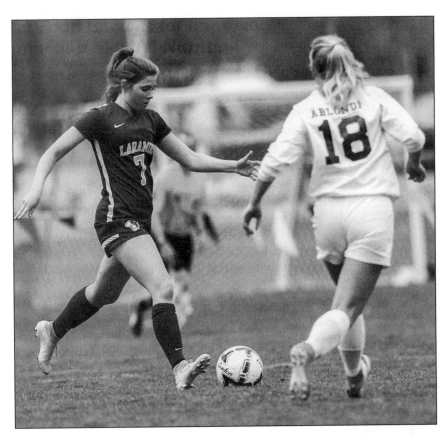

The amino acids needed for muscle development can be derived from soy protein and a variety of protein-rich plant foods.

Courtesy of the Lamarie Boomerang. Photographer: Shannon Broderick.

with carbohydrate before or during exercise or both (as will be discussed in chapter 9). Furthermore, athlete or not, your protein needs are likely to be higher if you intentionally restrict calories to promote weight or body fat loss (as further discussed in chapter 13).

Although no research suggests that protein recommendations are different for vegetarian athletes, it has been suggested that vegetarians may need to consume approximately 10 percent more protein than omnivores to account for the lower digestibility of plant protein compared with animal proteins. However, the additional requirement to account for lower digestibility is not true for all plant proteins. The protein in most soy products for example is readily digestible compared to protein from whole, cooked legumes, which is not as easily digested. Furthermore, in its release of the dietary reference intake (DRI) for protein, the Food and Nutrition Board of the National Academy of Sciences Institute of Medicine concluded that a separate recommendation for protein consumption was not required for vegetarians who consume complementary mixtures of plant proteins[3] and certainly eggs or dairy products.

Finally, it is important to mention that not all scientists believe that the protein needs of athletes are higher than those recommended for the general population. Although many studies show that protein use, and therefore requirements, increases with the initiation of exercise training, most of these studies have been short term and may not have allowed enough time for adaptation to the training regimen.[13] Hence, it is possible that the protein needs are only temporarily elevated and return to baseline at some point after training initiation and adaptation. For instance, a long-term study conducted in the early 1970s found that individuals starting a cycling program experienced a negative nitrogen balance with initiation of training, indicating that their protein needs were increased above that of their sedentary state, but this negative nitrogen balance returned to neutral after 20 days of training with no change in diet.[13] In the recent release of the DRIs, the scientists on the panel did not feel there was enough compelling evidence to suggest that additional protein is needed for healthy adults undertaking resistance or endurance exercise.[3] An abundance of research conducted since the previous edition of this book was published, however, has underscored the importance of additional, well-timed protein intake in athletes to help build and repair muscle protein, which includes both muscle fiber proteins and mitochondrial proteins. The specific timing of protein intake relative to resistance or aerobic exercise is discussed further in chapter 9. You can estimate your overall daily protein needs using the calculations in table 5.2.

TABLE 5.2   Estimating Daily Protein Needs

Enter your body mass (weight) in kilograms (weight in pounds divided by 2.2).	_____ kg *(line a)*
Enter estimated range of protein needed to support your current level of training and performance (see bullet points below). • 0.8 g protein/kg body mass (RDA for healthy adults) • 1.2 g protein/kg body mass (lower range recommended for athletes)* • 2.0 g protein/kg body mass (upper range recommended for athletes)*	_____ to _____ g/kg *(line b1) (line b2)*
Multiply *line a* by *line b1* to get your estimated lower range.	_____ g protein/day *(line c1)*
Multiply *line a* by *line b2* to get your estimated upper range.	_____ g protein/day *(line c2)*
Divide total range of protein by your typical number of meals or snacks to get an approximate amount of protein per meal. Note that consuming protein spread across three or more meals and snacks per day is thought to result in more effective muscle protein synthesis.	_____ to _____ g protein/ day ÷_____ meals and snacks/day

*Guidelines established by the American College of Sports Medicine, the Academy of Nutrition and Dietetics, and Dietitians of Canada.[8]

Meeting Protein Needs

Despite the controversy over the protein needs of vegetarians and athletes, you can easily meet your protein needs—even if they are in the upper level recommended—on a plant-based diet. This, of course, is provided that your diet contains both adequate energy and a variety of plant-based protein foods. The once-held belief that vegetarians needed to eat specific combinations of plant proteins in the same meal was dispelled in the 1990s, at least among nonathletic adults,[6] and replaced with the recommendation to simply consume a variety of plant-based protein-rich foods over the course of a day.[6,14] Emphasizing amino acid balance at each meal is not necessary because the limiting amino acids in one meal can be buffered (at least over the short term) by small pools of free amino acids in the gut, skeletal muscle, and blood. These amino acids come from the food consumed in the previous meal or snack and from the digestion of our own digestive enzymes and dead gut cells (which are sloughed off much like skin cells). Furthermore, although most plant foods tend to be low in certain amino acids (as discussed earlier), usual combinations of plant-based proteins consumed in the diets of most cultures—such as beans and rice—naturally provide complementary mixtures of the essential amino acids.[7] As such, many combinations of plant-based proteins provide a source of high-quality protein (see table 5.3). In addition, for vegetarians and semivegetarians, consuming small amounts of dairy, eggs, fish, or poultry can also provide complementary essential amino acids, which can enhance the quality of plant proteins.

TABLE 5.3   Natural Food Combinations That Provide All Essential Amino Acids

Single foods	Examples
Quinoa, soy foods, acorns	Tofu stir-fry, barbeque soybeans, tofu smoothie, texturized soy protein, marinated tempeh, quinoa with mixed vegetables, toasted acorns
Excellent combinations	**Examples**
Grains and legumes	Rice and beans, bean soup with vegetables and whole-grain crackers, tortillas with beans, peanut butter sandwich
Grains or vegetables with dairy or soy accent	Pasta with cheese, baked potato with dairy or soy sour cream, cream of vegetable soup, rice pudding
Legumes and nuts	Beans and nuts (particularly Brazil nuts),[a] hummus[a] made with chickpeas and tahini, lentil and nut "meat" balls
Other combinations	Sweet corn and tomatoes, sweet peppers or wheat germ,[a] coconut meat and apples,[a] soy protein isolate and sesame seed flour, sunflower seed flour or spirulina,[a] edamame and orange juice or medjool dates[a]

[a]Source: Woolf, Fu, and Basu (7).

That said, however, extensive research in the past 10 or so years suggests that athletes in intense training should consume a protein-containing snack or meal soon after exhaustive exercise, when amino acid pools may be compromised. Examples of high-quality proteins are soy protein[15](particularly with added sesame or sunflower seeds),[7] milk, yogurt, or egg protein and combinations of two or more vegetable proteins (table 5.3) such as hummus,[7] peanut butter on whole-grain bread, muesli with nuts and toasted grains, or a mini bean burrito. Most likely these are snacks you naturally select, maybe just not after exercise.

If you are concerned about your protein intake, don't be. Surveys of athletes have consistently found that most, simply by virtue of their high energy intake, on average meet or even exceed their protein requirements without trying. This is true for vegetarian and vegan athletes as well. Vegetarian diets generally derive 12.5 percent of energy from protein, whereas vegan diets derive 11 percent from protein. Therefore, according to these percentages, if you were a 176-pound (80 kg) male athlete consuming 3,600 calories, you would receive 1.41 grams of protein per kilogram of body weight from the average vegetarian diet and 1.2 grams per kilogram from the average vegan diet. If you were a 110-pound (50 kg) female gymnast consuming 2,200 calories, you would receive 1.38 grams per kilogram from a vegetarian diet and 1.21 grams per kilogram from a vegan diet.

Nevertheless, if you are concerned about your own protein intake, you can check yourself by counting your protein intake for a day or two using the information provided in tables 5.4 and 5.5. The information on the food labels should also be helpful. Remember also to count the protein in your bread, cereal, and grain foods, which can add up quickly. If you find your intake of protein is lacking compared to your estimated requirements, simply strive to add one to three servings of protein-rich vegetarian foods to your regular meals or snacks. For example, add soy milk to a fruit snack, lentils to spaghetti sauce, tofu to stir-fry, or chickpeas (garbanzo beans) to salad. Also don't forget to toss marinated tofu, beans or nuts when creating a Dragon Bowl or Breakfast Bowl. You can also experiment with cooking with chickpea flour or adding white or black bean puree to baked goods (see www.pulses.org for more ideas) and if necessary, sneak plant-based protein powder concentrates into smoothies, baked goods, and dips. However, the athletes who typically lack protein are often those who focus too much on carbohydrate (the bagel, pasta, banana athletes) or who consume too little food in general. Vegetarian foods that are particularly rich sources of protein are legumes, tofu, seitan, quinoa, soy protein isolate, pea protein isolate, and commercially available meat analogues, such as vegetarian hot dogs, burgers, and "chicken" made from soy or mycoprotein. Vegetarian athletes who are not particularly fond of many protein-rich plant foods or are allergic to them may also need to carefully monitor their protein intake or see a registered dietitian nutritionist knowledgeable about plant-based diets.

TABLE 5.4 Approximate Protein Content of Selected Food and Beverages

Food	Portion	Protein (g)
Bread, grains, rice, pasta	1 oz	2-3
Cheese, medium and hard	1 oz	7
Cheese, cottage	1/4 cup	7
"Cheese," soy or veggie	1 oz	6
Egg, whole	1 large	7
Edamame, shelled	1/2 cup	7
Hemp seeds	3 tbsp (30 g)	9.5
Hummus	1/3 cup	7
Legumes (most beans and peas), cooked	1/2 cup	7
Milk, almond	1 cup	1
Milk, cows'	1 cup	8
Milk, rice	1 cup	1
Milk, soy	1 cup	7
Pea protein isolate	2 tbsp	Varies by manufacturer
Nuts, most	2 tbsp	7
Peanut butter	2 tbsp	7
Quinoa, cooked	1 cup	11
Quorn (mycoprotein) Meat-Free Meatballs	4 meatballs (68 g)	14
Quorn (mycoprotein) Naked Cutlets	1 cutlet (69 g)	11
Quorn (mycoprotein) Turkey-Style Roast	1/5 roast (3 oz)	15
Plant-based protein bars	1 bar (varies)	8-20 (varies)
Plant-based protein powder (Vega and similar brands)	1 large scoop (33 g)	20
Seeds (e.g., chia, hemp, pumpkin, sunflower)	1 oz	6-9
Seitan	4 oz	21
Soybean-curd cheese	1/4 cup	7
Soy protein isolate	1 oz	21
Tempeh	1 cup	31
Textured vegetable protein (TVP), cooked	1/2 cup	8
Tofu, soft	1 cup	10

(continued)

TABLE 5.4   *(continued)*

Food	Portion	Protein (g)
Tofu, firm	1 cup	20
Vegemite sandwich spread	1 tsp	1.5
Veggemo (pea protein milk beverage)	1 cup	6
Vegetables, most, cooked	1/2 cup	2-3
Vegetarian "burgers"	1 patty (varies)	6-16
Vegetarian burger, Griller, Morning Star Farms	1 patty (96 g)	23
Vegetarian, Impossible Burger brand (made from soy, wheat, potato proteins, and leghemoglobin from genetically engineered yeast)[16]	1 patty (85 g)	20
Vegetarian "burger" crumbles	1/2 cup	7-11
Vegetarian "chicken" patties or nuggets	1 patty (~6 nuggets)	7-15
Vegetarian "dogs"	1 dog	9-12
Yogurt, dairy	1 cup	8
Yogurt, Greek	1 cup	20-24
Yogurt, soy	1 cup	8

Refer to appendix F for guidance on converting English units to metric.

Data compiled from the Diabetic Exchange List for Meal Planning, 2003; USDA National Nutrient Database for Standard Reference (https://ndb.nal.usda.gov/ndb/); and selected food labels, including those from Quorn, CalorieKing Australia, and Impossible Burger.

Role of Excess Protein

Improvements in both strength and muscle mass occur as a result of your training and are also dictated by your genetic makeup. Dietary protein simply provides the amino acid building blocks needed to make protein and facilitate neuroendocrine connections. Thus, you will not receive the training effects you deserve—muscle strength and muscle mass gains—if your diet is lacking in either energy or protein. On the other hand, you will not magically gain strength or functional muscle if you consume amino acid building blocks in excess. If this were true, your average male couch potato would look more like Arnold Schwarzenegger in his younger years. A classic study conducted at McMaster University in Canada in the early 1990s illustrates this point.[17] In this study, researchers randomly assigned both male strength athletes and sedentary subjects to receive one of three protein-modified diets for 13 days. One diet supplied approximately the U.S. RDA for protein (0.86 g protein/kg body mass/day), one provided close to the current recommendation for athletes (1.4 g protein/kg body mass/day), and one provided an excessive amount of protein (2.4 g protein/kg body mass/day). The researchers found

TABLE 5.5   Sample Log for Counting Protein

Food	Protein (g)
1-1/2 cups cornflakes (3/4 cup = 1 oz serving)	4-6
1 cup 1% milk	8
12 oz (1-1/2 cups) orange juice	0
White bread, 2 slices	4-6
2 tbsp peanut butter	7
1 can (~2 cups) fruit cocktail in light syrup	0
1 large handful (~1 cup) grapes	0
Jelly beans (~2 oz)	0
1/3 cup granola	2-3
1/4 cup almonds	14
2 cups vegetarian chili (contains ~1 cup beans and 1 cup onion, green peppers, and tomato sauce combined)	14
~2 oz cheddar cheese	14
15 saltine crackers	4-6
Total g	71-78
Total g/kg	1.11-1.22

Note: Reported daily carbohydrate intake for a 141-pound (64 kg) female volleyball player involved in off-season training. Her protein goal based on the RDA of 0.8 grams of protein per kilogram of body weight is 51 grams per day. Although she is likely to exceed her needs, she needs to increase protein intake during periods of more-intense training. This should happen naturally by increasing caloric intake. For example, she could add half a cup of beans and another grain serving (10 additional grams of protein) to the intake shown in the table.

Protein counting is most accurate if portion sizes are accurately measured and food labels are used to supplement the information presented in table 5.4. Refer to appendix F for guidance on converting English units to metric.

that the diet containing approximately the U.S. RDA for protein did not provide adequate protein for the strength athletes and impaired whole-body protein building compared to the other two diets. The diet providing 2.4 grams of protein, however, did not increase whole-body protein synthesis any more than the diet providing 1.4 grams of protein did. In contrast, the diet that followed the RDA recommendation supplied adequate protein for the sedentary men. Increasing protein intake in the nontraining men, however, did not increase protein synthesis. A recent meta-analysis and systematic review of data from 49 studies of over 1,800 participants found similar results.[18] Protein intakes of up to 1.62 grams per kilogram of body mass per day increased muscle size and muscle fiber area and increased strength (measured by one-repetition maximum) during periods of prolonged resistance training.

However, no further benefits were found with higher protein intakes (>1.62 g/kg). Another meta-analysis by Messina and colleagues found the gains in strength and lean body mass were no different when soy rather than whey was the source of protein.[19]

What happens to excess protein intake? Quite simply, if you consume more than you need, the nitrogen group is removed and it is either used for energy or stored as fat. This makes for an expensive source of energy, both from a personal metabolic and ecological viewpoint. Although it is not known whether habitually high protein intake (i.e., >~ 2 g protein/kg body mass/day) causes long-term detrimental effects, some medical professionals question whether such diets place added stress on the kidney[20] (which is the organ responsible for eliminating the excess nitrogen) and the liver, particularly when protein intake is from meat and dairy sources. One study found that an Atkins-style high-protein diet increased the risk for both kidney stones and calcium loss from bone.[21]

A final point, based on relatively recent research, is that spreading protein intake throughout the day—rather than in one or two big meals as many Americans typically do—may offer benefits for both athletes in heavy training and older individuals. These studies suggest that consuming 20 to 30 grams of protein (or 0.25-0.3 g/kg body mass/day) distributed evenly over three or four meals or snacks[18] is more effective at stimulating muscle protein synthesis over the course of a day than is concentrating protein intake into one or two large meals.[22,23] This means that including a significant source of protein in breakfast, lunch, and dinner meals and perhaps other snacks may be a beneficial pattern for many vegetarian athletes. Stay tuned for tips in chapter 12 on incorporating protein into a balanced eating pattern.

Considering Protein Supplements

Vegetarian and vegan athletes can meet their protein needs through diet alone. For convenience, however, many vegetarian athletes supplement their diets on occasion with protein-containing nutrition beverages or bars, which include soy protein isolate, pea protein,[24] hemp protein, or whey protein. Many brands and varieties are available from both large pharmaceutical companies and small or local "ma and pa" businesses. Although this is fine on occasion, these food products should not replace real food and real meals, despite some companies' marketing ploys to convince you otherwise. While some evidence suggests that heavily processed isolated proteins are more rapidly digested and promote greater protein retention (at least over the short term), evidence that this affects the gain of muscle or strength in well-trained athletes in the long run does not exist. In fact, a recent study in rats found that the slower-absorbed milk protein casein nicely complemented the faster-absorbed whey protein in prolonging the muscle protein synthesis response to exercise,[25] perhaps making milk protein in its natural form a better overall source of protein.

The idea of consuming isolated protein also interferes with my philosophy on healthy vegetarian eating because it ignores the way protein is typically consumed: in a mixed meal from whole foods. Even if there were a small grain of truth to the benefit of isolated-protein consumption, consistently giving up the pleasures of Thai-cooked tofu, savory split pea soup, or a bit of French cheese on a fresh baguette for a protein bar containing isolated soy, pea, or whey seems like a tragedy. These processed products serve their purpose but should not regularly replace the pleasures of eating real food. Many of us will also have to grapple with our acceptance of products such as the Impossible Burger that, because of genetic engineering, looks, tastes, and nearly bleeds like real meat.[16,26]

Indeed, adequate protein—which is easily provided by a vegetarian diet—is necessary for gaining muscle strength and muscle mass through athletic training. Excess protein intake in and of itself, however, will not promote muscle gain and, as we will learn in the next chapter, may even increase calcium needs. Read on.

6 | Optimizing Bone Health

Veronica, a vegan of many years, was interested in nutrition counseling because she was getting into running and had questions about how she could improve her diet. It came to light that she believed that the current recommendation for calcium intake of 1,000 milligrams a day is artificially high because of the influence of the dairy industry. She pointed to worldwide recommendations that are lower and was convinced that calcium and bone health are not significant issues for vegans. This thinking stems from a common myth in the plant-based world: that animal protein "pulls" calcium from bones and by avoiding meat and dairy, you are protected from poor bone health. This hypothesis was popular decades ago, but more recent research disproves it. Meanwhile, other studies point to the lower bone density of vegans who do not consume enough calcium.

Veronica and I discussed this research and looked at high-calcium plant foods that could help her meet the current recommendations. We also addressed the issue of oxalates and how some seemingly high-calcium foods like spinach are not reliable sources because of low absorbability. Lastly, we covered the multitude of factors and nutrients that affect bone health, all of which are important for people who limit or avoid animal foods. These topics are addressed in detail in this chapter. In the end, Veronica left our counseling sessions happy and with an evidence-based approach to bone health (and sports nutrition for her running, of course!) that works for her diet and lifestyle.

– Matt

It is not hard to argue the importance of bone health. As athletes, we know that we can't perform without a healthy skeleton and that our exercise training in turn helps us maintain healthy muscles and bone. Whether we are immediately concerned about the nutrients that promote healthy bone, however, is often another story. It seems that some athletes feel immune to bone problems, and others seem to think—as I once did—that getting adequate calcium is all that is needed. As vegetarians, many may also be antidairy—believing that calcium and bone-related research is tainted by the powerful dairy industry—which in the end could come back to haunt them. Results of research on long-term vegetarians and vegans, for example, has been mixed. Some studies show higher bone density in lactovegetarians and less bone loss after menopause,[1] and others indicate that vegetarians may be at risk for high bone turnover rates which can result in increased bone breakdown (resorption) and lower bone mineral density.[2-4] These differences among studies (and individuals) are most likely the result of overall eating patterns and lifestyle habits, which, depending on food choices, could include inadequate key nutrients. They could also be caused by a variety of factors that affect bone health and are not necessarily related only to being vegetarian or vegan. This chapter is directed at helping vegan and vegetarian athletes understand the basics of bone metabolism and bone health and how bone health can be optimized on a plant-based eating plan.

Bone Health Basics

Most of us think of bone simply as the rigid part of our skeleton that forms the levers on which our muscles contract. Bone, however, is a living tissue that is slowly yet actively broken down and rebuilt, a process scientists call *bone turnover* or *bone remodeling.* Bone turnover replaces existing bone structure with new bone structure and occurs in the developing skeleton of children and teens and in the nongrowing skeleton of adults. In fact, it is estimated that the adult skeleton is remodeled and replaced about every 10 years.[5] This remodeling is considered necessary for repairing microarchitectural damage and helping maintain healthy bone and normal calcium levels in the body. For example, one of the major functions of bone—apart from supporting our bodies—is to aid in maintaining blood calcium within the normal range. If bone could not be used as an immediate calcium reserve, the muscles in our body, including our heart muscle, would contract improperly, and many enzymes would operate uncontrollably. Obviously, the outcome would not be good. In addition, remodeling is probably also necessary for preventing the accumulation of microfractures, including stress fractures.

How bone remodeling occurs is fascinating. Two types of key bone cells, known as osteoblasts and osteoclasts, direct the process. Osteoclasts erode the bone surface—forming small cavities—through a set of reactions known as *resorption.* Osteoblasts act at the site of the cavities to synthesize the new bone matrix. This is referred to as bone *formation.* The new bone matrix is then mineralized with calcium, phosphorus, and other minerals, resulting in new bone tissue. Bone health is maintained if resorption and formation are tightly coupled, whereas bone loss ensues if bone resorption occurs at a rate greater than bone formation.

Structurally, bone tissue is made up largely of collagen—a protein that gives the bone its tensile strength and framework—and the calcium phosphate mineralized complex that hardens the framework. The combination of collagen fibrils and calcium phosphate crystals, commonly called *hydroxyapatite crystals*, makes bone strong yet flexible enough to bear weight and withstand stress.

Bone tissue, however, is not just bone tissue. Rather, adult bone is made up of two major types of tissue: cortical bone and trabecular bone. Trabecular bone makes up approximately 20 percent of your skeleton and has a faster turnover rate than cortical bone. This type of bone is found primarily in the axial skeleton (vertebrae, trunk, and head), the flat bones, and the ends of the long bones. It is estimated that as much as 20 percent of trabecular bone is undergoing active remodeling at one time. Cortical bone makes up the remaining 80 percent, but only 5 percent of its surface is in active remodeling at one time. Cortical bone is found primarily in the long bones, for example, those in the arms and legs. Common fracture sites are thought to have a high trabecular content. Trabecular bone has a faster turnover rate because it has more metabolically active cells and greater blood supply. Hence, trabecular bone is more sensitive to hormones that govern day-to-day calcium deposits and withdrawals, which means it more readily gives up minerals whenever blood calcium starts to drop. Loss of trabecular bone can occur whenever calcium withdrawal exceeds calcium deposits, but loss typically begins around age 30, even for people who exercise and eat a healthy diet. Although cortical bone also gives up calcium, this occurs at a slower and steadier pace. Cortical bone losses typically begin at about age 40 and continue slowly but surely thereafter.

Factors That Influence Bone Health

Many factors regulate bone health, mainly by influencing bone turnover and absolute bone content or density. These factors include physical activity, hormonal status, and nutrition. Participation in weight-bearing, impact-loading, and weight-training activities, which include running, racewalking, rope jumping, military marching, gymnastics, and weightlifting, promotes denser and stronger bones. Just how exercise does this is not completely understood, but a prevailing theory considers bone to react as a piezoelectric crystal that converts mechanical stress—from ground forces or powerful muscle contractions—into electrical energy. The electrical charges created then stimulate bone formation by stimulating osteoblast activity. The stimulatory effect appears to be related to the magnitude of the applied force and its frequency of application, but it can be inhibited by hormone signals or lack of them. We know, for example, that certain male and female athletes are at risk for low bone density and that those most at risk include females with altered menstrual function or low concentrations of the female hormone estrogen. Overall, higher bone-mineral densities are desirable because the incidence of fragility fractures is inversely proportional to bone-mineral content.

Hormones and More Hormones

The main hormones involved in bone remodeling and thus bone health include parathyroid hormone (PTH), vitamin D, calcitonin, and estrogen. The priority of several of these hormones, however, is not to maintain healthy bone but to keep blood calcium in check (as discussed earlier), which ultimately affects bone mineral content and density. PTH plays the major role in this effect, stimulating the release of calcium from bone into blood at the first sign of lowered blood calcium levels. PTH also activates vitamin D, signals the kidneys to retain more calcium and excrete less in urine, and indirectly signals the intestines, through vitamin D, to increase calcium absorption. Calcitonin, on the other hand, decreases rising blood-calcium concentrations by inhibiting osteoclast activity, thereby suppressing bone resorption and increasing both calcium and phosphorus loss in the urine.

The sex hormones estrogen and testosterone, or male androgens in general, appear to regulate bone turnover in both men and women. Both estrogen and androgens control proliferation of bone-building osteoblasts, whereas estrogen (and possibly androgens) inhibits the bone-degrading osteoclasts.[6] Estrogen deficiency increases the rate of bone remodeling and the amount of bone lost with each remodeling cycle[7] and menstrual dysfunction (characteristic of abnormal estrogen patterns) increases risk of stress and non-stress fractures in female athletes.[7,74] Both older and younger men with testosterone deficiency syndrome are at risk for low bone-mineral density and osteoporosis.[8]

Nutrition—More Than Just Calcium

Several nutrients play a critical role in bone health. Thanks to marketing by the dairy industry, most Americans are aware that calcium is important for bone health. If you are a vegan athlete, you are also probably aware that most Americans feel that if you don't "Got Milk," you don't "Got Calcium." Thus, in some sense, we have been brainwashed to equate bone health with cows' milk. Many dietary factors, however, affect bone health. Calcium, magnesium, a variety of vitamins (A, B_{12}, C, D, and K), flavonoids, and total protein favorably affect bone health, while phosphorus, caffeine, alcohol, and animal protein may negatively affect bone when overconsumed. Other factors, such as fluoride, are thought to optimize bone health but only if consumed in the right quantities. The next section reviews each of these nutrients and provides tips for choosing plant-based foods to optimize bone health.

Calcium

Calcium is the most abundant mineral in the body and is necessary for bone formation, muscle contraction, nerve-impulse transmission, and enzyme activation. Calcium intake plays a key role in bone health because it is the largest constituent of the bone crystals—made of hydroxyapatite—and has been found in many studies to be directly associated with a person's bone density. A recent review and meta-analysis, for example, found strong evidence that higher calcium intake during childhood or adolescence from dairy products, fortified foods, or supplements promotes bone-mineral content accrual and has the potential to increase peak bone mass.[5] In women who have already obtained peak bone mass, adequate calcium intake from food and supplements has also been shown to retard loss of bone-mineral content in early adulthood,[76] and dampen bone loss during menopause (to a mean −0.014% vs. 1% per year in controls).[9]

To this end, however, many athletes may not know that calcium balance is influenced by factors other than dietary calcium intake.[10] These include differences in calcium absorption in the intestines and calcium excretion in the urine and feces. On the intake side, 20 to 40 percent of the calcium consumed is absorbed by the intestines, but the absorption rate can vary considerably depending on the food source (as will be discussed later). On the excretion side, a small but well-designed study published in the early 1990s found that high dietary sodium and protein intakes increase calcium loss through urine.[11] Although the effect of dietary sodium and protein on increasing calcium loss is thought to be minimal, this study provided evidence that the combined effect of excessive animal protein and sodium can have a more pronounced effect.[11] In this study, eight nonathletic men consumed four different diets for one week each: 1) a low-sodium, low-protein diet (3,200 mg sodium, 1 g protein/kg body weight); 2) a low-sodium, high-protein diet (3,200 mg sodium, 2 g protein/kg body weight); 3) a high-sodium, low-protein diet (7,100 mg sodium, 1 g protein/kg body weight); and 4) a high-sodium, high protein diet (7,100 mg sodium, 2 g protein/kg body weight). Researchers found that urinary calcium loss on the high-sodium, high-protein diet—which is typical of the Western diet—was almost double (152 vs. 257 mg calcium lost per day) when compared to a diet lower in both nutrients and likely more reflective of a vegetarian diet. Consequently, to account for the additional 105 grams of calcium lost on the high-sodium, high-protein diet, it would be necessary to consume an additional 263 to 525 milligrams of calcium daily, assuming an absorption rate of 20 to 40 percent.

Based on these and other findings, it is often argued (as mentioned earlier) that vegans and vegetarians consuming little to no animal foods may have daily calcium requirements that are lower than those proposed by the dietary reference intake (DRI) for calcium.[12] The argument holds that because the vegan diet is lower in animal protein (and the sulfur-containing amino acids in general, which may be most responsible for the calcium-wasting effect) and most likely sodium, less calcium is lost in the urine and therefore less is needed in the diet. A related argument is that the potential renal acid load (which has been negatively associated with bone-mineral content in children)[13] is increased by high dietary intake of sulfur-containing amino acids found in concentrated form in meat protein and lowered by alkaline salts, which occur in plant foods.[14] Although this argument is indeed intriguing, little supporting evidence is available. Thus, your best bet as an athlete is to strive for the recommended DRI of 1,000 milligrams of calcium per day for adults ages 19 to 50. [12] Women older than 50 should strive for 1,200 milligrams per day, and those ages 9 to 18 should strive for 1,300 milligrams per day. Some evidence suggests that amenorrheic athletes (those who have not experienced a menstrual cycle for at least three months) may require 1,500 to 2,000 milligrams of calcium daily to optimize bone health.[15] Low calcium intake among athletes has been associated with an increased risk of stress fractures and decreased bone density,[16] particularly in amenorrheic athletes.[15] Exercise training, however, has not been shown to increase calcium requirements above that of the general population.

If you are a male or regularly menstruating female athlete, you can meet your calcium requirements by consuming several servings of dairy products[17] or five to six servings of calcium-containing plant foods daily.[12,18] Plant foods that are rich in easily absorbable calcium are listed in table 6.1 and include low-oxalate green leafy vegetables (kale, broccoli, Chinese cabbage, bok choy), tofu (set with calcium), tahini, certain legumes, fortified orange juice, almonds, and blackstrap molasses. Research has suggested that calcium absorption from most of these foods is as good as or better than milk,[19-21] which has a fractional absorption rate of 32 percent (see figure 6.1). Evidence shows, however, that the calcium-absorption rate from calcium-fortified orange juice (and likely other juices) varies by fortification system, with the fractional absorption being nearly 50 percent greater for calcium citrate malate than for tricalcium phosphate or calcium lactate.[22] On the other hand, the calcium in fortified soy milk, most legumes, nuts, and seeds is less well absorbed. The fractional absorption of these foods is 17 to 24 percent. Foods with a high-oxalate or high-phytate content, including rhubarb, spinach,[19-21] swiss chard, and beet greens, are poorly absorbed sources of calcium.

If after reading this section, you are still nervous about shaking the dairy habit, don't be. A clinical study conducted in Germany demonstrated that maintaining calcium balance was quite possible on a well-selected, diary-free diet. In this study, calcium balance and bone turnover were measured in eight young adults placed on energy-balanced vegan and vegetarian diets for 10 days each.[23] The researchers found that although calcium intake was lower on the vegan diet (843 ± 140 mg) compared with the lacto vegetarian diet (1,322 ± 303 mg), participants were able to maintain a positive calcium balance and appropriate rate of bone turnover on both diets. Interestingly, the calcium provided in the vegan diet was from natural, mostly well-absorbed foods and calcium-rich mineral water but did not contain calcium-fortified foods, blackstrap molasses, or kale. The inclusion of these foods would provide additional, convenient sources of calcium.

Although it is possible to maintain calcium balance on a plant-based diet,[12,18] some active vegetarians may find it more convenient to use fortified foods or

TABLE 6.1 Calcium, Calcium-to-Phosphorus Ratio, and Magnesium Content of Selected Vegetarian Foods

Food	Portion	Calcium (mg)	Calcium-to-phosphorus ratio	Magnesium (mg)
GRAIN EQUIVALENTS				
Bread, enriched	1 oz slice	43	1.5:1	7
Bread, whole wheat	1 oz slice	20	0.3:1 to 0.5:1	24
Cereal, calcium-fortified	1 oz	125-1,000	>1:1	Varies
VEGETABLES AND LEGUMES, INCLUDING SOY				
Beet greens	1 cup cooked	164	2.8:1	98
Black beans	1 cup cooked	46	0.2:1	120
Broccoli	1 cup cooked	62	0.6:1	32
Cabbage, Chinese (bok choy)	1 cup cooked	158	3.2:1	19
Cabbage, head	1 cup cooked	46	4.2:1	12
Chickpeas (garbanzo beans)	1 cup cooked	80	0.3:1	79
Collard greens	1 cup cooked	266	4.7:1	38
Kale	1 cup cooked	94	2.6:1	23
Lentils	1 cup cooked	38	0.1:1	71
Mustard greens	1 cup cooked	104	1.8:1	21
Okra	1 cup cooked, sliced	62	2.4:1	58
Pinto beans	1 cup cooked	79	0.3:1	86
Red kidney beans	1 cup cooked	50	0.2:1	80
Southern peas (black-eyed, crowder)	1 cup cooked	41	0.2:1	91
Soybeans	1 cup cooked	175	0.4:1	148
Sweet potato	1 medium, baked	43	0.7:1	31
Tofu, firm (calcium set)	1/2 cup	861*	3.6:1	73
Tofu, regular (calcium set)	1/2 cup	434*	3.6:1	37
Turnip greens	1 cup cooked	197	4.7:1	32
FRUITS				
Grapefruit juice, calcium fortified	1 cup	350	9.5:1	30
Orange juice, calcium fortified	1 cup	350	7:1-8:1	27

Food	Portion	Calcium (mg)	Calcium-to-phosphorus ratio	Magnesium (mg)
NUTS AND SEEDS				
Almonds	1 oz	70	0.5:1	78
Cashews, peanuts, pecans, pine nuts, sunflower seeds	1 oz	5-20	>0.1:1	22-71
Pumpkin seeds	1 oz	12	0.04:1	151
Tahini	1 tbsp	64	0.6:1	14
Walnuts	1 oz	28	0.3:1	45
MILK, PLANT-BASED MILKS, AND CHEESE				
Almond milk, calcium fortified	1 cup	482*	20:1	16
Rice milk, calcium fortified	1 cup	283*	2.1:1	26
Soy milk, calcium fortified	1 cup	368*	1.6:1	39
Veggemo (pea protein–based milk)	1 cup	585	N/A	N/A
Cows' milk, skim	1 cup	306	1.2:1	27
Cows' milk, 2%	1 cup	285	1.2:1	27
Cheddar cheese	1 oz	204	1.4:1	8
Mozzarella	1 oz	207	1.4:1	7
Swiss	1 oz	224	1.4:1	11
Vegan almond- and rice-based cheese alternatives	1 oz	225*	N/A	N/A
OTHER				
Mineral water	1 cup	24-40 (varies)	N/A	N/A
Molasses	1 tbsp	41	6.8:1	48
Blackstrap molasses, plantation	1 tbsp	200	N/A	N/S

Note: Refer to appendix F for guidance on converting English units to metric.

*Varies by brand.

Data from USDA National Nutrient Database for Standard Reference (https://ndb.nal.usda.gov/ndb/) and selected manufacturers.

calcium supplements to help meet their requirements. Calcium carbonate and calcium citrate are well-absorbed sources used in supplements, but calcium carbonate is generally less expensive. Long-term supplementation with calcium carbonate has not been found to compromise iron status in iron-replete adults[24] (as was once thought), but it is best to take calcium supplements several hours

Calcium absorption		Food
>50%		Bok choy, broccoli, Chinese/Napa cabbage, collards, kale, okra, turnip greens, TVP, blackstrap molasses
~30%		Milk, calcium-set tofu, calcium-fortified orange juice (with calcium citrate malate)
20%		Fortified soy milk, most nuts and seeds, most legumes, fortified orange juice (with tricalcium phosphate/calcium lactate)
≤5%		Spinach, Swiss chard, beet greens, rhubarb

FIGURE 6.1 Calcium absorption from vegetable and dairy sources. Values represent fractional absorption or percent of calcium intake absorbed in the intestines.

Data from Weaver and Plawecki (20), Weaver et al. (21), Heaney et al. (19), and Monsen and Balintfy (79).

after a meal, for example, at bedtime, rather than with meals.[25] Because vitamin D is also required for bone health, recent recommendations suggest that calcium and vitamin D should be supplemented together.[14]

Vitamin D

Healthy bones also depend on vitamin D, a versatile nutrient that functions both as a vitamin and a hormone. As you may know, vitamin D_3 can be made in the skin upon exposure to sunlight. Specifically, the ultraviolet B rays (which are highest in proportion at close to solar noon) convert a form of cholesterol that is found in the membrane of skin cells into vitamin D_3. Vitamin D_3 then circulates to the liver where it is converted to hydroxyl vitamin D_3 (calcidiol), the main storage form, and later activated as needed to its hormonally active form 1,25 dihydroxyvitamin D_3 (calcitriol) by the kidney and other body tissues. Calcitriol's main function is to maintain blood calcium, but in doing so, it also promotes intestinal calcium absorption, thereby helping to provide adequate quantities of calcium and phosphorus for bone formation. As an example, it has been estimated that only 10 to 15 percent of dietary calcium is absorbed when vitamin D is deficient, whereas more than 30 percent is absorbed when vitamin D is sufficient (serum 25-[OH]D concentration > 75 nmol/L).[26] Research from numerous randomly assigned clinical trials clearly suggests that adequate vitamin D and calcium are imperative for bone accrual[27] and the maintenance of healthy bone.[28] Evidence suggests that low vitamin D status is linked to increased risk for stress fractures in athletes. [16,29,30]

Numerous studies conducted in athletic populations have shown that some athletes are at risk for poor vitamin D status.[31] Vitamin D deficiency can manifest in unexplained muscle pain or weakness and compromised calcium balance. Those at risk include athletes with low intakes of fortified foods or supplements, limited sun exposure (especially in northern and extreme southern climates distant from the equator), indoor-only training schedules, dark-pigmented skin, excess body fat, and chronic use of sunscreen.[31] Vitamin D is found in a limited number of foods, which mainly include fortified cows' milk; certain brands of plant milk; calcium-fortified orange juice, breakfast cereals, and margarines; and in fatty fish (see table 6.2). Spending 5 to 30 minutes (depending on skin tone, and ease of burning) outside in your exercise shorts (with all or partial torso exposed) several times a week is enough to meet your vitamin D needs in the late spring, summer, and early fall if you are Caucasian.[32] However, taking in vitamin D in food or as a supplement is wise in the winter. This is also a wise idea if you are dark-skinned, because research shows that dark-skinned people may not produce adequate vitamin D from sunlight exposure.[78] Although evidence suggests that vegetarians and vegans may be at additional risk for deficiency because of lower dietary intake,[33] factors such as skin pigmentation, sun exposure intensity, and dietary supplementation seem to be more important predictors of vitamin D status than intake from food sources.[34]

How much vitamin D you should take as an athlete is not yet established. Recent guidelines from the International Olympic Committee suggest that the Endocrine Society's recommendation to consume 1,500 to 2,000 international units (IU) per day is a good starting point.[35] Athletes with larger

TABLE 6.2 Selected Vegetarian Sources of Vitamin D

Food	Portion	International units (IU)
Cereal, all varieties fortified with 10% daily value (DV)	3/4 cup	40-50
Cereal grain bar, fortified with 10% DV	1 bar	40
Egg	1 whole	25
Margarine, fortified	1 tbsp	60
Mushrooms, shiitake, sun dried	1 oz	400-500*
Milk, vitamin D fortified (nonfat, reduced fat, and whole)	1 cup	98
Milk, rice, vitamin D fortified	1 cup	100*
Milk, soy, vitamin D fortified	1 cup	100*
Orange juice, vitamin D fortified	1 cup	100

Note: The daily value (DV) for vitamin D is 600 IU. The Vitamin D Council, however, feels that the DV should be increased. Refer to appendix F for guidance on converting English units to metric.

*May be a source of D_2 rather than D_3.

total body or muscle mass, however, may need more. Because this value is much higher than what can be obtained from natural or supplemented food sources, a vitamin D supplement containing vitamin D_3 (cholecalciferol) is recommended, but may be needed only in the winter. If you are vegan you should know that the vitamin D_3 used in some supplements and fortified foods of animal origin. Look instead for vitamin D_3 derived from lichen (rather than lanolin) and D_2 produced from irradiation of yeast ergosterol.[12] Research has suggested, however, that the vitamin D_2 form (ergocalciferol)—often called vegetarian vitamin D—may be less effective than vitamin D_3 at increasing vitamin D status when taken at higher doses (>4,000 IU).[12] Evidence also suggests that vitamin D_2 supplementation may reduce circulating concentration of vitamin D_3.[36]

Magnesium

Magnesium is the third most abundant mineral in bone—after calcium and phosphorus—and is also involved in the bone mineralization process. As with calcium, magnesium in bone can act as a "bank" or reservoir to ensure that adequate magnesium is available to the body when needed. Both dietary intake of magnesium and the magnesium concentration in blood are found to be positively correlated with bone-mineral content, markers of bone strength, and overall bone health.

Concerning peak bone mass, a large, one-year, randomly assigned clinical trial conducted in Caucasian girls found that magnesium supplementation at close to the RDA (300 mg/day) increased bone mineral content in the hip and lumbar spine.[37] On the other end of the spectrum, a large study of more than 2,000 men and women enrolled in the Health, Aging, and Body Composition Study found that higher magnesium intake from foods and supplements was predictive of a higher bone-mineral density.[38] In this study, however, the researchers found that the relationship between dietary magnesium and bone health was apparent only in Caucasian but not black volunteers, which the researchers speculated was caused by differences in either calcium regulation or nutrient reporting.

Although true deficiencies of magnesium are rare, suboptimal magnesium status is thought to be widespread in the United States because of the limited intake of magnesium-rich whole grains, legumes, nuts, seeds, and leafy vegetables and excess intake of processed foods.[39]

Indeed, surveys of athletes find that intake of magnesium is often insufficient, particularly among athletes who restrict energy intake for sport (e.g., wrestling, ballet, gymnastics) or otherwise.[40] As a whole, however, vegetarian athletes may be at an advantage when it comes to dietary magnesium[41,42] because seeds, nuts, legumes, unmilled cereal grains, dark-green vegetables, and dark chocolate are high in magnesium. Refined foods or dairy products, on the other hand, tend to be low in magnesium. The magnesium content of selected foods is listed in table 6.1, along with the calcium content of these

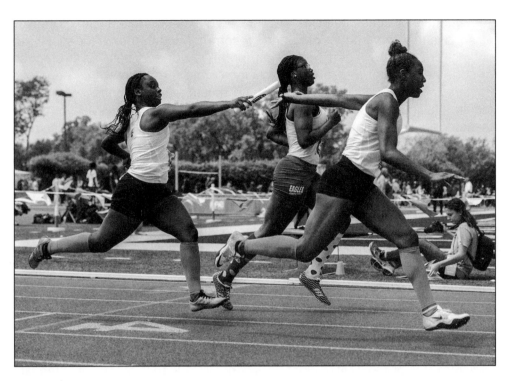

Although weight-bearing exercise promotes denser and stronger bones, it is important athletes consume adequate calcium, magnesium, and certain vitamins (A, B_{12}, C, D, and K). Dark-skinned athletes may be at greater risk for a vitamin D deficiency.

foods. A listing of the 20 best sources of magnesium is also found in chapter 11. The DRI for magnesium is listed in appendix E.

Fluoride

Adequate fluoride plays a critical role in the mineralization of bones and teeth.[43] In bone, fluoride is incorporated into the hydroxyapatite crystals, specifically replacing some of the chemical "hydroxyl" group, which is thought to make bones more resistant to breakdown (or osteoclast attack). In teeth, fluoride is incorporated into the developing tooth's mineralizing structure and helps increase resistance to acid demineralization. After tooth eruption, fluoride is incorporated into saliva and protects against development of cavities in children and adults. In fact, the Centers for Disease Control and Prevention (CDC) has named fluoridation of water one of the 10 most important public health efforts of the 21st century. The most significant sources of fluoride in the United States are green and black teas, seafood, and fluoridated water. Significant sources of fluoride are not found in other food sources; however, fluoridated toothpaste and oral health products can provide a source for teeth and bone if small amounts are swallowed. Although fluoride supplementation is shown to increase bone-mineral density in postmenopausal osteoporotic patients,[44] long-term treatment with fluoride for bone health is still considered experimental.[43] One of the key reasons is that the amount of fluoride recommended in the water supply for optimal oral health, 1 part per million (ppm), is not sufficient for promotion of bone cell growth (osteoblastic activity) or the prevention of osteoporotic fractures.[43] Intake of fluoride at amounts much higher (4 ppm) seem to be required to see significant increases in bone-mineral density (BMD), but even these doses do not appear to reduce risk of osteoporotic fractures. Such high doses may also be associated with side effects, including enamel fluorosis, which results in teeth discoloration, cosmetically unpleasant white spots, and weakened tooth structure. Similarly, excess fluoride at extremely high doses can also be detrimental to bone, inducing formation of large, abnormally placed mineral crystals that decrease bone strength and quality.

Although no hard-and-fast rules exist for ensuring that you get adequate, but not too much, fluoride, one of the first steps is to ensure that the water you drink or cook with contains appropriate levels of fluoride. In the United States, an estimated 72 percent of the public water supply is fluoridated, but this varies by state.[43] Within the United States, you can check the status of your area by contacting your local water utility company. You may also find helpful information about the fluoride content of your state's water supply on the CDC website. Fluoride concentrations are expressed as parts per million, which is equal to 1 milligram of fluoride per liter. Fluoride is generally added to tap water at the rate of approximately 1 part per million; however, the recent recommendations of the CDC are 0.7 parts per million to protect against dental cavities, while at the same time limiting risk of enamel fluorosis.[45] Thus, depending on the fluoride content of your water, you may want to adjust your water sources and even oral health product selection to ensure that your fluoride intake is close to the recommended adequate intake (AI) of 3 milligrams per day for adult women and 4 milligrams per day for adult men. For example, if your tap water contains 1.2 milligrams per liter and you consume 2 liters of tap water and tap water mixed with sport drink during your morning workout session (1.2 mg/l $\times$ 2 l = 2.4 mg), plus an additional 1.5 liters in coffee and drinking water throughout the day (1.2 mg/l $\times$ 1.5 l = 1.8 mg), you would easily be taking in more than the AI for fluoride and may want to avoid using fluoridated toothpaste. If you drink bottled water exclusively, remember that many do not contain fluoride. Some brands, such as Dannon Fluoride to Go, offer fluoridated versions of their water. Also, the fluoride content of water from home water-purification systems can vary widely.

Phosphorus

Phosphorus is the second most abundant mineral in bone and also plays a role in energy regulation and acid–base buffering. Unlike calcium, however, dietary phosphorus is readily absorbed at an efficiency of 60 to 70 percent, and too much phosphorus—rather than not enough—is a concern for bone health. Excessive phosphorus intake relative to calcium intake increases the hormones

PTH and calcitriol (active vitamin D), which ultimately results in removal of both calcium and phosphorus from bone.[46] Although research supporting the detrimental effect of excess phosphorus on bone is somewhat controversial, there is suggestion that high phosphorus intake over a long period may result in bone loss. One study of bone fractures in active teenage girls conducted by Harvard researchers found a strong association between phosphate-rich cola beverage consumption and bone fractures.[47] In the Framingham Osteoporosis study, cola drinkers were found to have an average hip BMD that was 4 to 5 percent lower than that of participants who did not drink cola,[48] but this relationship was not found for other sodas. Another epidemiological study in elderly vegetarian and omnivorous men and women found that excessive phosphorus negatively affected bone health.[77] Several studies have also looked at the specific effect of phosphorus-containing foods, including cola. Mixed results have been found in experimental trials involving young men and women asked to consume either low-calcium, phosphate-containing grocery foods for 28 days[49] or consume either 2.5 liters of cola per day or milk for 10 days. No change in markers of bone turnover were noted in the women consuming the processed food despite consistently elevated levels of parathyroid hormone, whereas markers of bone turnover and bone loss were quite apparent in the men consuming the cola.[50]

Although phosphorus is found in most foods, common sources in the Western diet include grains, meats, legumes, nuts, seeds, dairy products, soda, and phosphorus additives to foods (including meats)—mostly in the form of phosphates. Table 6.1 lists the calcium-to-phosphorus ratio of selected calcium-containing foods. This ratio is high in leafy greens, dairy, and calcium-fortified soy products and low in grains, nuts, and seeds. The ideal calcium-to-phosphorus ratio in the diet is not known, but is suggested to be 1:1 to 1.5:1 in favor of more calcium.[46,49] Because most Americans take in too much phosphorus, both from foods and soda, and many do not meet the recommendations for calcium, the calcium-to-phosphorus ratio of the average American diet tends to be less than ideal. Because this issue is still unresolved, the simple message may be to pack those leafy greens into your diet (a high calcium-to-phosphate ratio is just one more reason), avoid consuming too much soda (particularly cola) and other foods with phosphate additives, and strive to get your calcium from a variety of vegetarian sources.

Vitamins K, C, A and B$_{12}$

Vitamins K, C, A and B$_{12}$ also can affect bone health. Vitamin K has been gaining increasing attention because it is required for synthesis of a bone-specific protein called *osteocalcin*. Ostoecalcin is produced by bone-building osteoblasts and is involved in bone formation. Vitamin K represents a family of vitamins that include vitamin K$_1$ (phylloquinone) and K$_2$ (menaquinone). Like vitamin D, vitamin K can be obtained from food and nonfood sources, which in this case includes vitamin K$_2$ made by intestinal bacteria. It has been difficult to determine, however, just how much of the daily vitamin K needs can be obtained as a result of bacterial synthesis in the gut. Food sources of vitamin K_1 include green leafy vegetables, avocado, most cruciferous vegetables (broccoli, brussels sprouts, cabbage, and cauliflower) and plant oils and margarines.[10] Food sources of vitamin K_2 include fermented foods and certain cheeses. Although we still have a lot to learn about vitamin K and bone health, dietary vitamin K appears to be involved in peak bone formation and reducing the risk of bone fractures. In a study conducted on more than 70,000 women as part of the Nurses' Health Study, those who had low intakes of vitamin K (mainly from green vegetables) were at greater risk for hip fractures.[51] In children and adolescents, better vitamin K status is associated with decreased bone turnover[14,52] and increased total-body BMD.[53] More recent randomized, clinical trials, however, have not found that supplementation with vitamin K_1 or K_2 improves BMD at major bone sites.[54] Thus, the current thinking is that while evidence is insufficient to recommend routine supplementation with vitamin K for the protection of osteoporosis fractures, ensuring adequate intake of vitamin K (along with a flora of happy gut bacteria) is important. As an athlete, this may be one more reason to eat your green leafy vegetables and consider experimenting with fermented foods. Also, be aware that regular use of antibiotics decreases the number of vitamin K–producing bacteria in the gut. With that said, you may notice that many calcium supplements marketed to women now contain vitamin K as well as vitamin D.

Vitamins C and A play important—and often overlooked—backstage roles in bone health. Vitamin C is involved in the formation of collagen, which forms the matrix for all connective tissue in the body, including bones, teeth, skin, and tendons. Vitamin A's role is related to its function in cell growth, cell differentiation, and bone resorption, which is an essential step in bone growth and remodeling. Although it appears that only a severe deficiency of either vitamin is likely to affect bone health in adults, vegetarian athletes should consider bone health benefits another reason to meet the needs of both of these vitamins. Food sources of vitamin C are listed in table 7.4 on page 113 and sources of vitamin A in table 8.5 on page 132.

While vitamin B_{12} is rarely mentioned for bone health, it also appears to play an important role. Inadequate vitamin B_{12} status has been linked to low BMD in healthy adolescent[55] and elderly individuals[56] as well as increased fracture risk and osteoporosis in older individuals.[56] As will be discussed further in chapter 8, vegans and even vegetarians who do not regularly consume reliable sources of vitamin B_{12} are at particular risk of deficiency, and even mild to moderate B_{12} deficiency may result in increased bone resorption.[57] The mechanism appears to be caused by elevated concentration of a metabolite called *homocysteine*—a hallmark of vitamin B_{12} deficiency—that is also known to stimulate bone breakdown by osteoclasts and inhibit bone formation by osteoclasts.

Other Nutrients

Several other nutrients, including caffeine, alcohol, and isoflavones from soy and other plant foods, may also influence bone-mineral density and other aspects of bone health. Caffeine consumption was found to increase calcium excretion by the kidneys[14] and was associated with reduced bone-mineral density in epidemiological studies. The effect of lifetime caffeine intake, however, seems to be weak. For example, 10 cups (2,360 ml) of coffee every day for 30 years was associated with only a 1.1 percent reduction in bone mass.[58] In studies of postmenopausal women not on estrogen-replacement therapy, as few as two cups (472 ml) of coffee were found to accelerate bone loss in women who did not regularly drink milk[59] (or, let's just say, did not get adequate calcium). In young women aged 19 to 26, self-reported caffeine intake was not found to affect absolute bone-mineral density of the hip or spine after adjusting for other factors.[60]

In addition, too much alcohol is known to contribute to bone loss by inhibiting osteoblasts in their job of forming new bone.[75] Heavy drinkers may lose bone mass in just a few years. Similar to the case of caffeine, it is not clear how much alcohol is too much, but evidence indicates that people who have three to four drinks a day are at increased risk for bone loss. Small amounts of alcohol may have the opposite effect by actually promoting bone formation.

Flavonoids, including the isoflavonoids in soy products,[61] on the other hand, may have a beneficial effect on long-term bone health. Flavonoids are found in a variety of plant foods, including fruits, vegetables, herbs, spices, and essential oils. While it is fair to say that the isoflavonoids found in soy have been most studied, a large observational study of 50- to 60-year-old Scottish women found that total flavonoid intake of the diet was positively associated with overall BMD of the spine and hip and negatively associated with markers of bone resorption.[62] Interestingly, flavonoids in the catechin family—found in green tea, wine, cocoa, and dried plums—had the strongest association with bone mineral density.

Nevertheless, the flavonoids that have been most studied for their role in bone health are soy isoflavones. Isoflavones are structurally similar to estrogens and bind to estrogen receptors.[61] Observational studies suggest that soy consumption contributes to low rates of hip fractures in Asian populations, with seemingly better results in women who are early (<10 years) rather than late in menopause.[63] Clinical trials in Western women, however, have met with mixed results.[61] A meta-analysis of randomized control trials showed soy isoflavones (approximately 82 mg/day) increased spine BMD by 2.4 percent in the short term (6-12 months),[64] but randomized controlled trials lasting two to three years have shown no benefit on BMD of fracture-prone bone sites in postmenopausal women.[61] While the jury is still out, it is speculated that these differing results may be due to genetic differences or the form in which the isoflavones are consumed. Whole soy foods (associated with other phytochemicals) are typically consumed in Asian cultures, and isolated-soy isoflavones are consumed in Westernized cultures.

In addition to soy, flavonoids in other fruits and vegetables, including dried plums, blueberries, and vegetables of the onion family are also receiving attention for their possible bone-protective effects.[61] At the time of this publication, however, dried plums are the only food that has been tested in human clinical trials. Studies in postmenopausal women have found that consuming as few as five dried plums daily (50 g)[65] may inhibit bone resorption and dampen bone loss and may decrease loss of BMD at major fracture sites.[65-67] The conclusion for now might be simply to eat a variety of plant foods, including dried plums and soy foods if you enjoy them, but don't rely on one magic product to strengthen your bones. The isoflavone content of selected soy foods is presented in table 6.3. Please see the USDA database for the flavonoid content of selected foods (https://ndb.nal.usda.gov/ndb/).

TABLE 6.3   Total Soy Isoflavone Content in Selected Soy Products

Food	Portion	Value (mg)
Soybeans, cooked	1 cup cooked (172 g)	112
Soy cheese	1 oz (28.35 g)	1-2
Soy flour, full fat	2 tbsp (10 g)	18
Soy milk	1 cup (236 ml)	6
Soy protein concentrate (water extracted)	1 oz (28.35 g)	27
Soy protein concentrate (alcohol extracted)	1 oz (28.35 g)	3
Soy protein isolate	1 oz (28.35 g)	26
Soy bar	1 bar	Varies by brand and type
Soy chips	1 oz package	15
Soy dog	1 dog (70 g)	1
Tempeh, uncooked	1/2 cup (83 g)	50
Tofu, soft	1/2 cup (124 g)	28
Tofu, firm	1/2 cup (126 g)	29
Tofu, yogurt	1 cup (240 g)	80
Veggie burger, soy protein based	1 patty (70 g)	4

Total isoflavones (daidzein and genistein) extrapolated from S. Bhagwat, D.B. Haytowitz, and J.M. Holden, *USDA Database for the Isoflavone Content of Selected Foods, Release 2.0* (2008), accessed January 17, 2019, https://www.ars.usda.gov/ARSUserFiles/80400525/Data/isoflav/Isoflav_R2.pdf.

Bone Health and the Vegetarian Diet

Whether vegetarian athletes are at risk for poor bone health depends on many factors, including genetics, physical activity, exercise training, and dietary choices. Overall, limited research in groups of lacto-ovo vegetarians and vegans has found that the bone-mineral densities of vegetarians is similar to nonvegetarians if calcium intake is adequate and the diet contains good sources of protein (adequate protein is protective).[12] One cross sectional study in a small group of individuals on a raw-food vegetarian diet observed low bone mineral density along with low dietary protein (9% of calories) in raw food compared to matched controls following a standard American diet (Fontana 2005 at end). In contrast, a larger-scale investigation conducted on Seventh-day Adventists more than 30 years ago, a vegetarian diet appeared to be somewhat able to defend against bone-mineral loss in aging women[68] but not men.[69] The investigators found that although bone-mineral density was not different between younger lacto-ovo vegetarians and omnivores, increasing differences in bone mass appeared at age 50, and by age 89, nonvegetarians had lost 35 percent of their bone mass, whereas the vegetarians had lost just 18 percent.[68] A relatively recent meta-analysis of nine studies of over 2,700 men and women ages 20 to 79, however, suggests that little difference in bone density exists among vegetarians and vegans compared to omnivores.[70] Bone-mineral density was found to be approximately 4 percent lower in vegetarians and vegans at both the hip and spine, but these differences were not considered clinically meaningful. A recent study conducted on children and adolescents looked at the impact of vegetarian diets on peak bone mass and suggested that vegetarians may have a higher rate of bone turnover and subtle changes in bone regulatory markers that may be related to diet.[71] No studies have evaluated the impact of vegetarian diet on bone health in athletes. Collectively, however, research suggests that vegetarians should avoid a shortfall in overall energy and the nutrients that affect bone health—including calcium, vitamin D, and protein—while at the same time ensuring they consume enough protective nutrients, including magnesium, vitamin K, and phytochemicals.[12,72]

To maintain optimal bone health, your main concerns should be ensuring that you consume adequate calcium, receive a reliable source of vitamin D, and avoid taking in too much phosphate from soda and other processed foods. Tips for optimizing bone health are summarized in box 6.1. In addition, you should evaluate your training and—if you are female—ensure that you are menstruating regularly (see chapter 2). Weight-bearing activities like running, jumping, and resistance training promote bone density, which is great if you are a runner, ballplayer, dancer, gymnast, or power lifter, but not so great if you are a swimmer or cyclist. Athletes in these and other non-weight-bearing sports—no matter their performance or fitness level—need to incorporate regular weight-bearing activities into their in-season and off-season training, even if it is simply walking briskly a few miles or skipping rope several times a week. Speaking from experience, I forced myself to jog 6 to 10 miles (10-16 km) a week back in my days as a rather serious recreational long-distance cyclist. Although my motivation in part was to use weight-bearing activity to induce a piezoelectric effect as explained earlier, in the end, I found it was great cross-training. The rest of the story is that I eventually became a runner, but that's another topic of discussion.

Indeed, a vegetarian diet packed with appropriate foods can adequately support bone health—with or without dairy products—just as it can maintain a normal iron status, which is discussed in the next chapter.

Box 6.1

Tips for Optimizing Bone Health

- Consume an overall healthy diet that is adequate in energy and dietary protein and contains an abundant variety of fruits, vegetables, herbs, and spices.

- Focus on consuming well-absorbed, calcium-rich foods daily from a variety of plant and, if appropriate, dairy sources.

- Maintain adequate levels of vitamin D in the blood by spending 5 to 30 minutes outside in your exercise shorts several times a week if you are Caucasian. In the winter, or year-round if you are dark skinned, consume foods fortified with vitamin D or take a vitamin D supplement. The Endocrine Society recommends 1,500 to 2,000 IU (more than the RDA) of vitamin D_3 for those whose exposure to sunlight is inadequate.[35]

- Incorporate leafy greens into the diet regularly, if not daily. Most leafy greens are well-absorbed sources of calcium and also contain vitamin K and vitamin A. Leafy greens also are low in phosphorus.

- Reduce the phosphorus content of your diet by limiting the intake of regular and diet soda and foods with added phosphates. However, do not limit plant foods high in phosphates in an effort to improve the calcium-to-phosphate ratio because many of these foods, such as nuts, seeds, grains, and legumes, are excellent sources of other nutrients, including magnesium.

- Check that the water you drink and cook with contains adequate fluoride. And remember that both too little and too much fluoride can compromise bone health.

- Consume adequate energy. Low intake of energy and protein can compromise bone and also compromise intake of important nutrients, including calcium and magnesium.

- As will be discussed in chapter 8, consume a reliable source of vitamin B_{12} daily.

- Limit caffeine intake to 1 to 2 cups (236-472 ml) of caffeine-containing beverages per day. Even this amount may increase calcium loss if calcium intake is not adequate. Replacing some coffee beverages with catechin-rich green tea may provide benefit to overall bone health.

- Consume a diet rich in fruits, vegetables, herbs, spices, and green tea. Consider consuming whole soy foods containing isoflavones as part of your diet. Although research is inconclusive, the flavonoids in these foods may benefit bone health.

- If you drink alcohol, do so in moderation. Excessive intake of alcohol not only keeps you from performing your best, but may also impair bone health.

7 | Boosting Iron Intake and Absorption

Elaine is a professional dancer and a yoga instructor who first adopted a vegetarian diet, then vegan, and then moved onto mostly raw foods. Despite her active lifestyle, she started to incorporate water fasts into her routine, some lasting several days. At first she felt energized and light, and her abilities in dance and yoga persisted. But after fighting a cold for over a week, her energy levels didn't return. She focused on eating more fruit, knowing vitamin C might be helpful, but unknowingly, she wasn't meeting other nutrient needs, including iron, and had depleted her body's iron stores.

Elaine reached out for help after getting labs that showed very low serum ferritin (an iron-containing protein that serves as a key marker of iron status in blood) levels. Thankfully, she was open to adding more foods to her diet. We discussed iron-rich plant foods and her needs as an exceptionally active woman. She was willing to take a supplement to get her iron stores back up quickly, as long as we developed a plan to meet her future needs with food only. With supplementation, she bounced back quickly and now sustains her activity level through high-iron foods like lentils, spinach, swiss chard, edamame, blackstrap molasses, and figs. Her vitamin C intake was already quite high, so she did not need to make a specific effort to consume these foods to boost absorption and help her maintain adequate iron levels.
– Matt

You have probably been informed at least once during your athletic career that you need to watch your iron consumption either because you are vegetarian or because you are an athlete. Indeed, nearly every source you read implies that vegetarians and athletes need to take a supplement or include a little flesh foods in their diet to achieve normal iron status. Although you should take warnings about poor iron status seriously, you should rest assured that is it quite possible to maintain adequate iron stores by consuming a vegetarian diet alone—hold the fish, chicken breast, and supplements. This chapter reviews the basics of iron metabolism and why iron is important to athletes, and provides suggestions for boosting iron intake and absorption on a vegetarian diet.

What Is So Important About Iron?

Every living cell—whether plant or animal—contains iron. Most of the iron in your body is found as part of two proteins called hemoglobin (found in red blood cells), and myoglobin (found in muscle cells). Hemoglobin in blood carries the oxygen you breathe from your lungs to the tissues throughout the body, and myoglobin in muscle holds and stores oxygen for use during exercise. Myoglobin is particularly important for muscle fibers used in aerobic exercise: slow-twitch red (or type I) fibers. In fact, it is the myoglobin that makes muscles used in endurance activities reddish in color and may help explain why chickens, with white muscle in their breasts, can fly only a few feet, but ducks, with dark muscle in their breasts, can fly for hours. Also, just in case you were curious, myoglobin is also important for diving birds and mammals, such as ducks and my favorite, the loon. It allows them to dive underwater for extended periods without taking a breath.

The iron in hemoglobin and myoglobin is key because it has special chemical properties that allow hemoglobin to carry oxygen and then release it to the tissues as needed, and myoglobin to store oxygen and release it within muscle when needed for aerobic metabolism. As discussed in chapter 2, cells—particularly working muscle cells—need a regular supply of oxygen to produce energy. Iron-containing hemoglobin is also needed to assist in the elimination of carbon and hydrogen atoms released during the use of carbohydrate and fat fuels for energy, forming carbon dioxide and hydrogen. Thus, having adequate iron stores is particularly important during exercise when the hemoglobin-rich red blood cells shuttle between the lungs and exercising muscle, bringing in fresh oxygen and eliminating carbon dioxide.

In addition to its vital role in oxygen and carbon dioxide shuttling, iron helps many enzymes in the energy-generating pathways. Iron is also needed to make new cells, hormones (such as thyroid hormone), neurotransmitters, and amino acids and also helps make new DNA.

Iron is so important to your body that is has been referred to as the body's gold: a precious mineral to be hoarded. Following absorption in the intestines, a protein called *transferrin* escorts it to the many tissues in our bodies. Only a very small amount of iron is found unescorted in the blood. Iron is stored primarily in the liver and bone marrow as part of two other proteins called *fer-*

Vegan View: Getting Iron Without Animal Foods Is Easier Than You Think

Vegans are likely to achieve adequate iron intake, although the research suggests their iron stores are in the low-normal range.[1,2] As we discuss in this chapter, low but adequate iron storage is not necessarily a problem because it is associated with lower risk of some diseases. The concern is that if iron intake dips, there is less opportunity to prevent deficiency. Vegans may have an advantage over lacto-ovo vegetarians in this instance because eggs and dairy contain virtually no iron and, in fact, they may inhibit absorption of iron consumed from other sources at the same meal.[3] Replacing egg and dairy calories with whole plant foods is likely to increase total iron intake. A 2017 systemic review found that people eating a vegan diet had higher iron intake than people eating vegetarian and omnivorous diets.[4]

Meeting iron needs is possible when animal foods are excluded, and some components of plant foods improve iron absorption, which is a crucial step beyond intake. It is clear that vitamin C, which is found in virtually all fruits and vegetables, increases absorption of nonheme iron by as much as five times.[5] Additionally, vitamin A and carotenoids appear to enhance iron absorption by reducing the inhibiting effect of polyphenols and phytates (found in whole grains) on iron absorption. Adding vitamin A to an iron supplement reduces anemia more than iron alone.[6] Combining iron-rich foods with a variety of fruits and vegetables is an important step in ensuring adequate intake and increased absorption.

ritin and *hemosiderin*. Some storage also occurs in the spleen and muscle. A small amount of the storage protein ferritin also circulates in the blood. Serum ferritin can be used to assess iron storage (or status) because levels in serum typically reflect iron stores in the liver.[7] Ferritin, however, can be increased in blood when inflammation is present due to intense or exhaustive exercise or illness.[7] Therefore, ferritin does not always paint a true picture of iron status in athletes undergoing intense training regimens because low ferritin levels can be falsely elevated by inflammation, making an iron-depleted athlete appear to have normal status.

Iron is incorporated into the hemoglobin molecules during the formation of red blood cells, which occurs mostly in bone marrow. Your red blood cells typically live for three to four months. When they die, the spleen and liver salvage the iron and send it back to the bone marrow for storage and reuse. In this way, iron is truly hoarded and recycled. Small amounts of iron, however, are lost daily through the shedding of cells in your skin, scalp, and gastrointestinal (GI) tract and through sweat during exercise. The greatest loss of iron, however, occurs through bleeding and menstrual cycle losses. Normal average daily iron loss is approximately 1 milligram for men and nonmenstruating women, and 1.4 to 1.5 milligrams for menstruating women because of the higher losses from monthly menstrual bleeding.[5] These daily losses, therefore must be replaced through the diet.

Athletes in training may lose iron through GI bleeding, the destruction of red blood cells, urinary loss, and heavy sweating. GI bleeding is a recognized problem that occurs in endurance runners, cyclists, and triathletes[8-11] and is thought to be related, at least in part, to regular use of aspirin and anti-inflammatory medications. These medications may have a toxic effect on the gut lining, leaving it raw and bleeding.[12-14] Red cell destruction, called *hemolysis*, may be induced by the stress of repetitive foot contact with the ground during prolonged running or marching,[13,14] or by the rapid propulsion of blood cells through the blood vessels as a result of intense muscular training. This excess force can then rupture some of the red blood cells, which, although not dangerous, can increase iron loss. Loss of hemoglobin in urine, called *hematuria*, usually follows hemolysis because the kidneys' capacity to hoard the hemoglobin released from ruptured blood cells is temporarily overwhelmed. Iron loss in urine can also occur if muscle cells are ruptured during intense training, resulting in the release of stored myoglobin, or if the inner lining of the bladder becomes irritated, resulting in loss of red blood cells in the urine. Blood loss in urine may occur in any athletic situation that places stress on the bladder and may include prolonged running and running during pregnancy. Finally, iron loss through sweat is also thought to be significant for some athletes during prolonged effort, although not all experts agree. Research in this area suggests that iron loss through sweating may be significant (as high as 0.3 to 0.4 milligrams of iron lost per liter [4 cups] of sweat) in the first hour of exercise[15] but decreases with increasing duration.[15,16] It is estimated that iron losses during two hours of exercise represents approximately 3 percent of the RDA for men and 1 percent for women.[16] Although few studies have cumulatively assessed total iron losses in athletes, data collected from endurance-trained athletes indicate that iron losses from feces, urine, and sweat were approximately 1.75 milligrams for men and 2.3 milligrams for women.[17] These losses are higher than the estimated average losses of 1.0 and 1.4 milligram for nonathletic men and women respectively.[5]

Additionally, recent research has discovered the importance of an iron-regulating hormone called hepcidin. This hormone is released when iron concentrations are high and in response to inflammatory stimuli associated with exercise training, and it reduces dietary iron absorption. While hepcidin release is thought to help explain why some athletes are prone to poor iron status during heavy training (in addition to possible increased losses discussed above), a recent study from Peter Peeling's lab in Australia[46] found that an athlete's iron status influences both the baseline level of hepcidin and the magnitude of its response after training. This suggests that hepcidin release may be the body's underlying mechanism for controlling iron absorption and iron recycling in response to iron demand. It is not currently known whether hepcidin is lower in athletes following plant-based compared to traditional American diets. A study in vegetarian children found no differences between vegetarian and non-vegetarian children.[45]

Iron Needs of Athletes

Daily iron requirements for healthy people in the United States vary by sex and age and are shown in appendix E. Overall, iron requirements are higher for women than men and are elevated during times of growth in both sexes. The RDA is 8 milligrams for adult men and 18 milligrams for adult menstruating women. The recommended intake is roughly 10 times the estimated average daily loss discussed earlier to account for the low absorption of iron by the intestines. On average, only 10 percent of the iron in the diet is absorbed from a diet providing both animal and plant sources of iron.[5] The recommended intake for iron, however, does not account for either the additional loss that may occur in athletes during heavy training (as discussed earlier) or for the lower iron absorption from a diet of plant sources only. Absorption from food will be discussed later but is estimated to be 15 to 35 percent from animal flesh foods and 1 to 23 percent from plant foods.[1] The U.S. RDA states that the iron requirement for athletes in training may be 30 to 70 percent greater than for those who do not participate in regular strenuous exercise[5] to account for their increased daily loss, whereas those of vegetarians may be 80 percent greater than those of nonvegetarians to account for the lower absorption rate of iron from a vegetarian diet.[5]

Although it is impossible to extrapolate these recommendations to a recommended value for vegetarian athletes, you should consider that your iron needs may be higher than the daily recommendation—particularly during intense training—but that your needs are likely to vary depending on your food choices (also discussed later). You should also recognize that some degree of adaptation occurs in athletes and vegetarians, which over the long run enhances your ability to absorb and retain iron. A few studies provide examples of this phenomenon. One study found that men placed on a mostly plant-based diet with low iron bioavailability for 10 weeks were able to partially adapt by increasing iron absorption and decreasing iron loss in the feces. Another study of male runners found that iron absorption was significantly higher in male distance runners compared to a control population,[8] which was assumed to be an adaptive response. Iron absorption is also known to be affected by iron status and is higher in people with lower iron stores[2,18]—although this is not an optimal way to enhance the body's ability to absorb more iron. Whether hepcidin plays a role in this adaptation is yet to be established.

As a final note, iron needs may also be temporarily increased by high-altitude training and rapid growth in young athletes.[1] Inadequate iron intake during the initial phase of high-altitude adaptation may also lengthen the adaptation period, ultimately reducing training quality at altitude. While training at altitude, the body must adapt to the reduced air pressure by increasing production of hemoglobin-rich red cells, whereas a growth spurt significantly elevates iron requirements. Both situations can draw upon body iron reserves and result in iron deficiency if iron intake is not adjusted.

Results of Iron Deficiency

Quite simply, if you don't get enough iron in your daily diet to replace your losses, your ability to transport adequate oxygen for energy generation will be impaired. Ultimately, this is felt as a lack of "get up and go" both on and off the playing field.

As you would expect, athletic performance is impaired if the body becomes so deficient in iron that hemoglobin production is halted and its concentration in the blood drops below the normal range—a condition called *anemia*. It is imperative, however, to also recognize that impairments in aerobic capacity, athletic performance, and aerobic training adaptation can occur[19-23] even in the early stages of iron deficiency when iron stores in the liver and body tissues are lowered, but blood hemoglobin is still within the normal range (see box 7.1). For instance, one study conducted at Cornell University followed 42 iron-depleted, but not anemic, women for six weeks.[24] The women, who were initially untrained, first cycled 9.3 miles (15 km) to determine how quickly they could complete the bout. Tissue iron status was assessed through a technique that measures the concentration of serum transferrin receptors, which becomes elevated as tissue stores become depleted. Half then took an iron supplement containing 100 milligrams of ferrous sulfate per day, and the other half took a placebo. After four weeks of bicycle training, the women cycled the 9.3-mile distance again. Interestingly, the women who had had low tissue iron stores but normal blood hemoglobin levels at the beginning of the training—and were not allowed to replenish these stores with an iron supplement—failed to improve their cycling time. This clearly shows that iron depletion can prevent the normal fitness improvements that occur with training. The group who had had normal tissue iron stores experienced the expected training improvement whether they received the iron supplement or the placebo.

An earlier study, conducted at Pennsylvania State University, additionally indicates that cognitive function may be impaired with moderate iron depletion.[25] In this study, young, nonathletic women who had low iron stores were tested for several cognitive functions both before and after supplementation with iron or a placebo for 16 weeks. Iron supplementation in this group resulted in significant improvements in attention, memory, and learning during a variety of cognitive tasks. Taking the placebo did not. This has implications for real life as well as athletic situations.

The performance impairment associated with iron depletion without anemia is thought to be caused by the lowered levels of iron-containing enzymes in various tissues. Many of these enzymes are involved in the energy-generating pathways of muscle and brain cells. What is important to you as a vegetarian athlete is to recognize that even mild iron deficiency may impair both physical and mental performance. Mild iron deficiency (body tissue depletion) is not detected by measuring the hemoglobin concentration, which your doctor might do at a standard visit, but by measuring additional markers of iron status. Mild

Box 7.1

Stages of Iron Deficiency

Iron deficiency occurs when the body's iron stores are depleted and a restricted supply of iron to various tissues becomes apparent. If not corrected, iron deficiency can lead to iron deficiency anemia, which is a condition defined by a low hemoglobin concentration in the blood. Iron deficiency commonly occurs in three stages.

Stage 1: Diminished total-body iron content. This stage is identified by a reduction in serum ferritin. Serum ferritin concentration typically correlates well with total-body iron stores. However, within this stage, there may be varying degrees of depletion. Typically, a reduction in athletic performance is not apparent when iron stores in the liver are low but may likely occur when iron stores are depleted in the skeletal muscle or other tissues. If you suspect your iron is low, ask your health care provider to measure the concentration of your serum transferrin receptors as well as serum ferritin. Keep in mind, however, that serum ferritin is often elevated in endurance athletes[7] and is not by itself a good indicator of body iron stores in athletes.

Stage 2: Reduced red blood cell formation. This stage occurs when the iron supply is insufficient to support the formation of red blood cells. High levels of a blood marker called zinc protoporphyrin (ZPP) can indicate this stage. When iron is not readily available, zinc is used in its place, producing ZPP. To help diagnose this stage, your physician might measure your transferrin saturation along with ZPP. Transferrin is a protein that carries iron in the blood. This test indicates iron deficiency if less than 15 percent of this protein contains iron.

Stage 3: Iron deficiency anemia. In this final stage, hemoglobin concentration is affected and drops below the normal range, which is typically 12 to 15 grams per deciliter for women and 14 to 16.5 grams per deciliter for men. This prevents synthesis of red blood cells and results in anemia. The normal range, however, will be slightly higher for athletes living at higher altitudes.

iron deficiency also may not present with classic symptoms of iron deficiency anemia, which include fatigue, weakness, lethargy, abnormal temperature regulation, and impaired immune function. Many of these classic symptoms typically are not apparent until the hemoglobin concentration drops and the athlete becomes anemic.

Risk Factors for Iron Deficiency

Quite frankly, almost everyone is at risk for iron deficiency. Iron deficiency is the most common nutrition deficiency worldwide—particularly in women of childbearing age—and is the only nutrient deficiency that is significantly prevalent in industrialized countries, including the United States. The World Health Organization estimates that a staggering 800 million women and children are anemic, with close to half because of iron deficiency.[26] The athletes considered at greatest risk for iron deficiency include female athletes, distance runners and triathletes, vegetarians, and regular blood donors.[7,27,28]

Limited studies, however, are available on vegetarian athletes. Therefore, we do not know whether vegetarian athletes are at greater risk for iron deficiency, with or without anemia, than their meat-eating teammates. A recent meta-analysis, which combined data from 24 studies in the general population, found significantly lower serum ferritin concentrations in vegetarians compared to nonvegetarian controls.[29] Similar results were noted in a study conducted on female runners.[30] In this study, the athletes who followed a modified vegetarian diet had lower iron status than their meat-eating teammates, despite reporting similar iron consumption in the diet. Several smaller studies specifically measuring blood markers of anemia found that iron deficiency anemia is no more common among vegetarians than among the general population.[30-33] Certainly, any athlete or vegetarian can be prone to iron deficiency anemia if he or she restricts food intake (approximately 6 mg of iron is consumed per 1,000 kcal) or makes poor food choices.

With that said, it has been my professional and personal experience as a sports dietitian and vegetarian athlete for over 30 years that achieving normal iron status is possible through selection of a healthy diet without dependence on iron supplements or an occasional chicken breast (unless of course you are on the semivegetarian plan). I have not taken an iron-containing supplement for over 25 years, except on rare occasions for just a few weeks. I discovered—after the embarrassing situation of becoming anemic *during* my dietetic internship—how to boost my iron intake and absorption. This has included maintaining normal iron status—on a plant-based diet alone—while averaging 150-plus miles (241 km) a week on a bicycle, training for two marathons, and running during pregnancy with a singleton and twins. Yes, I refused the prenatal vitamin, but I was confident I was eating well and had my iron status checked regularly—just in case. I should clarify, however, that I have been fortunate to have never experienced heavy iron losses through gastrointestinal bleeding, hematuria, or excessively heavy menstrual cycles. My two vegetarian, athletic daughters passed through childhood without a need for iron supplements. Both, however, have taken a short course of an iron supplement (yes, prescribed by their mother) after experiencing low ferritin concentrations and declining running performance associated with their adolescent growth spurts. Both periodically take an iron-containing multi-vitamin during heavy periods of training. The key, I believe, is eating well (specifics are coming in the next section), not restricting energy intake, and supplementing only when and if the body has additional iron needs or losses. Of further note, it is important to clarify, again based on the literature and my own experience, that vegetarian athletes on a healthy diet seem to maintain serum ferritin concentrations (i.e., iron status) that fall within the range clinicians often call low normal (or slightly greater than borderline), but that this is not a bad thing. Maintaining iron stores on the lower end of normal may be one factor that contributes to a reduced risk of cancer and other chronic diseases in vegetarians. In having borderline stores, however, vegetarian athletes may need to supplement occasionally, for example after giving blood, experiencing a growth spurt, experiencing an excessively heavy menstrual cycle, or relocating from sea level to 7,220 feet (2,200 m). This is because their storage reserves are lower on average than regular meat-eating athletes.

Ensuring Sufficient Iron Intake and Absorption

In athletes, iron depletion is most commonly attributed to insufficient energy and low iron intakes, but it can also be influenced by excess loss in some athletes,[27] as discussed earlier. In vegetarians, lower status is thought to be the result of a lower bioavailability of dietary iron rather than absolute iron intake because research collectively shows that vegetarians generally consume as much iron as, or slightly more than, omnivores.[1] Thus, to avoid the pitfalls of poor iron status, include a variety of iron-rich foods in your daily diet and ensure that the iron you consume is well absorbed. To get started, you need education on plant sources of iron and on the dietary factors that enhance and inhibit iron absorption. After that, you just need to make sure you make good choices and, as always, that you meet your energy intake needs.

First, good sources of iron are typically found in whole and enriched grains, cereals and pasta, root and leafy-green vegetables, dried fruits, legumes, and nuts and seeds. These are listed in table 7.1. Chances are that if you are eating a well-balanced vegetarian diet and are not restricting your calories, you are already getting enough iron. If you think your diet may be lacking, add more iron-rich foods. You can also try cooking in an old-fashioned iron skillet or tossing an iron "egg" or "stone" into soups and sauces. The iron obtained from the skillet or stone can add to the iron content of cooked foods, particularly when the foods cooked are slightly acidic, such as tomato sauce. This is an old trick used by populations throughout the world living on a plant-based diet. Iron eggs, however, are difficult to find in the United States but may be available online.

Next, ensure that the iron you have consumed is absorbed. As you most likely know, the iron found in plant foods, eggs, and dairy is in a form called nonheme, or elemental, iron, which is not absorbed as well (1-23% that is consumed is absorbed)[1,34] as the heme iron form found in meat (approximately 25% that is consumed is absorbed).[5,34] *Heme* refers to iron in the form of myoglobin and also hemoglobin (just like in the body), which is why dark meat has a higher iron content than whiter meat. In fact, heme iron is better absorbed because it is treated as a protein and is not affected by meal composition or gastrointestinal secretions. Nonheme iron, on the other hand, must be released from its binding to various plant structures by digestive enzymes and enters the small intestine in a specific chemical form (Fe^{2+}). Nonheme iron is subject to "attack" by many different chemical reactions, including oxidation and binding with other dietary components, which reduces absorption. The one exception to this may be iron found in the leghemoglobin (a hemelike protein naturally found in soybean roots) that gives the Impossible Burger its "meaty taste" thanks to some fancy genetic engineering.[35]

TABLE 7.1   Approximate Iron Content of Selected Plant Foods

Food	Portion	Iron (mg)
GRAIN EQUIVALENTS		
Bread, enriched	1 slice or 1 oz	0.7-1.2
Bread, whole wheat	1 slice	0.8
Cereal, ready to eat and fortified	1 serving (1 oz)	2.0-22.4
Brown rice and wild rice	1 cup cooked	1.0
Oatmeal	1 cup cooked	1.6
Pasta, enriched	1 oz uncooked	0.7-1.2
Quinoa	1 cup cooked	2.8
VEGETABLES AND LEGUMES		
Beet greens*	1 cup cooked	2.7
Black beans	1 cup cooked	3.6
Broccoli*	1 cup cooked	1.1
Brussels sprouts*	1 cup cooked	0.7
Cabbage, Chinese (bok choy)	1 cup cooked	1.8
Collard greens*	1 cup cooked	2.2
Chickpeas (garbanzo beans)	1 cup cooked	4.7
Kale	1 cup	1.2
Lentils	1 cup cooked	6.6
Mustard greens*	1 cup cooked	1.0
Peas, green*	1 cup cooked	2.4
Pinto beans	1 cup cooked	3.6
Potato*	1 medium, baked	2.2
Red kidney beans	1 cup cooked	5.2
Southern peas (black-eyed, crowder)	1 cup cooked	4.3
Soybeans	1 cup cooked	8.8
Spinach	1 cup cooked	6.4
Sweet potato*	1 medium, baked	1.1
Swiss chard	1 cup cooked	4.0
Tofu, firm (calcium set)	1/2 cup	3.4
Tofu, regular (calcium set)	1/2 cup	6.7

Food	Portion	Iron (mg)
VEGETABLES AND LEGUMES *(continued)*		
Tomato*	1 cup raw	0.5
Turnip greens*	1 cup cooked	1.2
Veggie burger, Garden Burger	1 patty (100 g)	1.5
Veggie burger, Griller	1 patty (96 g)	3.7
Veggie burger, Impossible Burger	1 patty (85 g)	3
Winter squash*	1 cup cooked	0.9-1.4
FRUITS		
Apricots	5 halves, dried	0.9
Raisins	1/4 cup	0.7
Raspberries, frozen*	1 cup	1.6
Strawberries*	5 large	0.4
Watermelon*	1 wedge	0.7
NUTS AND SEEDS		
Almonds	1 oz	1.2
Cashews	1 oz	1.7
Chia seeds	1 oz, dried	2.2
Peanuts	1 oz	0.6
Pecans	1 oz	0.7
Pine nuts	1 oz	1.6
Pumpkin seeds	1 oz	4.2
Sunflower seeds	1 oz	1.1
Tahini	1 tbsp	1.3
Walnuts	1 oz	0.8
OTHER		
Molasses	1 tbsp	0.9
Blackstrap molasses	1 tbsp	3.6

Note: Refer to appendix F for guidance on converting English units to metric.

*Also a good source of vitamin C.

Data from USDA Food Composition Databases (https://ndb.nal.usda.gov/ndb/).

Iron absorption from plant sources can be both enhanced and inhibited by various dietary factors (see tables 7.2 and 7.3). By far the most potent plant-based factor is vitamin C, which aids in the absorption of iron from most plant sources.[36] Research has shown that ingesting 25 to 75 milligrams of vitamin C—roughly the amount in half a cup (118 ml) of most fruit juices—increases the absorption of iron from foods consumed in the same meal threefold to fourfold.[37] Consuming other organic acids, such as citric, malic, tartaric, fumaric, acetic, and lactic acids, may also increase iron absorption,[38] but their effects are not as powerful as vitamin C's.

On the other hand, iron absorption from plant sources can be inhibited by excessive intake of plant phytates, plant polyphenolics, bran, cocoa, coffee, tea (including some herbal teas), soy, and milk protein, and foods with high dietary concentrations of calcium, zinc, and other minerals. Fortunately, much of the natural processing that happens to foods, including soaking beans and fermenting soy products, helps reduce the inhibitory effects of many of these factors (see tables 7.2 and 7.3). Also fortunate is that many vegetables and fruits that are high in iron are also high in vitamin C (see table 7.4). In addition, commonly eaten combinations, such as beans with tomato-based sauce, stir-fried tofu and broccoli, and orange juice with toast or cereal, also result in generous levels of iron absorption. Not so fortunate is the fact that many of the foods and beverages we enjoy tend to inhibit iron absorption. Tea consumed hot or cold is a great example. The tannins in tea bind tightly with iron in the intestines so less iron is available for absorption. The way around this is to consume these and other iron inhibitors between meals. Alternately, beverages that contain fruit juices, including lemonade,[34,39] may enhance iron absorption. See box 7.2 for a summary of how to boost iron intake and absorption.

TABLE 7.2   Dietary Factors That Enhance Iron Absorption

Factor	Source
Vitamin C	Citrus fruits and juices, melons, berries, pineapple, tomatoes, bell peppers, broccoli, potatoes (see table 7.4)
Organic acids such as acetic, citric, fumaric, malic, and tartaric acids	Fruits, vegetables, and vinegars
Lactic acid	Sauerkraut
Retinol and carotenoids (not yet proven)	Dark-green, red, and orange fruits and vegetables
Specific food-processing methods	Leavening and baking bread; soaking and sprouting beans, grains, and seeds; fermentation process for making some soy foods (miso, tempeh, natto); coagulation with a gluconic acid derivative in making silken-style tofu
Sulfur-containing amino acids	Many plant protein foods
Tissue-protein factor (TPF) (also called meat protein fraction)	Flesh foods (TPF is a factor other than heme found in meat, poultry, and fish that promotes the absorption of nonheme iron from other foods consumed in the same meal.)

TABLE 7.3   Foods and Their Factors That Affect Iron Absorption

Food	Hindering factor (if known)	Enhancing factor (if known)
Bran, whole grains, legumes, nuts, and seeds	Phytates	Leavening and baking bread (hydrolyzes phytates); soaking and sprouting beans, grains, and seeds
Soy products	Soy (phytate or protein)	Fermentation process for making some soy foods (miso, tempeh, natto); coagulation with a gluconic acid derivative in making silken-style tofu
Tea, coffee	Polyphenols (tannins)	—
Some vegetables, some herbal teas, red wine	Polyphenolics	—
Calcium-rich antacids, calcium phosphates, supplements	Calcium, zinc, magnesium, supplemental doses of other minerals	—
Eggs, milk	Egg or milk protein; factor not known	—
Spices	—	Enhancing factors not established

TABLE 7.4   Approximate Vitamin C Content of Select Foods

Food	Portion	Vitamin C (mg)
Asparagus	1 cup cooked	44
Beet greens	1 cup cooked	36
Broccoli	1 cup cooked	101
Brussels sprouts	1 cup cooked	71
Cabbage, all varieties	1 cup cooked	20-45
Cantaloupe	1 cup	59
Cauliflower	1 cup cooked	56
Collard greens	1 cup cooked	35
Cranberry juice cocktail	1 cup	90
Grapefruit	One half	39
Grapefruit juice	1 cup	94
Honeydew	1 cup	31
Kale	1 cup	53

(continued)

TABLE 7.4 *(continued)*

Food	Portion	Vitamin C (mg)
Kiwi	1 medium	71
Kohlrabi	1 cup cooked	90
Lemon juice	From 1 lemon	31
Mango	1 cup	46
Mustard greens	1 cup cooked	35
Okra	1 cup cooked	26
Orange juice	1 cup	97-124
Orange	1 medium	70
Papaya	1 cup	87
Peas, fresh or frozen	1 cup cooked	77
Peppers, green	1 cup cooked	120
Peppers, red	1 cup cooked	233
Pineapple	1 cup	56
Plantain, raw	1 medium	33
Potato	1 medium	19
Raspberries	1 cup	32
Strawberries	1 cup	98-106
Tangerine	1 medium	22
Tomato or vegetable juice	1 cup	44-67
Tomato sauce	1 cup	66
Tomato, raw or canned	1 cup	22-23
Turnip greens	1 cup cooked	40
Watermelon	1 wedge	23
Winter squash	1 cup cooked	19

Note: Refer to appendix F for guidance on converting English units to metric.

Data from USDA Food Composition Databases (https://ndb.nal.usda.gov/ndb/).

Considering Iron Supplements

Athletes concerned about their iron status should first try to boost their intake and absorption of iron from foods. However, there are times when vegetarian athletes may require iron supplements to maintain or slightly replenish iron stores. An athlete allergic to or who dislikes legumes, nuts, and seeds, for example, will likely struggle to take in enough iron. A female endurance athlete with excessive menstrual blood loss on top of heavy endurance training may also find it difficult to maintain iron status during the preracing and racing seasons. Certainly if iron deficiency or iron deficiency anemia is diagnosed, iron supplements should be taken (usually for several months) as directed by the physician.

If you want to supplement, you should first check with your personal or team physician or talk with a registered dietitian to ensure that you are indeed iron depleted or iron deficient. Your physician can determine whether your iron status is truly compromised by checking your serum ferritin level or serum iron-binding capacity (see box 7.1). Some physicians may also be willing to check your zinc protoporphyrin or serum transferrin receptor concentrations, which may be better indicators of iron status in athletes, pending their cost and availability. This

---

Box 7.2

Tips for Boosting Iron Intake and Absorption

- Inventory the iron-rich foods in your diet. If your diet lacks such sources, include more iron-rich foods daily (see table 7.1). If desired, cook in an iron skillet or use an iron "egg" or "stone." Remember, as an athlete who eats a plant-based diet, your iron needs may be elevated. Consult the USDA Food Composition Databases for the iron content of foods not listed in the table.

- Include a source of vitamin C or other organic acids in most meals. Consider foods that are good sources of vitamin C and iron as well as food combinations that provide both. You can rarely go wrong by adding a small glass of citrus juice or topping foods with chopped peppers, tomatoes, tomato salsa or sauce, or a splash of flavored vinegar. One recent study found that iron absorbed from tofu increased significantly when it was consumed with 10 ounces (295 ml) of orange juice.[40] Another found that iron absorbed from wheat flour products was increased by drinking 5 ounces of lemonade (150 ml).[39] In contrast, the low iron absorption from lentil dal[18] could be easily enhanced by incorporating vitamin C foods into the recipe or the meal.

- Assess your regular consumption of inhibitors. Try to limit their consumption or consume them between meals. For example, instead of drinking milk or iced tea with a bean burrito or lentil soup, replace the beverage with citrus juice to enhance the iron absorbed from that meal. Or, drink water and top the meal with chopped tomato or a splash of vinegar. Enjoy your tea or milk with a between-meal snack that is lower in iron. Also, consume tofu with vegetables or fruit. At breakfast, don't drink tea or coffee while eating iron-rich cereal, whole grain toast, or a bran muffin. Instead, drink a glass of orange juice or eat a bowl of fresh melon to enhance the iron absorption. Depending on your training schedule and preference, morning tea or coffee should then be consumed an hour or so before or after your iron-rich breakfast.

is important to mention because I have learned over the years that iron is not responsible for "all things fatigue." Low iron status is one of many factors linked to fatigue and poor performance, yet is the one athletes and coaches usually blame. Again, reduced hemoglobin, hematocrit, and red blood cell levels are not sensitive or specific markers of iron status in endurance athletes because of the exercise-induced plasma volume expansion[41] (see box 7.3). Taking iron supplements on your own, except in the form of a multivitamin, is not advised. Unnecessary iron supplements could result in gastric distress (one of the side effects of iron supplementation) or unknowingly lead to hemochromatosis, an iron overload disease, in genetically susceptible people. It may also promote inflammation—but more research is needed to prove the latter.

If iron supplementation is needed, low-dose iron supplements may be the best bet because they are less likely to cause side effects. The side effects of taking iron tablets are not pleasant and include stomach upset, burning gut, constipation, and diarrhea. Many doses and preparations of iron are available, however. Athletes who have difficulty tolerating oral supplements should discuss the issue with their doctor. Often times, athletes may better tolerate the supplement if they start with a lower dose (and progress to the target dose) or take their supplement with or after meals or at bedtime. Changing to a different form or preparation is also an option, as is iron injections if your physician feels this is appropriate. After you have replenished the depleted stores—which may take several months—you can switch to a multivitamin and begin focusing on diet. Eventually, you can drop the multivitamin. Alternatively, you may be able to take a low-dose iron supplement intermittently when needed—for example during menstrual bleeding or after giving blood—rather than regularly. The main advantage of intermittent supplementation is that it reduces side effects associated with high doses of iron.[42] Intermittent supplementation is controversial among some practitioners, however, and specific protocols are not yet available.

Problems With Too Much Iron

Research suggests that high levels of iron in the blood are associated with an elevated risk of many chronic diseases, including heart disease, Parkinson's disease, cancer, and cancer mortality.[43] Iron may stimulate production of free radicals (discussed in the next chapter), which can attack many of the stable molecules in the body. Attack by free radicals is thought to promote the formation of oxidized low-density lipoprotein (LDL) particles (elevating the risk for cardiovascular and other vascular diseases, tumors, and even nerve cell death). In addition, the prevalence of hereditary hemochromatosis, an iron storage disease, is high in the United States and many countries but is not well recognized.[43] Excess supplementation even in athletes can increase risk of iron overload in those with hereditary hemochromatosis.[44] The storage of excess iron in these individuals can be the underlying cause of liver disease,

Box 7.3

Is It Really Anemia?

You are feeling fine and stop by your physician's office for another matter only to learn—surprisingly—that your hemoglobin is low. You are told you are anemic.

If you are an endurance athlete or athlete who has just initiated the season, chances are you are experiencing something called *dilutional anemia, sports anemia,* or *athletic anemia.* This type of anemia is not really anemia and is caused by normal expansion of the volume of plasma fluid that occurs with training. Dilutional anemia is noted in endurance athletes during the precompetition or competition season (particularly when the weather is hot). It is also commonly noted at the beginning of the season for some athletes but then disappears when red blood cell formation catches up with fluid volume expansion. In this case, many markers of iron status, including hemoglobin, hematocrit, and red blood cell concentrations are falsely lowered and are therefore not accurate indicators of iron status.[41] On the other hand, serum ferritin may be elevated in endurance athletes and also inaccurately reflect iron storage.[7]

Dilutional anemia is not something to worry about because it will not impair performance or health. You should, however, determine that you are indeed experiencing dilutional rather than true anemia. You can do this by having your serum ferritin concentration checked or, better yet, by repeating the test after you have taken two or three days off from training. The training effect of volume expansion is short lived and will return to normal if you rest for several days. Don't worry, your plasma volume expands again as soon as you resume exercising and is beneficial. It helps you maintain your fluid volume for longer while sweating during exercise. Often, athletes experiencing volume expansion notice its effects in funny ways. For example, the ring you picked out during the off-season suddenly becomes tight, or the strap on your sport watch has to be loosened one or two slots.

increased skin pigmentation, diabetes, heart disease, arrhythmias, arthritis, and hypogonadism. Clearly, excess iron in the diet or in the body is nothing to mess with. And unless you supplement, it is something a vegetarian may be immune to.

We hope that after reading this chapter you understand how you can boost iron absorption and achieve normal iron status on a vegetarian diet—without the need to supplement. The next chapter addresses how you can make better choices to avoid dependence on vitamin and mineral supplements in general.

8 | Breaking Free of Multivitamin Dependence

A collegiate tennis player came to see me about the nutritional quality of his diet. He had been a vegetarian in Germany as a teenager, but his parents encouraged him to eat meat after a blood test revealed some abnormal values. He admitted he had recently quit eating meat and was ready to be vegetarian again. "But this time I want to do it properly," he added. An assessment of his diet suggested it contained adequate energy and carbohydrate (mainly from grain products), some vegetables, and an occasional piece of fruit. At the time he was still eating fish, had tried a few meat analogues (mainly vegetarian burgers), but was not eating many legumes (other than processed soy). He was also religiously taking a multivitamin. Overall I felt his diet was not too bad but could be improved by increasing the variety of his food choices. We discussed the importance of eating an assortment of plant foods, including colorful fruits and vegetables, as well as legumes and nuts. I sent him off with "Vegetarian in a Nutshell" (a handout published by Vegetarian Resource Group, www.vrg.org/nutshell/nutshell) and the immediate goal of increasing his fruit and vegetable intake and trying dishes that contain legumes. My long-term plan was to help him discover new foods and ways to incorporate them into his diet so that he would feel more confident in his food choices and less dependent on his multivitamin supplement.

– Enette

As an athlete following a plant-based diet, you may be the target of the message that you need to take a vitamin and mineral supplement of some sort in order to maintain nutritional status. This may also be true if you are an athlete or getting older, because manufacturers now love to target the aging boomers (and anyone who feels they are getting older). Why such claims? Vegetarians, as the claims go, need vitamin and mineral supplements because of their meatless diet. Athletes need supplements because of purported excessive nutrient losses caused by increased breakdown and excretion of nutrients during training, and aging individuals need supplements to well, prevent aging. Such claims, however, neglect the simple fact that vegetarians (and many semivegetarians) are more likely than omnivores to choose diets rich in a wider variety of plant foods packed with vitamins and minerals, particularly if they make good food choices. They also ignore the fact that athletes are more likely to meet their vitamin and mineral needs than less active people simply because they eat more calories and have a higher volume of food intake. In general, there is little evidence that athletes have higher vitamin and mineral requirements than inactive people, with the possible exception of iron, riboflavin, vitamin C, and sodium. Although some vegetarian athletes should monitor certain "red flag" nutrients with a watchful eye, this need is based more on food choice and energy intake than on eating a plant-based diet.

This chapter provides an overview of how to meet your vitamin and mineral needs through a well-balanced diet rather than depending on unnecessary vitamin and mineral supplements. Although you may not be comfortable completely giving up your daily multivitamin and mineral supplement, the information presented in this chapter should help you understand how vitamins and minerals affect your general health and performance and how your requirements for the major vitamins and minerals can be met by making better food choices. Iron and the nutrients involved in bone health are not emphasized here because they were the focus of previous chapters.

Vitamin and Mineral Primer

Getting adequate amounts of vitamins and minerals is important for health and performance. Both vitamins and minerals are key regulators of numerous bodily functions, many of which are critical for exercise and performance.[1] Vitamins and minerals are classified as micronutrients—in contrast to the macronutrients carbohydrate, protein, fat, and water—because the body needs them in much smaller quantities. Macronutrient requirements are expressed in grams, whereas micronutrient requirements are expressed in microgram to milligram quantities. Micronutrients also perform different functions than macronutrients do. Macronutrients provide sources of energy, maintain cellular hydration, and provide the body structure for performing work. Micronutrients aid in the body's use of macronutrients during many processes, including energy generation and maintenance of skeletal health. Many vitamins and minerals also play a role in immune function and help protect cells from oxidative damage.

Our daily requirements for macronutrients and micronutrients depends on whether the nutrient is used up or conserved for use and reuse, and whether the nutrient is stored in the body and in what quantity. For example, carbohydrate is used for energy, whereas iron is hoarded and reused. Thus, the daily carbohydrate need for athletes is close to 500 grams per day, and the daily requirement for iron is 18 milligrams per day for menstruating women and 11 milligrams per day for adult men. Because only a small percentage of the minerals consumed are absorbed into the body, nutrient requirements are also influenced by how efficiently the intestines can absorb them.

So what is the difference between vitamins and minerals? Vitamins are organic substances found in food. Organic means that they contain the elements carbon, oxygen, and hydrogen. Vitamins aid in many essential biochemical reactions by catalyzing, or speeding them up. Without vitamin catalysts, many chemical reactions would occur too slowly to allow us to live. Vitamins are needed regularly in the diet because the body cannot make them. There are 14 known vitamins: 4 fat-soluble vitamins (A, D, E, and K) and 10 water-soluble vitamins (vitamin C, and the eight B-complex vitamins).[2] In general, the body is able to store enough fat-soluble vitamins to last for months but only enough water-soluble vitamins to last no more than a few weeks.

Minerals, on the other hand, are not organic and serve more as structural or helper components of enzymes rather than as catalysts. Fifteen minerals—calcium, phosphorus, magnesium, iron, sodium, potassium, chloride, zinc, iodine, copper, selenium, chromium, manganese, fluoride and molybdenum—are considered essential.[2] There is also evidence that arsenic, boron, nickel, silicon, and vanadium play a role in physiological processes, but we know so little about them that there is no established dietary reference intake (DRI), only a suggested upper limit.

Getting Your Vitamins and Minerals on a Vegetarian Diet

Most vegetarian athletes can meet their need for vitamins and minerals by consuming a diet that provides adequate energy and consists of a variety of wholesome foods, including whole grains, legumes, leafy greens and other vegetables, fruit, and, if acceptable, dairy products and eggs. Because of hectic training and work or school schedules, however, some athletes make poor food choices, resulting in a deficient intake of many vitamins and minerals. Others may be at risk for deficiencies simply because they restrict food intake to maintain low body weight and also make poor food choices.[3] This is often the case with athletes involved in sports such as gymnastics, dancing, diving, figure skating, wrestling, and even distance running. Collective evidence in athletes has suggested that intake of iron, calcium,[3] zinc,[4] and magnesium[5] are often insufficient, particularly among female athletes.[6] Similar information in vegetarian and vegan populations has found that vitamin B_{12}, iron, zinc, vitamin D, calcium, and iodine status are occasionally compromised.[7-9]

Better Food Choices for Improved Vitamin and Mineral Nutrition

Despite what supplement companies and vitamin gurus want you to believe, it is always best to improve your nutritional status through better food choices. The exception is vitamin D, which is obtained more efficiently from sensible exposure to sunlight rather than from the diet (see chapter 6). The reason is simple. Mother Nature wanted us to eat food. Food is packed not only with vitamins and minerals but also with many known and unknown factors that aid in nutrient absorption and use. These factors—often called phytochemicals—may even reduce the risk of chronic diseases. Great examples include the bioflavins found in citrus fruits and vegetables that help the body absorb vitamin C, and the many anticancer substances such as isoflavones, indole, polyphenols, isothiocyanates, lycopene, quercetin, ellagitannins, resveratrol, sulforaphane, and organosulfur compounds that trap free radicals (see box 8.1) and interfere with cellular processes involved in cancer progression.[10]

Isolating one compound from a fruit or vegetable and putting it in a pill is probably appealing to people who would rather skip the spinach and swallow a supplement, but it defies nature. In fact, we have learned that supplementing with isolated vitamins[11-14] often does not yield the same protective benefits of simply eating fruits and vegetables.[10,15,16] Taking beta-carotene supplements, for example, has been shown to increase rather than decrease the risk of lung cancer and cardiovascular disease,[11-13] promoting particularly adverse effects in smokers and people exposed to asbestos.[11,13] In a large meta-analysis of 68 randomized studies, dietary supplementation with beta-carotene and vitamins A and E was found not only to have no benefit on health outcomes but also to possibly increase mortality. Taking folic acid supplements quite surprisingly was also found to increase the risk of artery reclogging in heart patients following coronary stenting, an operation that unclogs arteries.[12] Eating plenty of fruits and vegetables high in these and other nutrients, on the other hand, appears to protect against most chronic diseases.[17] Supplements made from concentrated fruit and vegetable extracts also do not provide the full benefits of whole foods. These supplements lack soluble and insoluble fiber and other structural components that help keep bowel functions regular and have a protective influence on gut health and blood sugar regulation.

Tackling Vitamins With Less Reliance on Supplements

The bottom line is that supplements—even if they are pure extracts of real foods—do not provide the same benefit as consuming the real thing. Indeed, the nutrient content of whole real foods can be lost or destroyed through cooking, processing, or improper storage—either on your part or the growers' and food distributors'—but these factors can be minimized. To retain the nutrient content of food, purchase more locally grown foods, and eat fresh foods shortly after purchase. When cooking, don't overcook. Cook or sauté in

Box 8.1

Free Radicals and Antioxidants

Free radicals are produced by normal bodily processes that include the oxidation reactions required for energy generation from carbohydrate, fat, and protein (as described in chapter 2) during rest and particularly during exercise. Environmental factors such as ultraviolet light, air pollution, and tobacco smoke also produce free radicals. Free radicals are problematic because they are unstable and can attack and damage cellular proteins, unsaturated fatty acids located in cellular membranes, and even DNA. Their ability to damage DNA and genetic-related material explains why they may play a role in cancer promotion. In addition, free radicals are hypothesized to be responsible for exercise-induced protein oxidation and to possibly contribute to muscle fatigue and soreness.[1,18-20]

Dietary antioxidants can stabilize free radicals and protect against oxidative stress. In this role, they may have a protective effect on cognitive performance, aging, cancer, arthritis, cataracts, and heart disease. Although high intake of fruits and vegetables has been shown time and time again to have a protective effect on many age-related diseases, including cancer and heart disease,[15,17,21] the specific factors responsible are not yet understood. Known vitamin and mineral antioxidants include beta-carotene, other carotenoids, vitamin C, vitamin E, copper, and selenium. Research has also identified an assortment of chemicals in plants (termed phytochemicals) that may be involved in cancer prevention.[10,22] Although the specific mechanisms are being investigated, it is well recognized that antioxidant vitamins actively scavenge and quench free radicals, often becoming oxidized and inactive themselves in the process. Vitamin C is particularly important for the parts of the body that consist of water, whereas vitamin E is important in the cell membrane. Copper and selenium, on the other hand, serve as important cofactors for enzymes involved in the body's own free radical–defense system.

It is not yet known whether antioxidants influence muscle recovery and enhance performance. Although studies have found that antioxidant supplements may reduce lipid peroxidation, they do not appear to enhance exercise performance.[18-20] Research is needed, however, to determine whether a plant-based diet naturally high in a variety of antioxidants and phytochemicals[21,23,24] would enhance recovery and dampen the oxidative damage that occurs with heavy training. One study for example found that consuming a drink containing black grape, raspberry, and red currant concentrates before a bout of strenuous exercise reduced oxidative stress and possibly also muscle damage.[25] Several other studies have found that consuming other fruit and vegetable juices, including tart cherries,[26-28] pomegranate,[29,30] and black currant[31] juice or concentrates, reduced exercise-induced oxidative stress and possibly also muscle soreness and damage. So keep eating those whole grains and colorful fruits and vegetables.

a minimal amount of water or oil and with as low a heat as possible. Storing fresh produce and grains in a dark, cool place away from direct sunlight, and in airtight containers, if appropriate, also preserves their nutrient content. Finally, educating yourself about good sources of the major nutrients and consuming a variety of foods containing these nutrients should help you meet your nutrient needs and maybe even lead you to feeling secure enough in plant-based eating to eliminate your dependence on supplements. The following section briefly discusses the vitamins that either are important to active vegetarians or that may be low in poorly selected vegetarian diets.

B Vitamins

The B-complex vitamins are a set of eight vitamins: thiamin, riboflavin, niacin, biotin, pantothenic acid, vitamin B_6, folate, and vitamin B_{12}. Collectively, these vitamins function as catalysts (coenzymes) in the release of energy from carbohydrate, fat, and protein, and also in the development, growth, and repair of all body cells. Therefore, requirements for some, but not all, B vitamins are tied to energy intake.

Surveys of athletes in general have noted that riboflavin, folate, and vitamin B_6 are frequently low in the diet of some female athletes,[32] most likely because of inadequate consumption of fruits, green leafy vegetables, legumes, and dairy products. Clinical studies have also noted that active people who restrict their energy intake or make poor dietary choices are at risk of poor thiamine, riboflavin, and vitamin B_6 status.[33]

Athletes who follow vegetarian diets and do not restrict energy intake should easily be able to meet their requirements for most B vitamins, which are widely distributed in plant foods (see table 8.1). In fact, many of the best sources of B vitamins, such as folate, are provided by plant rather than animal foods. However, vitamin B_{12} and possibly also riboflavin are potential exceptions. Both vitamins are of special interest to athletes and intake of both tends to be low in vegetarian diets that contain little or no dairy or animal products.

Riboflavin Riboflavin is important for the formation of enzymes known as flavoproteins, which are involved in energy production from carbohydrate and fat. Research suggests that riboflavin needs increase with the initiation of an exercise program and possibly also with an abrupt increase in training volume,[32-34] such as at the beginning of the preseason. Although riboflavin is widely distributed in foods, major sources include milk, other dairy products, meat, and eggs. An 8-ounce (236 ml) glass of milk, for example, contains 20 percent of the RDA for riboflavin. Because some studies have found that vegans take in less riboflavin than nonvegetarians and may be at greater risk of deficiency,[35-37] vegan and vegetarian athletes who consume little or no dairy foods should make an effort to consume riboflavin-containing plant foods. This is particularly important when increasing training volume or when restricting energy intake.

Good plant sources of riboflavin include whole-grain and fortified breads and cereals, legumes, tofu, nuts, seeds, bananas, asparagus, dark-green leafy vegetables, avocado, and sea vegetables, such as seaweed, kombu, arame, and dulse (see table 8.2). A recent double-blind, placebo-controlled trial study in ultramarathoners completing the 100-mile (161 km) Western States Endur-

TABLE 8.1   B Vitamins and Vitamin C for Vegetarian Athletes

Vitamin	Recommended intake for athletes	Major vegetarian sources	Noted problems with excessive consumption
Thiamin (B$_1$)	DRI = 1.2 mg men, 1.1 mg women; recommendation of 0.6 mg/1,000 kcal may be more appropriate for athletes	Whole-grain products, enriched breads and cereals, legumes	No known toxicity
Riboflavin (B$_2$)	DRI = 1.3 mg men, 1.1 mg women; recommendation of 0.6 mg/1,000 kcal may be more appropriate for athletes	Milk and dairy products, enriched grain products, green leafy vegetables, legumes (see table 8.2)	No known toxicity
Niacin	DRI = 16 mg men, 14 mg women; recommendation of 6.6 mg/1,000 kcal may be more appropriate for athletes	Whole-grain products, enriched breads and cereals, legumes	Headache, nausea, flushing of face, burning and itching skin from nicotinic acid supplementation
Biotin	Adequate intake (AI) = 30 mg for adults	Legumes, milk, egg yolk, whole-grain products, most vegetables	No known toxicity
Pantothenic acid	AI = 5 mg for adults	Milk, eggs, legumes, whole-grain products, most vegetables	No known toxicity
Vitamin B$_6$	DRI = 1.3 mg for adults ages 19-50; athletes may need values higher than the DRI because of increased protein intakes	Protein foods, legumes, green leafy vegetables (see table 8.4)	Loss of nerve sensation, impaired gait
Folic acid	DRI = 400 mcg	Green leafy vegetables, legumes, nuts, enriched grain products (see table 8.3)	Prevents detection of B$_{12}$ deficiency
Vitamin B$_{12}$	RDA = 2.4 mcg	Animal foods only: fish, milk, eggs; also nutrition support formula and fortified vegan products	No known toxicity
Vitamin C	DRI = 90 mg for men, 75 mg for women; athletes may need 100 mg	Fruits and vegetables, particularly bell peppers, citrus fruits, broccoli (see table 7.4 on page 113)	Diarrhea, kidney stones, scurvy (when ceasing megadoses), reduced copper absorption

ance Run found that two single, high doses (100 mg) of riboflavin supplements decreased muscle pain and soreness and improved recovery.[38] While more research is certainly needed, short-term use of this nutrient may prove to be of interest to some athletes.

TABLE 8.2 Riboflavin, Zinc, and Copper Content of Selected Vegetarian and Dairy Foods

Food	Portion	Riboflavin (mg)	Zinc (mg)	Copper (mcg)
GRAIN EQUIVALENTS				
Bread, enriched	1 oz slice	0.09	0.20	70
Bread, whole wheat	1 oz slice	0.06	0.55	80
Cereal, fortified	1 serving (1 oz)	0.42	1.20-3.80	Varies
VEGETABLES AND LEGUMES, INCLUDING SOY				
Asparagus	1 cup cooked	0.25	1.10	370
Avocado	1/4 avocado	0.06	0.30	100
Beet greens	1 cup cooked	0.42	0.72	360
Black beans	1 cup cooked	0.10	1.90	360
Broccoli	1 cup cooked	0.10	0.35	95
Cabbage, Chinese (bok choy)	1 cup cooked	0.11	0.30	40
Collard greens	1 cup cooked	0.20	2.50	70
Chickpeas (garbanzo beans)	1 cup cooked	0.09	0.30	580
Kale	1 cup cooked	0.09	0.30	200
Lentils	1 cup cooked	0.15	2.50	500
Mustard greens	1 cup cooked	0.09	0.15	120
Peas, green	1 cup cooked	0.24	1.90	280
Pinto beans	1 cup cooked	0.11	1.70	370
Red kidney beans	1 cup cooked	0.10	1.90	430
Southern peas (black-eyed, crowder)	1 cup cooked	0.10	2.20	460
Soybeans	1 cup cooked	2.00	0.50	700
Tofu, firm (calcium set)	1/2 cup	0.13	2.00	480
Tofu, regular (calcium set)	1/2 cup	0.06	1.00	240
Turnip greens	1 cup cooked	0.10	0.20	360
FRUITS				
Banana	1 medium	0.09	0.20	90
NUTS AND SEEDS				
Almonds	1 oz	0.23	0.95	330
Cashews	1 oz	0.06	1.60	630

(continued)

TABLE 8.2   *(continued)*

Food	Portion	Riboflavin (mg)	Zinc (mg)	Copper (mcg)
NUTS AND SEEDS *(continued)*				
Peanuts	1 oz	0.03	0.90	190
Pecans	1 oz	0.04	1.30	330
Pine nuts	1 oz	0.06	1.80	380
Pumpkin seeds	1 oz	0.09	2.10	390
Sunflower seeds	1 oz	0.07	1.50	520
Tahini	1 tbsp	0.07	0.70	240
Walnuts	1 oz	0.04	0.90	450
MILK, SOY MILK, AND CHEESE				
Soy milk, calcium fortified	1 cup	0.53	0.50	200
Cows' milk, skim	1 cup	0.45	1.00	30
Cows' milk, 2%	1 cup	0.45	1.10	30
Cheddar cheese	1 oz	0.11	0.90	9
Goat cheese, hard	1 oz	0.34	0.45	180
Mozzarella, low moisture	1 oz	0.09	0.90	8
Parmesan, hard	1 oz	0.09	0.80	9

Note: Values for most vegetables and legumes are for those that have been cooked, boiled, and drained and without salt. Values for most nuts are for dry-roasted varieties without added oil or salt. The RDA is 1.6 mg for riboflavin, 15 mg for zinc, and 900 mcg for copper. Refer to appendix F for guidance on converting English units to metric.

Data from USDA Food Composition Databases (https://ndb.nal.usda.gov/ndb/).

Vitamin B$_{12}$ An adequate supply of vitamin B$_{12}$ is essential for athletes. Vitamin B$_{12}$ functions as part of a coenzyme complex that is essential in the synthesis of DNA (the body's genetic code) and red blood cells and in the formation of the protective sheath (called *myelin)* that surrounds nerve fibers. Vitamin B$_{12}$ is of particular importance to vegan and near-vegan populations because cobalamin, the active form, is found exclusively in animal products.[9,39] Thus, both vegan athletes and those consuming little dairy or eggs are at risk for low vitamin B$_{12}$ status.[40,41] Vegan athletes should consume vitamin B$_{12}$-fortified foods daily or take a vitamin B$_{12}$-containing supplement or multivitamin. Vegetarian athletes should also consider a supplemental source if their intake of dairy products or eggs or both is limited. For example, an 8-ounce (236 ml) glass of milk provides approximately 40 percent of the RDA for vitamin B$_{12}$ while an egg and 1 ounce (28 g) of low-moisture, part-skim mozzarella cheese provides 20 to 25 percent (see https://ndb.nal.usda.gov/ndb). Vegan sources include Red Star T6635 nutritional yeast, and fortified plant-based milks, breakfast cereals, margarines, and some meat analogues. Korean laver is also reported to be a B_{12} source.[42] Athletes are encouraged to carefully check the labels of their favorite brands or contact the manufacturers for nutritional information.

A comprehensive list of fortified foods is not included in this book (as it is for other nutrients) because the B_{12} content varies by brand and product and may change periodically. For example, according to the USDA Food Composition Database, Morningstar Farms Grillers currently provide close to 100 percent of the daily value (DV) for B_{12} and their Veggie Breakfast Sausage Links provide 50 percent of the DV (neither are vegan), while their Garden Burger vegan burger lists no B_{12} (USDA Food Composition Databases). Red Star T6635 nutritional yeast, however, is a reliable source. Two teaspoons (10 ml) supply nearly the adult RDA of 2.4 micrograms and is delicious sprinkled on many foods. Contrary to information recently published in the public press and elsewhere,[43] nori and chlorella seaweeds are not a reliable source of well-absorbed B_{12}.[9]

Because of the irreversible neurological damage that can occur with vitamin B_{12} deficiency, vegans (and near vegans) should consider having their B_{12} status monitored regularly[39] by their personal or team physician. Senior athletes, who may be at risk for vitamin B_{12} deficiency because of the reduced absorption rate of this vitamin in the gut that occurs with aging, may also want to have their status monitored. The typical symptoms of B_{12} deficiency (usually apparent in the red blood cells) can be masked by high intake of folate, which is abundant in plant foods.

Other B Vitamins   Maintaining adequate levels of other B vitamins is generally not a problem for vegetarian athletes, unless, of course, they restrict energy intake or avoid grains and pulses (beans, peas, and lentils), which are excellent sources of most of the B vitamins. Nevertheless, a brief discussion of folate and vitamin B_6 may be of interest, particularly to female athletes.

Although folate is most likely abundant in the diet of vegetarians and vegans,[8,35,44] it is worth discussing because of its importance in the prevention of cancer, cardiovascular disease, and birth defects in the fetus during pregnancy. Dietary folate is a generic term that includes both the naturally occurring form termed *folate* (or polyglutamated folate) and the folic acid that is used in fortified foods and dietary supplements.[2] Like vitamin B_{12}, folate is an essential factor in DNA synthesis and new-cell formation. Because many American adults do not get enough folate, the government now mandates that 140 micrograms of folic acid be added to every 100 grams of enriched grain products such as pasta, breakfast cereals, and flour. Dietary folate, however, was first found in leafy green vegetables, which is how it got its name. The word folate is derived from the Latin word for leaf: *folium*.

The richest sources of naturally occurring folate are legumes and dark-green leafy vegetables. (See table 8.3 for a list of the top 21 vegetarian sources of folate.) Various amounts of folate, however, are found in most fruits and vegetables, with oranges serving as a common source in the U.S. diet. The most abundant sources of folic acid are fortified grain products, including ready-to-eat breakfast cereals, bread, rice, and pasta, which provide 15 to 100 percent of the DV. Although vegetarian athletes are likely to meet folate requirements easily, even without including fortified foods,[45] athletes should keep in mind that folate is easily destroyed by heat and oxidation (for example after cutting) and interactions with medications, including antacids and aspirin. Results from a study conducted in the Slovak Republic—which also likely apply to

TABLE 8.3   Top 21 Natural Vegetarian Sources of Folate

Food	Portion	Value (mcg)
Edamame, from frozen	1 cup cooked	482
Lentils	1 cup cooked	358
Southern peas	1 cup cooked	358
Pinto beans	1 cup cooked	294
Okra	1 cup cooked, sliced	269
Spinach	1 cup cooked	263
Black beans, navy beans	1 cup cooked	256
Asparagus	1 cup cooked	243
Red kidney beans	1 cup cooked	230
Green soybeans	1 cup cooked	200
Great northern beans	1 cup cooked	181
Collard greens	1 cup cooked	177
Turnip greens	1 cup cooked	170
Broccoli	1 cup cooked	168
Chickpeas	1 cup cooked	161
Brussels sprouts	1 cup cooked	157
Lima beans	1 cup cooked	156
Beets, red	1 cup cooked	136
Split peas	1 cup cooked	127
Papaya	1 cup chopped	116
Corn, canned	1 cup cooked	115

Note: The DRI for folate is 400 mcg for adults. Many ready-to-eat breakfast cereals are fortified with close to the RDA for folate. Refer to appendix E for guidance on converting English units to metric.

Data from report by single nutrient for total folate, USDA Food Composition Databases (https://ndb.nal.usda.gov/ndb/nutrients/index).

the United States—further suggest that folate intake may be seasonal, with a higher prevalence of deficiencies observed in winter and early spring among omnivores but not vegetarians.[44] Additionally, synthetic folic acid appears to be better absorbed (85-100% bioavailable) compared to natural folate (50% bioavailable) which may be important to consider during pregnancy or to the rare vegetarian athlete who avoids fruits, vegetables, and legumes.

Vitamin B_6 is also worth further discussion. Both active and inactive women often take in insufficient amounts of this vitamin if they restrict energy or make poor dietary choices,[32,33] and B_6 is commonly targeted as a vitamin to supplement. Evidence suggests that exercise may increase the requirement for vitamin B_6.[32] Vitamin B_6 has been purported to benefit people with mental depression, premenstrual syndrome (PMS), arthritis, carpal tunnel syndrome, sleep disorders, and asthma, but supplementing with vitamin B_6 has received mixed and mostly negative reviews. Unlike some of the other B vitamins, however, regular supplementation with doses higher than two to three times the RDA may cause neurological symptoms. Thus, your best bet is to forget B_6 supplements and strive for adequate B_6 intake through the diet. Vitamin B_6 is widely distributed in foods; the best sources are protein foods, including vegetarian protein sources (see table 8.4).

Vitamin C

Vitamin C provides many important health and performance functions. Vitamin C is probably best known for its roles in collagen synthesis and the prevention of scurvy, a disease caused by vitamin C deficiency and characterized by spongy gums and weak muscles.[1] As such, collagen is necessary for the formation and maintenance of the connective tissues of the body, such as cartilage, tendon, and bone. Vitamin C is needed for the synthesis of carnitine, which transports long-chain fats into the mitochondria for energy generation, as well as several hormones produced during exercise, including epinephrine, norepinephrine, and cortisol. As discussed in chapters 7 and 11, vitamin C also aids in the absorption of nonheme iron and is a potent antioxidant that helps trap free radicals and keep vitamin E in its active form.

Vitamin C depletion can induce fatigue, muscle weakness, and unexplained bruising and bleeding around the hair follicles and gums, and can decrease the ability to train because of recurrent injuries to connective tissue.

Vegetarian athletes are likely to have an abundance of vitamin C in their daily diets. Vitamin C is found in most fruits and vegetables, including bell peppers, tomatoes, potatoes, berries, and citrus fruits (see table 7.4 on page 113), and is an additive in many fruit and juice products. Surveys of nonactive individuals have found that vegetarians typically consume close to twice the current recommendation for vitamin C—with vegans having the highest intake[8]—and display plasma concentrations of vitamin C higher than those of omnivores.[21,23] Although some suggest that athletes may need more vitamin C because of their increased use of vitamin C to fight damage to body cells from smog,

TABLE 8.4 Top 20 Vegetarian Sources of Vitamin B_6

Food	Portion	Value (mg)
Ready-to-eat cereals, fortified	1 oz (3/4 to 1-1/3 cup)	0.50-3.60
Chickpeas	1 cup cooked	1.14
Chocolate malted drink mix, fortified	3 heaping tsp	0.92
Rice, long grain, parboiled, enriched	1 cup cooked	0.84
Hash browned potatoes	1 cup prepared	0.74
Baked potato	1 medium	0.63
Prune juice	1 cup	0.56
Banana	1 cup sliced	0.56
Stewed prunes	1 cup	0.54
Plantain	1 medium	0.54
Mashed potatoes, home prepared	1 cup	0.52
Carrot juice	1 cup	0.50
Sweet potatoes, canned	1 cup cooked	0.48
Brussels sprouts	1 cup cooked	0.45
Scalloped potatoes, home prepared	1 cup	0.44
Spinach	1 cup cooked	0.44
Peppers, red	1 cup	0.43
Marinara sauce, commercially prepared	1 cup	0.43
Soybeans	1 cup cooked	0.40
Pinto beans	1 cup cooked	0.39

Note: The DRI for vitamin B_6 is 1.3 mg for adults ages 19 to 50. Refer to appendix F for guidance on converting English units to metric.

Data from report by single nutrient for vitamin B_6, USDA Food Composition Databases (https://ndb.nal.usda.gov/ndb/nutrients/index).

environmental pollutants, and free radicals produced during exercise, little evidence supports a generally higher requirement for athletes.[2,46] The recommended intake in the United States is 75 milligrams per day for adult females and 90 milligrams per day for adult males.[2]

Many athletes take vitamin C supplements in the belief that it will prevent colds and other acute illnesses and aid in the recovery from exercise. This may be particularly important after endurance or ultraendurance events. One commonly quoted study conducted by researchers in South Africa randomly assigned endurance-trained men to received either 600 milligrams of vitamin C or a placebo for the three weeks before a 26-mile (42 km) running race.[47]

The baseline vitamin C intake of both groups was over five times the RDA, or approximately 500 milligrams. During the 14 days after the race, the runners who supplemented with vitamin C had fewer upper-respiratory-tract infections than did those without the supplement (33% compared to 68%). A recent meta-analysis assessed the effect of vitamin C supplementation at doses greater than 200 milligrams for preventing and treating the common cold.[48] The study, which involved 29 trial comparisons of over 11,000 participants, determined that high-dose vitamin C supplementation does not reduce the occurrence of the common cold, but does reduce the length of cold symptoms. Among nearly 600 athletes undergoing short periods of extreme physical stress (marathon runners and skiers) in five separate studies, however, vitamin C supplementation cut the risk of colds by 35 to 64 percent.[48] These findings are not consistently reported; however, and an earlier study of ultramarathon runners did not find that vitamin C supplementation (1,500 mg/day for 7 days) influenced oxidative and immune responses during or after a competitive race.[49]

Vitamin C may also facilitate recovery from intense training by enhancing collagen repair and trapping the free radicals produced during exercise. Studies demonstrating that vitamin C supplementation prevents muscle damage or oxidative stress, however, are scarce. One study conducted at the University of North Carolina at Greensboro found that supplementing with either 500 or 1,000 milligrams of vitamin C per day for two weeks reduced blood markers for oxidative stress following a 30-minute run at moderate intensity in a group of relatively fit nonathletic men.[50] Another recent study which used both rats and humans subjected to endurance training, found that daily supplementation with vitamin C (1,000 mg in human participants) prevented some of the expected cellular adaptations to exercise and dampened the training-induced responses.[51] Although more studies are needed, the conclusions for vegetarian athletes may simply be to keep eating fruits and vegetables, particularly during periods of high-volume training, and avoid the supplements.[18] Evidence suggests that daily consumption of 200 milligrams (easily obtainable on a plant-based diet) leads to full saturation of plasma and white blood cells, indicating that additional intake would not lead to further benefit.[1]

Vitamin A and the Carotenoids

Vitamin A is important for normal vision, gene expression, growth, and immune function. Technically, vitamin A is found only in animal products, but it can be made easily from beta-carotene and several other carotenoids, which form the beautiful red, orange, and yellow pigments in fruits and vegetables. Some dark-green fruits and vegetables also contain carotenoid pigments, but their color is masked by the green color of chlorophyll. Although surveys of various athletic groups have indicated that most athletes easily consume enough vitamin A, athletes who restrict energy intake may be at risk of insufficient vitamin A levels. Vegetarians as a group typically take in adequate amounts of vitamin A and have high blood levels of beta-carotene[23] and likely the other carotenoids as well. Because of their heartier appetites, vegetarian athletes are also likely to meet, if not exceed, the RDA for vitamin A and have an abundance of healthy carotenoids circulating in their blood. You can meet the RDA for vitamin A just by consuming one carrot, and carrots are not even the richest source (see table 8.5).

No evidence suggests that marginal intake of vitamin A or the carotenoids influence exercise performance.[1] Nevertheless, the carotenoids found naturally in plant foods likely reduce the risk of many types of cancer[10,52] and several age-related diseases, including macular degeneration, a degenerative eye disease that leads to blindness.[53,54] A diet high in carotenoids and other anti-oxidants in fruit and vegetables may also lessen the severity of the oxidative damage associated with heavy training (see box 8.1). The best strategy for ensuring adequate intake is to eat dark-green and red-orange fruits and vegetables daily. Good sources of beta-carotene, lutein, and zeaxanthin include leafy greens, pumpkin, sweet potatoes, carrots, and winter squash. Eggs may also be a significant source. Good sources of lycopene are tomato products, watermelon, and pink grapefruit. Taking a daily antioxidant supplement may provide some of the carotenoids, but it is not likely to provide as much nutritional impact as getting them straight from the source. In fact, as is often the case, antioxidant supplements seem to have no effect on factors such as the development and progression of macular degeneration, as intake of foods rich in these nutrients do. Taking doses greater than the RDA of vitamin A is not recommended because vitamin A can cause headache, nausea, fatigue, liver

TABLE 8.5   Top 10 Vegetarian Sources of Vitamin A

Food	Portion	RAE* (mcg)
Sweet potato, boiled with or without skin	1 cup mashed	2,581
Carrot juice	1 cup	2,256
Pumpkin, canned	1 cup	1,906
Carrots, frozen	1 cup cooked	1,235
Butternut squash, baked	1 cup	1,144
Carrots, raw	1 cup chopped	1,069
Spinach, canned, chopped	1 cup cooked	1,049
Collards, frozen, chopped	1 cup cooked	978
Kale, frozen, chopped	1 cup cooked	956
Turnip greens, frozen, chopped	1 cup cooked	882

Note: The DRI for vitamin A is 900 micrograms RAE per day for men and 700 micrograms per day RAE for women (3,000 and 2,333 IU respectively). Refer to appendix F for guidance on converting English units to metric.

*RAE = Retinol activity equivalents are used to account for preformed retinol and beta-carotene.

Data from report by single nutrient for RAE, USDA Food Composition Databases (https://ndb.nal.usda.gov/ndb/nutrients/index).

and spleen damage, peeling skin, and joint pain. Supplementation with the carotenoids does not have the same toxic effect.

Vitamin E

Vitamin E is a nutrient we still don't know much about. Vitamin E is a generic term for eight naturally occurring compounds of two classes designated as alpha-tocopherols and gamma-tocopherols.[2] The most active is in a form called RRR-alpha-tocopherol. Vitamin E's main function is to protect the polyunsaturated fats found in the cells from oxidative damage by free radicals. This includes protecting the membranes surrounding the muscle cells and the cells' energy-generating powerhouse, the mitochondria.

As far as scientists know, vitamin E needs do not increase with physical training. It is suggested, however, that some athletes may need more vitamin E because of their higher intake of polyunsaturated fats, which increases with increased energy expenditure. Athletes may also benefit from higher intake in the initial stages of training to increase vitamin E stores in the muscle cells. The principal sources of dietary vitamin E (both the gamma and alpha forms) include vegetables, nut and seed oils, wheat germ, and whole grains (see table 8.6). Some nuts are high in one form but not the other, which highlights the importance of variety. Animal products are generally poor sources of vitamin E.

Studies assessing both the dietary intake of vitamin E and the levels of vitamin E in the blood of nonathletes strongly suggest that vegetarians are likely to have both a higher intake and a higher blood level than omnivores.[23] However, it is suggested that vitamin E status should be assessed by looking at the ratio of tochopherol to cholesterol in blood because a significant portion of the alpha-tocopherol is transported as part of the low-density lipoprotein (LDL), or bad cholesterol, (and vegetarians typically have lower LDL cholesterol concentrations).[23] Studies indicate that vegetarians have a much higher ratio of alpha-tocopherol to cholesterol in the plasma, which protects against LDL oxidation.[21,23] Research also indicates that absolute vitamin E concentrations in the blood of vegetarians often exceed the suggested value deemed optimal for cancer prevention.[23] Hence, you are likely to get ample vitamin E in its naturally occurring forms if you eat a well-rounded diet containing whole grains, nuts, seeds, and vegetable oils.

Whether you could benefit from taking a vitamin E supplement that provides levels far greater than the RDA is quite a different story. Because of its role as an antioxidant, there is some thought that taking supplemental doses of vitamin E may reduce the risk of heart disease and certain cancers and even reduce muscle damage and soreness associated with exercise. Currently, the evidence supporting vitamin E supplementation is not at all compelling. Collective analysis of vitamin E supplementation studies suggests that consuming high levels of vitamin E has a negligible effect on reducing the risk of heart disease[55,56] or protecting against exercise-induced lipid peroxidation or muscle damage.[57] It is possible, however, that an acute dose of vitamin E supplementation may be important for athletes training or competing at higher altitudes.[58-60] One

TABLE 8.6 Top 20 Vegetarian Sources of Vitamin E (Alpha Tocopherol)

Food	Portion	Value (mg)
Ready-to-eat cereals (Total and Product 19)	1 oz (3/4 to 1-1/3 cup)	13.5
Sunflower seeds	1 oz	7.4
Almonds	1 oz	7.3
Spinach, frozen	1 cup cooked	6.7
Turnip greens, frozen	1 cup cooked	4.4
Hazelnuts or filberts	1 oz	4.3
Dandelion greens	1 cup cooked	3.6
Soy milk	1 cup	3.3
Nuts, mixed	1 oz	3.1
Carrot juice	1 cup	2.7
Turnip greens	1 cup cooked	2.7
Pine nuts	1 oz	2.7
Beet greens	1 cup cooked	2.6
Pumpkin or sweet potato, canned	1 cup cooked	2.6
Broccoli, frozen	1 cup cooked	2.6
Canola oil	1 tbsp	2.4
Pepper, red	1 cup	2.4
Mango	1 fruit	2.3
Papaya	1 fruit	2.2
Peanuts	1 oz	2.2

Note: Refer to appendix F for guidance on converting English units to metric.

Data from report by single nutrient for vitamin E (alpha-tocopherol), USDA Food Composition Databases (https://ndb.nal.usda.gov/ndb/nutrients/index).

study in mountain climbers found that supplementation with 200 milligrams twice daily for 10 weeks reduced cellular damage and helped maintain physical performance.[60] In general, however, the best bet is to obtain vitamin E though a healthy vegetarian diet.

Tackling Red Flag Minerals: Are You Getting Enough?

The following section discusses the minerals that may be insufficient in the diets of active vegetarians and vegetarian athletes (other than those discussed in chapters 6, 7, and 11) and briefly touches on others that are likely of little concern in the diet of vegetarian athletes.

Zinc

Zinc is a component of many enzymes in the body, including those involved in protein synthesis, DNA synthesis, reproductive function, and immune function. Several of these enzymes are also involved in the major pathways of energy metabolism, including lactate dehydrogenase, which is important for the rapid generation of energy from carbohydrate through fast glycolysis (often incorrectly called anaerobic metabolism).

Zinc is commonly suggested as a red flag nutrient for vegetarian athletes,[3,9] because zinc intake is often low in both athletes and vegetarians in general,[4,9] and its absorption rate is lower in a vegetarian diet than in a mixed omnivorous diet.[2,9] Zinc is less well absorbed from a vegetarian diet because of the higher phytate concentrations in plant foods (phytates bind zinc and limit its absorption) and the lower intake of animal proteins, which tend to enhance zinc absorption. As such, the dietary requirement for zinc may be elevated by as much as 50 percent in vegetarians, particularly in those whose major food staples are unrefined grains and legumes.[2] In addition, lower zinc concentrations, which are thought to indicate zinc status, are consistently observed in vegetarian and nonvegetarian athletes during heavy training.[4,5]

Just because zinc is a red flag nutrient, however, does not mean that you cannot meet your zinc needs without supplements on a vegetarian diet. Rather, you should ensure you are taking in enough absorbable zinc. In fact, ensuring that you obtain enough zinc is similar to ensuring you get enough iron. A study from the U.S. Department of Agriculture found that nonathletic women were able to maintain normal zinc status on a lacto-ovo vegetarian diet, even though this diet was lower in total zinc and higher in phytate and fiber than the control meat-containing diet.[61] The key to their success at maintaining zinc as well as iron status was the incorporation of legumes and whole grains.[62] Athletes in training should find it easier than their sedentary vegetarian counterparts to regularly consume enough legumes, whole grains, and other zinc-rich foods to maintain zinc status without supplementation, unless, of course, they are restricting energy intake. Other plant sources of zinc include fortified cereals, nuts, soy products, meat analogues and some hard cheeses (see table 8.2). Check the label on your favorite meat analogues because zinc content varies considerably. As happens with iron, some food preparation techniques, such as soaking and sprouting beans, grains, and seeds; the leavening of bread; and the consumption of zinc-rich foods with other organic acids such as citric acid can reduce the binding of zinc by phytate and increase the absorbability of zinc.[9,63]

The significance of the low or slightly compromised zinc status noted in athletes during training[64-66] is not yet understood. In fact, some studies have found that zinc supplementation does not influence zinc levels during training[64,67] and appears to have no benefit on athletic performance.[67] This may suggest then that lowered serum zinc levels do not indicate zinc status in athletes, but reflect altered storage sites. For example, zinc storage may shift from the blood into skeletal muscle or other tissues during training. Nevertheless, to

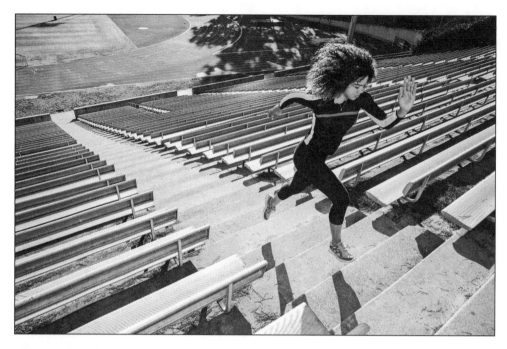

Zinc and iron status is often low in vegetarian athletes, especially during training, but a diet that includes legumes, whole grains, nuts, and soy should provide enough of both nutrients to preclude supplementing.

Peathegee Inc/Blend Images/Getty Images

ensure that your zinc level is not compromised, strive to meet or exceed the dietary recommendations for zinc of 11 milligrams per day for adult men and 8 milligrams per day for adult women. A well-controlled clinical trial conducted at the United States Department of Agriculture's Grand Forks Human Nutrition Research Center found that inadequate zinc intake of approximately 4 milligrams per day for nine weeks significantly impaired submaximal cycling and peak oxygen uptake in men.[68]

Iodine

The body's main use for iodine is as a component of thyroid hormone. Thyroid hormone is an important regulator of energy metabolism, heart rate, and protein synthesis and is the hormone best known for preventing a sluggish metabolism.

A handful of studies[37,63,69-75] have noted that iodine may be a red flag nutrient for some vegans and vegetarians. Although iodine status is not generally a concern for athletes living in industrial countries—because of the fortification of table salt—these studies found a high prevalence of iodine deficiency among vegans and vegetarians compared to nonvegetarians. This deficiency was related to the consumption of plant foods[70] grown in soil with low iodine levels,[73] limited consumption of cows' milk,[72] limited intake of fish or sea products,[70] and reduced intake of iodized salt.[70,73] In one of these studies conducted near Bratislava, Slovakia, an area where the iodine content of soil is likely low, a striking 80 percent of vegans and 25 percent of vegetarians were found to be deficient in iodine compared to 9 percent of those on a mixed diet.[70] What is additionally problematic—and perhaps a growing concern—is that perchlorate pollutants in the food and water supply can inhibit iodine uptake by the thyroid and the synthesis of thyroid hormone. Perchlorate comes from solid fuels used to power high-energy devices such as rockets, flares, fireworks, and air bags and appears to be a problem only in people with low iodine intake.[76]

Because vegetarian athletes can get by with and, in fact, may need more sodium and salt than is recommended for sedentary people (as discussed in chapter 11), vegetarian athletes can ensure adequate iodine status by regularly using iodized salt in cooking and baking. Half a teaspoon (3 g) of iodized salt provides close to the RDA for iodine of 150 micrograms per day (along with 1,163 milligrams of sodium or the amount found in about 1 liter of sweat). Unfortunately, the iodine content of plant foods varies depending on the soil content. And processed foods, most sea salts, and gourmet salts are not reliable sources of iodine because the salt used in processing and sea salt generally are not iodized. Reliance on iodized salt, on the other hand, is probably not necessary if you regularly include sea vegetables in your diet.

Copper

Copper is an essential mineral that—like many minerals—we need to better understand. Copper plays a role in iron metabolism and hemoglobin production and like iron is also important for energy metabolism. Unlike iron, however, copper is an antioxidant rather than a prooxidant and is a cofactor for superoxide dismutase, one of the body's enzymes that protect cells against oxidative damage. Copper is also thought to be important in collagen formation.

Copper may be a red flag nutrient for some vegetarian athletes. An earlier study in the Slovak Republic suggested that both copper intake and blood markers of copper status may be low in vegetarians compared to omnivores,[77] which may be because copper from plant foods is not as well absorbed.[78] Several studies in athletes have found insufficient copper intake and status among endurance runners[79] and athletes actively attempting to lose weight.[80] In contrast, other studies in athletic populations have found no indication that low copper status is of notable concern.[81,82]

A vegetarian diet has the potential to supply adequate amounts of copper (see table 8.2), and, in fact, vegetables, nuts, seeds, and whole grains are a major source of dietary copper.[2,78] Copper, like zinc and iron, can also be made more readily available by soaking, fermenting, or sprouting copper-containing foods.[78] As with iron, mineral-to-mineral interactions, especially competitive binding between zinc and copper, can decrease copper availability, whereas organic acids (except vitamin C) can increase availability. Unlike iron absorption, high intake of vitamin C impairs copper absorption, which is one reason vitamin C supplementation above 1,000 milligrams is not recommended.

Although it is not known whether marginal levels of copper influence performance or health, a recent study in copper-deficient adults found that supplementation improved functional activities of daily living. Overt copper deficiency, which is rare, however, can lead to anemia. Selected vegetarian sources are listed in table 8.2. The recommended intake for copper is 900 micrograms per day for adults.

Other Key Minerals

Although several other minerals are required for health and possibly for performance (see table 8.7), deficiencies in these minerals typically do not pose a problem for the general population or for vegetarian athletes. The content of several of these minerals, including selenium, copper, and iodine, however, varies in the food supply depending on soil conditions. While most soil conditions are generally favorable, you may want to check conditions in your area, particularly if you purchase locally grown produce or grow your own. Selenium is of interest to scientists because of its role as a cofactor in one of the body's internal defense systems, glutathione peroxidase, and is also imperative for the synthesis of thyroid hormone (along with iodine, iron, and zinc). Selenium supplementation, however, is not recommended unless you live in an area with selenium-deficient soil (e.g., areas in China, New Zealand, and Africa). General supplementation of any of the other minerals is also discouraged.

TABLE 8.7 Trace Mineral Intake for Vegetarian Athletes

Mineral	Recommended intake for athletes	Major function	Major vegetarian sources	Problems with excessive consumption
Magnesium	420 mg men; 320 mg women	Involved in protein synthesis, oxygen delivery, energy metabolism, and muscle contraction; also a component of bone	Whole-grain products, legumes	Nausea, vomiting, diarrhea
Chromium	35 mg men; 25 mg women ages 19-50	Enhanced insulin action (part of glucose tolerance factor)	Whole grains, nuts, beer, egg yolks, mushrooms	Not known
Selenium	55 mcg for adults	Defends against oxidation; regulates thyroid hormone; may protect against certain types of cancer	Whole grains, nuts, and vegetables grown in selenium-rich soil	Hair and nail loss, skin rash, fatigue, irritability
Manganese	2.3 mg men; 1.8 mg women	Cofactor for several metabolic reactions, including bone formation; deficiencies are rare	Widespread in food supply	Weakness, nervous system problems, mental confusion
Molybdenum	45 mcg for adults	Works with riboflavin in enzymes involved in carbohydrate and fat metabolism	Whole-grain products, legumes	Rare

Considering Vitamin and Mineral Supplements

To date, no evidence suggests that extra vitamins or minerals taken either as a multivitamin and mineral supplement or alone will enhance athletic performance, increase endurance or strength, or build muscle, unless, of course, you are deficient to begin with. Certainly, a vitamin or mineral deficiency can impair performance, but deficiencies generally occur in athletes who restrict energy intake or make poor food choices.[83] Deficiencies are not common in athletes with robust appetites. The exceptions to the rule include vitamin B_{12} for vegan or near vegan athletes, iodine (and selenium) for people obtaining food grown in deficient soils, and vitamin D for people exposed to insufficient amounts of sunlight.[84] More research is needed to determine whether supplemental intake of the antioxidant vitamins beyond what can be obtained in a normal diet is beneficial during training, but according to a recent review by the International Olympic Committee, the evidence is not promising.[85,86] Scientific evidence is insufficient to recommend vitamin or mineral supplements as a way to prevent cancer or heart disease.[1]

In certain cases, however, a multivitamin and mineral supplement may be necessary or prudent to improve overall micronutrient status. Typically, supplementation with a multivitamin is recommended for "dieters" or people consuming fewer than 1,200 calories a day, those with food allergies or intolerances, and those who are pregnant or planning to get pregnant. With respect to the latter, the Centers for Disease Control and Prevention recommend that every woman who could possibly get pregnant take 400 micrograms of folic acid daily in a multivitamin or in foods that have been enriched with folic acid, in addition to a healthy diet, to prevent neural tube defects.

In addition, athletes who find it necessary to supplement may be better off supplementing with a standard multivitamin and mineral supplement than with individual nutrients. The multivitamin and mineral supplement should provide no more than 100 percent of the RDA for the essential nutrients and should contain only components that are universally accepted by nutritionists. Although in most cases, the local store brand is as good as, and costs less than, a nationally recognized brand, competitive athletes should consider paying a little more for a product that is certified for sports by NSF International. This certification not only ensures the product contains the nutrients listed on the label but that it is also free from contaminants and tested for banned substances. In all cases, vegetarian athletes should strive to improve eating habits and avoid relying on the multivitamin; supplementation should not provide an excuse to choose tortilla chips over fresh kale for dinner. Also keep in mind that because many products are enriched and fortified in the United States and other countries, taking vitamin and mineral supplements may be unnecessary. In the end, however, there is probably nothing wrong with taking a general multivitamin if it makes you feel more secure during heavy stages of training, as long as you strive to eat a healthy diet.

Food—The Best Source

I am a firm believer that vegetarian athletes should stay as independent from vitamin supplements as possible. Food is the way you were meant to get your vitamins, minerals, and phytochemicals. To accomplish this, you must ensure that you meet your energy needs and select a variety of wholesome foods, including whole grains, legumes, leafy greens and other vegetables, fruit, and, if acceptable, dairy. The information presented in chapters 12 and 14 put these recommendations into practice. The information presented in this chapter (as well as chapters 6 and 7) should help you inventory your intake of the red flag vitamins and minerals and understand how easy it is to meet the vitamin requirements that increase with training, such as vitamin C and riboflavin. Although there are times when you regularly or occasionally need a supplement—such as vitamin B_{12}, vitamin D, or iron—you will be a much better advocate of the vegetarian diet if you live, train, and perform as free from multivitamin and mineral dependence as possible. In the next chapter we talk about the importance of nutrition and nutrient timing before, during, and after exercise.

9 | Prioritizing Food and Fluids Before, During, and After Events

About a year after our twins were born, my husband and I decided to run a marathon to help us get back into shape. The trouble was, we had a lot less time than we had been used to. But as it goes with athletes, we somehow managed to keep decent training schedules that included regular long, tempo, and marathon-paced runs. I even maintained higher weekly mileage than I did for my first (prechildren) marathon. And my husband managed to sneak in weekly grueling interval runs. Overall, our training went well, and we arrived in the marathon city the day before the event—both feeling as if we might set personal records.

Our mistake, however, started with our ignoring the basics of preevent nutrition planning. Rather than hitting a grocery store to stock up on high-carbohydrate foods and reading through our race packet information to learn where the water and sport drink stops would be, we went sightseeing with the kids and the in-laws, who were along to help. When deciding what to do for our premarathon breakfast, I told my husband we could grab something from the coffee shop near the hotel, which was two blocks from the starting line, and supplement it with the two bananas I had brought and a few glasses of the race's "official sport beverage" that I assumed would be available at the starting line. I made too many assumptions.

Race morning, our hungry early-rising twins ate the bananas, we discovered that the bakery did not open until after the marathon start time, and that there was no official sport beverage at the starting line. A volunteer told us, however, that there would be plenty available at mile 5 (8 km) and at every water station thereafter (information that was most likely covered in our race packet). I also could not find the sport gels I thought I had packed. Nevertheless, we ran, but we had kissed our chances of personal records goodbye. I began feeling zapped just after the 10-mile mark (16 km) and crawled in 22 minutes slower than my anticipated time. My husband, who has two previous finishes in less than three hours, finished in 3:22.

–Enette

Consuming the right food and fluid before, during, and after exercise is important for optimal training and performance. Nutrition during these times provides fuel for the brain and exercising muscles, helps prevent dehydration, and provides the building blocks for recovery. This is so important that neglecting proper nutrition during these times can negate all your hard training and all your efforts to eat healthy at other times. Thus, this chapter will help you optimize your performance by teaching you how to take in the right amount of the right foods at the right time before, during, and after your training and competitions. It also reviews exciting sport science that has evolved concerning nutrition before, during, and after an event and what these results mean to a vegetarian athlete.

Prioritizing Preevent Nutrition

The meal you eat before exercise is as important during your regular training and practice sessions as it is before your most important game or race of the season. This meal should provide just the right amount of carbohydrate, fluid, and protein to prevent hunger, low blood sugar, and stomach or intestinal discomfort, and it should also be relatively low in fat and fiber. The nutrition provided by the preevent meal may also optimize your training and performance. If consumed three to four hours before exercise, a high-carbohydrate meal can restock glycogen stores in the liver (which have been lowered by the overnight fast) and even top off glycogen stores in the muscles.[1] If consumed half an hour to two hours before exercise, the ingested carbohydrate may serve as a supplemental fuel in addition to your muscle and liver glycogen stores. The only potential disadvantages to consuming a meal too close to exercise is that it may cause stomach discomfort or, in sensitive athletes, lead to a condition called rebound hypoglycemia (low blood sugar), which can result in fatigue in the early periods of exercise. However, you may be able to prevent rebound hypoglycemia by avoiding the consumption of carbohydrate 20 to 60 minutes before you start to exercise (see box 9.1) or selecting preevent carbohydrate foods with a low glycemic index (see chapter 3 and appendix D).

Box 9.1

Special Concerns for Preevent Meals

Rebound hypoglycemia. Although rare, some athletes experience a condition called rebound hypoglycemia (low blood sugar) during exercise when carbohydrate foods are consumed 15 to 75 minutes before exercise.[6] This is caused by elevated levels of the hormone insulin (released in response to the carbohydrate-containing meal), whose job it is to facilitate the entry of glucose into the muscle and other body tissues. Symptoms specifically associated with low blood sugar include lightheadedness, fatigue, tiredness, and shakiness. Sensitive athletes who experience rebound hypoglycemia should consume their preexercise meal 90 to 120 minutes before exercise. Selecting mostly carbohydrate foods with a low glycemic index before exercise may also help. In addition, two cups (472 ml) of a carbohydrate-containing fluid replacement beverage can also be consumed 5 to 10 minutes before exercise without ill effects.

Hunger. Fluid-replacement beverages, or sport drinks, consumed 10 minutes before practice or competition may delay feelings of hunger and provide benefits similar to those of carbohydrate consumption during exercise. These beverages are readily absorbed and appear in the bloodstream 5 to 10 minutes after ingestion. When consumed in this fashion, fluid replacement beverages do not contribute to rebound hypoglycemia.

Nausea. Preevent emotional tension or anxiety may delay digestion and contribute to nausea and even vomiting before a practice or competition. Liquid meals may be better tolerated and more easily digested under these conditions.[1] Beverages with lower concentrations of sugar, such as fluid-replacement beverages rather than fruit juice, and that are low in fructose may also be better tolerated. Athletes who experience preexercise nausea should attempt to consume one or two cups (236-472 ml) of a liquid supplement or smoothie as tolerated instead of a regular meal 45 to 90 minutes before exercise. These athletes should also avoid foods and beverages containing high amounts of fructose and possibly also specific fermentable carbohydrate or FODMAPs (molecules found in food that can be difficult to digest and absorb, as reviewed in chapter 3).[7-9] Sipping slowly rather than gulping these beverages may prevent swallowing excessive air, which is thought to contribute to nausea. Finally, a few soda crackers or a piece of dry toast are also options. Consume water as tolerated.

Heartburn. Athletes, particularly those involved in stop-and-go sport activities, often experience heartburn, or gastrointestinal reflux. Heartburn is caused when the ring of muscles located at the bottom of the esophagus, called the lower esophageal sphincter, becomes too relaxed. These sphincter muscles keep the food you have swallowed into your stomach from being regurgitated back up. Coffee, chocolate, peppermint, and high-fat meals have consistently been found to relax the sphincter muscles and contribute to heartburn. Other foods such as milk; raw sulfur-containing vegetables such as onions, garlic, and

(continued)

Special Concerns for Preevent Meals *(continued)*

green peppers; and even bananas are believed to cause reflux in some people. To prevent heartburn, avoid high-fat meals and culprit food products before exercise. *(Note: these culprit foods do not induce heartburn in everyone)*

Diarrhea, intestinal cramping, and bloating. Noninfectious diarrhea and cramping and bloating during exercise can be caused by eating high-fiber, high-residual, or gas-producing foods (which include whole grains, fruits with skin, small seeds, legumes, lactose-containing dairy products, and poorly absorbed sugars such as FODMAPs[9]) too soon before exercise. It can occur when regular defecation habits are hindered by travel, stress, or competition. Athletes who experience such problems during exercise should monitor their intake of whole grains and cereals, legumes, high-fiber fruits, olestra, lactose, sugar alcohols, and FODMAPs in general in the preevent meal.[8,9] Sensitive athletes should avoid these foods in the days leading up to major competitions or events or longer if necessary (although it may be important to see a registered dietitian if symptoms are persistent). See appendix C for a list of foods containing FODMAPs. Ensuring that defecation habits are regular is also imperative. However, because games, races, or even training sessions are not always held at the same time, drinking half to three-quarters of a cup (118-177 ml) of coffee, tea, or plain hot water with the preevent meal may promote defecation before exercise initiation and thereby prevent intestinal problems.

Improved Performance Through a Preexercise Meal

Just how much improvement you can expect from eating a preevent meal depends on many factors, including how long and intensely you exercise, how well you have eaten in the preceding days, whether you plan to supplement during exercise, and your choice of carbohydrate. Earlier studies in cyclists (one of the easiest sports to research) have estimated that carbohydrate-rich meals consumed three to four hours before exercise can improve race time (during a lab-simulated race) by about 15 percent,[2] prolong time to fatigue by approximately 18 percent,[3] and improve work output toward the end of exercise by approximately 24 percent.[4] For athletes involved in stop-and-go or team sports, a study in runners found that a carbohydrate-rich meal consumed three hours before exercise improved endurance during an interval-running protocol that involved moderately paced running interspersed with 30-second sprints every five minutes until exhaustion.[5]

Carbohydrate-containing meals consumed 30 to 90 minutes before exercise also have been shown to improve endurance performance by 7 to 27 percent.[10-12] However, research has not shown the consistent performance-enhancing effects when carbohydrate is ingested during this window as compared to three to four hours before exercise. Nevertheless, consuming a carbohydrate-containing preexercise meal is most practical during this time frame if you participate in early-morning practices or training sessions, and it should not hinder performance unless you experience stomach upset or rebound hypoglycemia (see box 9.1). A limited amount of research has also found that consuming preexercise foods with a low glycemic index (GI), such as lentils, bran cereal, steel-cut oats, peaches, or apples may sustain blood sugar levels during extended exercise better than foods with a high GI, including white bread, mashed potatoes, and cornflakes and also may improve endurance performance.[10-12] A benefit of selecting carbohydrate-rich, low-GI foods in the preexercise meal, however, has not been universally found.[1] In theory, consuming low-GI foods in the hour or so before exercise should provide a slower release of glucose for use during exercise, as compared to high-GI foods, and may make personal sense for many plant-based athletes despite the lack of consistent evidence. A list of the glycemic index of common foods can be found in appendix D.

When and What to Eat Before Exercise

Exactly how much carbohydrate and fluid you should consume and at what time depends on your sport and individual tolerances. The general guidelines for both fluid and carbohydrate intake are summarized in table 9.1 and suggest that athletes drink 5 to 10 milliliters of fluid per kilogram of body weight (1 oz = ~ 30 ml) two to four hours before exercise and consume either a large carbohydrate meal (providing 3-4 g of carbohydrate per kilogram of body mass) three to four hours before exercise or a smaller meal or snack (providing 1-2 g of carbohydrate per kg of body mass) one to two hours before exercise.[1] As an example, a 198-pound (90 kg) male track athlete who eats breakfast 90 minutes before exercising should consume 90 to 180 grams of carbohydrate and 450 to 900 milliliters (15-30 oz) of fluid in the preevent period. A 132-pound (60 kg) female cyclist should consume 60 to 120 grams of carbohydrate one to two hours before an early-morning training ride, and 180 to 240 grams four hours or so before a late-afternoon training ride and aim to consume 300 to 600 milliliters (10-20 oz) of fluid three to four hours before her rides. A sample preevent meal that provides 90 grams of carbohydrate and focuses on low-GI foods is provided in table 9.2. In addition, evidence shows that consuming a well-tolerated carbohydrate source, such as a fluid-replacement beverage or piece of fruit with a few sips of water, 5 to 10 minutes before exercise will further benefit performance during prolonged or intense exercise. Carbohydrate consumed with adequate water immediately before exercise provides benefits similar to carbohydrate consumption during exercise.

Concerning fluid intake in the pre-event meal, other research has suggested the benefit of high-sodium containing fluids such as broth-based soups to help maintain fluid balance during exercise. A study conducted at the Pennington Biomedical Research Center found that consumption of about a cup and a half (355 ml) of chicken noodle soup which provided just over 1300 mg sodium before a 90-minute bout of moderate exercise improved fluid balance both during and

TABLE 9.1   Carbohydrate and Fluid Recommendations Before, During, and After Exercise

	Carbohydrate	Fluid
Before exercise: 24 hrs	Consume a carbohydrate-rich diet that provides 5-10 g carbohydrate/kg body weight. 7-12 g carbohydrate/kg recommended when preparing for endurance events > 90 min in duration.	Drink generous amounts of fluid to ensure that you are well hydrated. Monitor the color of your urine, which should be pale to light yellow.
Before exercise: 1-4 hrs	Consume a meal or snack that provides 1-2 g carbohydrate/kg body mass if taken 1-2 hrs before exercise OR 3-4 g carbohydrate/kg body mass if taken 3-4 hrs before exercise.	Drink 5-10 ml/kg of fluid 2-4 hrs before exercise. This should allow enough time for excess fluid to be excreted as urine before starting exercise.
Before exercise: 5-10 min	If desired, 15-30 g carbohydrate may be consumed with water or as part of a fluid-replacement beverage.	If possible, drink 150-350 ml (~ 3/4 to 1-1/2 cups) immediately before or at the start of exercise.
During exercise	Consume 30-60 g/hr for exercise lasting 1 to 2.5 hours or longer. Initiate this shortly after the start of exercise. New evidence suggests that intake of up to 90 g/hr may be beneficial during intense, prolonged effort if the sugar sources are varied (i.e., multiple transporter carbohydrates).	Drink enough fluid to maintain body weight. If you cannot accomplish this, drink as much as you can tolerate but enough to prevent losses >2% of body weight. In general, optimal hydration can be facilitated by drinking small amounts every 15-20 min as dictated by sport rules and practicality. Knowing individual sweat rate helps individualize goals. You should never gain weight during exercise because this indicates you are drinking too much fluid.
After exercise	Consume a mixed meal providing carbohydrate, protein, and fat soon after a strenuous competition or training session. Carbohydrate intake of 0.7 g/kg is recommended to promote muscle glycogen restoration. If speedy refueling is required (events < 8 hours apart), consume 1.0-1.2 g carbohydrate/hr for the first 4-6 hrs. If muscle building or muscle recovery is desired, aim for 0.25-0.3 g protein/kg body weight.	Drink up to 1.5 l for every kg of body mass lost during exercise (or 3 cups for every pound lost). Including sodium in or with the fluid prevents urinating much of this water intake.

Summarized from Thomas, Erdman, and Burke (1).

after exercise by increasing ad libitum water intake and reducing the amount of ingested fluids lost during the 90-minute exercise.[42] Yes, it is certainly likely veggie noodle soup would do the same thing and be useful under conditions that may include prolonged exercise in hotter environments.

Other somewhat commonsense guidelines for the preevent meal are to consume only familiar, well-tolerated, high-carbohydrate foods that are low

TABLE 9.2   Preexercise Meals Providing 90 Grams of Carbohydrate

Early morning	Estimated carbohydrate (g)
1 cup oatmeal, Irish or steel cut	30
1 tbsp raw or brown sugar	15
1 cup fresh peaches	30
1 cup soy milk	12-15
2 cups water (472 ml)	—
Total	87-90
Later in the day	
Macaroni salad made with 1 cup macaroni, 1/3 cup chickpeas, mixed vegetables, and a light vinegar and oil dressing	40-55
1 slice bread	15
1 thin slice (3/4 oz cheese or soy cheese)	—
1 large apple	30
2 cups water (472 ml)	—
Total	85-100

Note: Based on the approximate carbohydrate content of foods provided in table 3.2 on page 36. The carbohydrate content of foods per serving listed on food labels is also useful in planning a preevent meal. Refer to appendix F for guidance on converting English units to metric.

in simple sugars, and fiber[1] and don't contain excess spice and are typically higher sodium. Experimenting with a new food or new sport product is fine as long as you experiment during training or practice and preferably not before an important one. If you are accustomed to eating gas-producing foods such as legumes and they offer no ill effects—go for it! Again, these and other low-GI foods may offer a performance advantage over higher-GI foods by providing a slowly released form of glucose during exercise. On the other hand, gas-producing and high-fiber whole-grain foods may not be as readily emptied from the gut and may contribute to nausea or diarrhea. This is particularly a concern if you get a "nervous stomach" or typically have problems defecating before competitions. Guidelines for special circumstances, such as rebound hypoglycemia, heartburn, nausea, gas, and diarrhea, are presented in box 9.1.

Fasting and Early-Morning Workouts

It would be unfair to leave you with the idea that your performance will be absolutely impaired if you skip breakfast before an early-morning workout. Indeed, it is crazy to think you should get up at 4 a.m. to eat before your 5 a.m. training run (at least many of the athletes I have worked with tell me it is). Oh, better make that 3 a.m. so you can have time to adequately hydrate.

In truth, eating before an early-morning workout is not always necessary and at times, fasting may be desired as part of your training strategy. Research and intuition hold that the preevent meal is more likely to make a difference the longer and more intense your training session or race and if you paid little attention to your nutrition for a couple of days before the event.[1] Recent work has also found that glycogen plays an important role in regulating the muscle's adaptation to higher-intensity training.[13] Strategies that restrict carbohydrate availability, such as exercise during the fasting state, can, on the other hand, enhance training of certain endurance systems that rev up fat-burning machinery.[14] Thus, there may be times when eating is imperative for training and other times when a workout in the fasting state is the best strategy.

I have personally established what I call the three-to-four flat rule for my early-morning runs. If I have eaten well the day before and am adequately hydrated, I can run an easy 3 to 4 miles (5-6 km) on just a few sips of water and feel fine. If I run a little harder, a large glass of a fluid-replacement beverage or diluted fruit juice or half a banana holds me over. But if I run 4 miles or more, I need to get out of bed a little earlier so I have time for a light carbohydrate breakfast 45 to 60 minutes before I run. The same goes for hilly workouts. Figuring out a similar rule or set of personal guidelines might be beneficial. It lets you know your limitations and may even give you a few extra moments of valuable sleep.

Carbohydrate Loading and Nutrition the Week Before Competition

No chapter discussing preevent nutrition would be complete if it failed to discuss carbohydrate loading. *Carbohydrate loading,* or *glycogen supercompensation,* as it is also called, is practiced by many endurance athletes and sometimes other athletes for the purpose of elevating their muscle glycogen stores above normal before a major competition or event. Indeed, this practice has been found to improve performance in male athletes performing endurance exercise lasting more than 90 minutes. Performance improvement in female athletes has also been observed, but not as consistently as in male athletes.

Glycogen supercompensation is different from simply eating a high-carbohydrate diet before competition in that it requires the athlete to follow a diet-and-exercise protocol for several days before the chosen competition. The early classic carbohydrate-loading protocol of the 1960s and 1970s included a depletion phase that required the athlete to exercise until near exhaustion the week before competition and then eat a diet very low in carbohydrate (<10% of energy) for three days. This was followed by three days of a high-carbohydrate (approximately 80-90% of energy) diet. While this protocol was quite effective at supercompensating glycogen stores above those found on even a normally high-carbohydrate diet, the low-carbohydrate phase produced negative side effects including weakness, irritability, carbohydrate cravings, and susceptibility to infection. Modified protocols suggest a training taper and a typical carbohydrate diet (55-60% of energy) up until three days before competition and then switching to an extremely high carbohydrate diet. Although omitting the depletion phase and simply following a high-carbohydrate diet, compared to a lower-carbohydrate diet, for several days before competition has been noted to improve performance during running,[15] soccer,[16] and other sports, this type of regimen is not truly carbohydrate loading because it simply ensures that glycogen stores are adequate rather than supercompensated at the start of exercise.

If you are an endurance athlete, then, how do you carbohydrate load? Unfortunately, there is no definitive answer. Despite numerous studies, there is no set and agreed-on protocol for glycogen supercompensation. Two fairly recent studies have produced nearly conflicting conclusions about the correct diet and training regimen for glycogen loading. One study found that an exhaustive taper is necessary in order to maximize the glycogen supercompensation effects. In this study, male athletes performed either a glycogen-depleting exercise (120 min of moderate cycling followed by 1-min sprints to exhaustion) or a nondepleting exercise (20 min of moderate cycling) before consuming a high-carbohydrate diet (9 g of carbohydrate per kg of body weight) for seven days.[17] The muscle-glycogen content of the athletes in the glycogen-depleting exercise group was elevated by 138 percent of baseline on day three and by 147 percent on days five through seven; whereas, the muscle glycogen in the group that exercised for 20 minutes was elevated by 124 percent of baseline on day three and declined between days three and seven to a value similar to baseline. A second study found that a short-term bout of high-intensity exercise followed by a high carbohydrate intake enabled athletes to attain supercompensated muscle glycogen levels within 24 hours.[18] In this study, male athletes performed a short sprinting regimen on a stationary bike and then consumed a high-carbohydrate diet (10.3 g of carbohydrate per kg body weight) that emphasized high-GI foods. The sprinting regimen consisted of above maximal effort followed by 30-seconds of all-out cycling effort. Muscle glycogen stores were found to increase on the order of 80 percent in all muscle fibers during this 24-hour regimen. This was comparable to or higher than those reported during two- to six-day regimens.

As you can see from these two studies—one stating that a long taper is necessary for glycogen supercompensation and the other stating that supercompensation can be achieved in 24 hours after intense exercise and high carbohydrate intake that it is difficult to make specific suggestions. Because both protocols seem to have an influence on supercompensating glycogen stores, athletes may want to start with the most convenient protocol and switch to the alternate if expected results are not obtained. However, it is still believed that athletes should not perform true glycogen-loading regimens more than a few times a year. This is because the enzymes in the body seem to adapt and lose their ability to respond to the loading protocols by packing in extra glycogen. Thus, you should use glycogen loading only before your most important competitions. Furthermore, because glycogen loading can result in a small amount of water retention and weight gain (0.5-1 kg [1-2 lb]), it may not help athletes in events where even a small amount of excess body weight can impair performance, for example, during shorter running events. The weight gain concern does not apply during endurance events because benefits gained from the extra fuel offset any negative effects from the small weight gain, which is usually lost as exercise progresses.

Prioritizing Nutrition and Fluids During Exercise

The goals of your nutrition strategy during practice, training, or competition are to consume enough carbohydrate (if necessary) to optimize performance and to consume an appropriate amount of fluid to maintain hydration.[1] Research suggests almost unequivocally that consuming 30 to 75 grams of carbohydrate per hour during exercise will benefit performance during both prolonged and intermittent, high-intensity activities. Carbohydrate supplementation extends endurance and improves race time during simulated endurance races or trials and also improves sprinting ability and power output at the end of the race. Although less is known about team sports, accumulating research suggests that carbohydrate ingestion before and during a game is likely to enhance intermittent exercise capacity during a variety of sports such as soccer, rugby, field hockey, basketball, American football, and racquet sports.[19] As with endurance events, carbohydrate ingestion appears to have the greatest effect toward the end of the game. In one of these studies, university soccer athletes showed an improvement in performance during dribbling, agility, and shooting when a carbohydrate-containing sport beverage was ingested instead of a placebo.[20] In another, carbohydrate supplementation improved tennis stroke quality during the final stages of prolonged play.[21] Carbohydrate ingestion most likely exerts these performance benefits by maintaining blood glucose concentration, thereby ensuring a continuous source of carbohydrate for the working muscle, or by activation of the reward centers in the brain.[1] These benefits are most noted during the latter stages of a race or after half-time, when liver and muscle glycogen are compromised. During prolonged events, these benefits are in addition to those gained by consumption of a preexercise carbohydrate meal.[3,22]

Research in the last decade suggests that use of carbohydrate mouth rinses, also known as carbohydrate mouth sensing, may have performance benefits before or during exercise. This practice—which involves holding or swishing carbohydrate-containing solutions in the mouth for several seconds—has been observed to result in performance improvements of typically 2 to 3 percent during exercise lasting approximately one hour, with the most profound effects noted after an overnight fast.[23] The contact of carbohydrate with the sensors of the mouth and oral cavity are thought to induce performance benefits through stimulation of parts of the brain and central nervous system that enhance perceptions of well-being and increase self-selected work output.[24] Nonetheless, studies suggest that carbohydrate ingestion may offer more performance benefit than carbohydrate rinsing.[25]

Fluid intake, with or without carbohydrate, also ensures optimal performance. Historically, research in this area has shown—without a doubt—that fluid ingestion during exercise improves endurance performance and that the performance-enhancing effects of carbohydrate and fluid are independent but additive. For example, one study conducted in the United Kingdom in the late 1990s found that male and female runners ran 33 percent longer before exhaustion when they consumed 180 milliliters (0.75 cup) of water every 15 minutes compared to when they consumed no fluids.[26] Their actual time to exhaustion during the treadmill test was 133 minutes when they consumed water and 78 minutes when they did not. Another study conducted at the University of Texas in Austin found that male athletes experienced a 6 percent improvement in sprinting performance when they consumed 1,330 milliliters (5.6 cups) of water, enough to replace about 80 percent of their fluid lost through sweat, compared to when they ingested just 200 milliliters (0.85 cup) of water.[27] In this study, the athletes cycled for 50 minutes at a relatively intense effort before completing a sprint to the finish that took approximately 10 minutes. Not surprisingly, the athletes experienced a 12 percent improvement in performance when they consumed 1,330 milliliters of carbohydrate-containing sport drink rather than water.

Although dehydration from inadequate fluid consumption can impair performance[27], both dehydration and overhydration can result in severe, life-threatening health consequences that are important to mention. Briefly, varying degrees of dehydration are common during exercise because athletes typically drink enough to satisfy their thirst but do not drink enough to offset the fluid losses that occur during sweating. This is primarily because thirst is not an adequate guide to fluid replacement, but it is also caused by factors such as water availability; game rules and regulations; intense focus on playing, training, or racing; and even drinking skill during exercise. The American College of Sports Medicine, Academy of Nutrition and Dietetics, and Dietitians of Canada recommend that athletes avoid fluid deficits of greater than 2 percent of body weight during exercise.[1] Fluid deficits at this level can compromise cognitive function and aerobic exercise performances, particularly in hot weather. Greater fluid loss (3-5% of body weight) impairs performance of anaerobic high-intensity activities and sport-specific technical skills. Dehydration can also be life threatening and lead to increased core temperature, headache, dizziness, gastrointestinal discomfort and poor concentration. All of these symptoms are a result of decreased blood flow, which reduces the escape of heat through the skin and the absorption of ingested fluid and foods. If not corrected, dehydration can lead to heat injury, exhaustion, heatstroke, and death. See box 9.2 for information on calculating your degree of fluid deficit during exercise.

In contrast, hyponatremia, or "water intoxication," has emerged in the sports medicine world as a cause of life-threatening illness and race-related death in endurance competitions such as the marathon and ultramarathon.[1,28] Hyponatremia occurs when excess water, relative to sodium, accumulates in the blood and is defined by an abnormally low concentration of plasma sodium (<135 mmol/l).[1] In athletes, hyponatremia typically results from drinking an excessive amount of low-sodium fluids during prolonged endurance exercise. A report found that hyponatremia occurred in approximately 13 percent of runners completing the 2002 Boston Marathon, and of those, slightly less than 1 percent experienced severe hyponatremia (sodium concentration <120 mmol/l).[29] In this event, the strongest indication of hyponatremia was weight gain during the race of 1 kilogram to almost 5 kilograms (2.2-11 lbs) caused by fluid intake that far exceeded the sweat rate. This and other studies also indicate that those at greatest risk for hyponatremia are female and slower athletes who finish toward the back of the pack, but hyponatremia does occur in male athletes and appears to increase with the use of nonsteroidal anti-inflammatory medication during competition. To avoid becoming hyponatremic, athletes should know their approximate sweat rate (see box 9.2) during all training events in which they participate and drink only enough to replace their losses. Drinking sodium-containing fluids such as

---

Box 9.2

Estimating Individual Sweat Rate and Fluid Requirements During Exercise

- Determine nude body mass in kilograms (after using the restroom). Scale must be accurate to at least 0.1 kilogram or 0.2 pound.
- Perform regular exercise or training for one hour without consuming fluids. You can also exercise for 30 minutes and multiply the answer by two.
- Towel off and determine nude body mass.
- Subtract postexercise body mass from preexercise body mass.
- Body mass loss is directly proportional to fluid loss; 1 kilogram lost equals 1 liter of fluid, and 1 pound lost equals 2 cups of fluid.
- Calculate fluid deficit by dividing fluid loss by starting weight and multiplying by 100.

Example:
An athlete weighs 90 kilograms before exercise and 88.6 kilograms after exercising for one hour.

- 90.0 – 88.6 = 1.4 kilogram
- 1.4 kilogram = 1.4 liters or 1,400 milliliters
- Sweat rate = 1,400 milliliters/hour
- Fluid deficit = 1.4 kilogram/90 kilogram = 1.6 percent

If this athlete replaces the fluid lost through sweat by consuming a 6 percent carbohydrate fluid replacement beverage, he or she will consume 84 grams of carbohydrate per hour, which is greater than the current recommended intake of 30 to 60 grams per hour.

higher-sodium fluid-replacement beverages or ingesting sodium-containing foods during events lasting more than two hours may also be prudent. General symptoms of hyponatremia are nonspecific and include fatigue, nausea, and confusion. Severe cases can result in grand mal seizures, respiratory arrest, acute respiratory distress syndrome, coma, and death.

In addition to carbohydrate and fluid, it is a good idea to ingest sodium during exercise of prolonged duration (>2 hrs) and if you sweat heavily (>1.2 liters/hr) or are a "salty sweater."[1,30] The average concentration of sodium in sweat is about 1 gram per liter, but this varies among athletes. You are a salty sweater if you notice salt residue on dark-colored workout gear or clothing.

When and What to Eat During Training and Competition

The general guidelines for both fluid and carbohydrate intake during exercise are presented in table 9.1. As a general rule, carbohydrate ingestion should be a priority during competition and on days you train at a relatively intense effort for longer than 60 to 90 minutes. Remember, however, that carbohydrate may also be helpful for shorter interval sessions or when you are unable to eat an adequate preevent meal. This includes mouth sensing protocols. The recommendation is to aim for 30 to 60 grams of carbohydrate per hour with a focus on high-GI choices. For best results, consume carbohydrate at regular intervals (if allowed by the rules of your sport) and begin shortly after the onset of exercise.

Additional evidence, however, suggests that higher carbohydrate intake—up to 90 grams per hour—may be beneficial during endurance and ultraendurance events such as marathon and ultramarathon runs, century and double century (160 and 320 km) bicycle races, and adventure racing.[1] Athletes striving for higher hourly intake of carbohydrate should ingest carbohydrate that has several rather than a single sugar source, i.e., glucose and fructose. This is referred to as multiple-transporter carbohydrate. Although scientists used to think that muscle was able to take up and use a maximum of 1 gram of dietary carbohydrate per minute—regardless of body size—relatively new research suggests this is not the case.[31,32] The limiting factor apparently lies in the intestines, where different carrier molecules are responsible for escorting different sugars, such as glucose and fructose, across the intestinal wall. If only one type of simple sugar is consumed, we can only absorb about 60 grams of sugar per hour, but if more than one type is consumed, we can recruit different carriers and absorb and oxidize up to 100 grams per hour. Fortunately, the carbohydrate found naturally in fruits and fruit juices is made up of a variety of sugar sources (see figures 9.1 and 9.2), as is the carbohydrate provided by many fluid-replacement products such as Gatorade.

Like carbohydrate intake, fluid intake during exercise should be closely monitored on days you train or compete for more than an hour. This of course is provided you are well hydrated at the start of exercise; otherwise, fluid intake is even more important. To prevent dehydration, the American College of Sports Medicine, Academy of Nutrition and Dietetics, and Dietitians of Canada recommend that athletes drink enough fluid during exercise to replace what is lost through sweat.[1] A typical sweat rate is 300 to 2,400 milliliters per hour and varies according to exercise intensity and duration, fitness level, and environmental conditions.[1] It is best, however, to have an idea of your own fluid requirements, which can change throughout your training season and in response to different types of exercise and different environments. Preliminary evidence indicates that tattooed skin produces less sweat that has a much

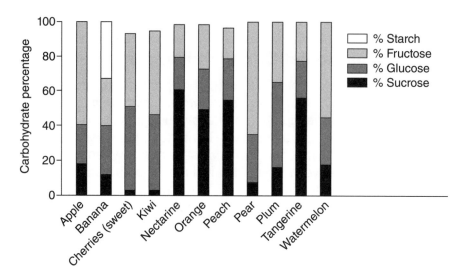

FIGURE 9.1   Types of sugar in selected fresh fruit.
Data from the United States Department of Agriculture (USDA).

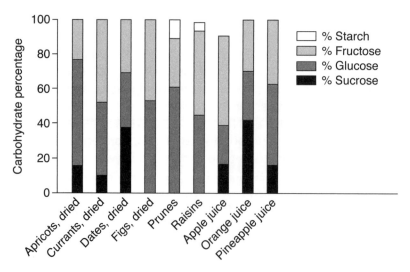

FIGURE 9.2   Types of sugar in selected dried fruit and juice.
Data from the United States Department of Agriculture (USDA).

higher composition of sodium than the sweat produced by nontattooed skin,[33]; this may have important implications for athletes with significant areas of tattooing. See box 9.2 for information on calculating sweat rate and determining personal fluid requirements. Regularly measuring your weight before and after exercise also helps you determine whether you are hydrating enough or too much. You should never gain weight during exercise. If you do, it means you are overhydrating and may be placing yourself at risk for hyponatremia.

Understanding your own fluid needs during exercise will help you establish a personal fluid intake plan according to the rules and rigors of your sport, and help ensure that you do not go overboard and consume too much fluid. For example, I typically aim to consume about one liter of fluid every hour, which is close to my sweat rate during moderately intense running. When I run a long race, I estimate how much fluid (in small cups) I need to drink at each water station based on the distance between stations and my estimated pace. If the stations are too far apart, such as in a marathon with water stations every 5 miles (8 km), I have to decide whether to ask a relative to supply water or to carry my own. During a training run, ride, or cross-country ski event, I might have the option of stashing water along a predetermined route or planning a route where I can get water at gas stations or from a friend's outdoor hose. If I played a team sport, I would estimate how much fluid I would need to consume during regularly scheduled breaks, bench time, and time-outs and balance that with my anticipated playing and bench time. This may sound like a bit of work, but improperly hydrating can impair performance and have life or death consequences.

Tips for Meeting Fluid and Carbohydrate Guidelines

Both water and sport drinks such as Gatorade and Powerade can replace fluid losses. In general, sport drinks that are labeled as a fluid-replacement beverage should contain 6 to 8 percent carbohydrate by volume along with a small amount of sodium and potassium (see box 9.3). They should not be carbonated because carbonated beverages are more difficult to drink and not as well tolerated while exercising. The advantage of sport drinks is that they are convenient and provide an easily absorbed source of carbohydrate and fluid that tastes good to most people during exercise. Alternatively, some sport gels pack 20 to 25 grams of carbohydrate in a small packet that can be carried easily. These are a good option if water is available along the route or on the sideline. Products such as Clif Shot Bloks and Sport Beans (made by Jelly Belly) which taste somewhat like gummy bears, and regular jelly beans also provide carbohydrate, sodium, and potassium and must be consumed with water. Sport drinks and gels that contain protein along with carbohydrate are also available. The sport drink should be easily absorbed, and the gel should be consumed with water.

As a vegetarian, however, you may prefer more natural or noncommercial sources of carbohydrate. In this case, diluted fruit juices (4 oz [118 ml] of

Box 9.3

What's Magic About 6 to 8 Percent?

The goal for athletes when drinking a carbohydrate-containing beverage is to get the fluid, sugars, and electrolytes into the body as quickly as possible without causing gastrointestinal upset. Therefore, it's important to know that the amount of sugar in a beverage strongly influences both how quickly the beverage empties from the stomach and also how rapidly it is absorbed by the intestines. Research has shown that solutions containing 2 to 8 percent carbohydrate by volume from various sources (glucose, fructose, maltodextrins) are generally emptied quickly from the stomach and absorbed as well as or better than water. Their better absorption is attributed to the sugar and electrolyte content, which pulls water molecules beside them upon absorption in the intestines. Thus, beverages with 6 to 8 percent carbohydrate by volume do not compromise fluid replenishment during exercise and also provide an additional energy source. Some athletes may tolerate beverages with higher carbohydrate content by volume (up to 10%), but these beverages typically delay gastric absorption and may cause intestinal discomfort and diarrhea.

Although most fluid-replacement beverages such as Gatorade or Powerade fit the bill, most juices, fruit drinks, "energy drinks," and sodas are too concentrated to be rapidly absorbed without incident during exercise. You can determine the percent of carbohydrate by volume of carbohydrate-containing beverages as follows:

$$\frac{\text{Grams of carbohydrate per serving of beverage} \times 100}{\text{Total volume of serving}}$$

For example, 1 cup (236 ml) of apple juice contains 29 grams of carbohydrate.* The percent of carbohydrate by volume in apple juice would be calculated as follows:

$$\frac{29 \text{ grams} \times 100}{236} = 12.3 \text{ percent}$$

Thus, apple juice needs to be diluted slightly to be well absorbed and used during exercise.

This calculation does not work properly in protein-containing beverages such as milk. Note, the percentage of carbohydrate by volume is different from the percent of energy from carbohydrate.

*Values obtained from USDA Food Composition Databases (https://ndb.nal.usda.gov/ndb/).

juice in 4 oz of water produces a solution of approximately 6%), low-sodium vegetable juices such as carrot juice (7% solution), and solid foods such as fruit or bread ingested with water are appropriate. Honey, particularly in small packets, may also be of interest to some vegetarians for use instead of a sport gel. Several studies have shown that both honey and easily digested solid food are as effective as liquids in increasing blood glucose and enhancing performance, provided that they are ingested with water.[6,34,35] The guideline is to drink approximately 8 ounces (236 ml) of water with every 15 grams of carbohydrate ingested to create a 6 percent solution. Be creative and develop your own recipe for a homemade, fruit-based, fluid-replacement beverage. See box 9.4 for ideas.

A Special Note for Prolonged Endurance and Ultraendurance Events

If you participate in exercise events lasting more than five hours, you need to pay particular attention to your intake of carbohydrate and fluid, as well as sodium, potassium, other electrolytes, and maybe even protein. And remember that variety is key! An interesting phenomenon experienced by endurance and ultraendurance athletes is that they can get sick of carbohydrates—particularly sweet carbohydrates—right about the time they need them the most. Taking a variety of carbohydrate sources along in your jersey pocket, waist pack, or in your own cooler (if applicable) may help prevent the "sick of carbohydrate" trap. Things to bring along include different flavors of fluid-replacement beverages, whole and sliced fruit, trail mix, sport bars, baked potatoes with salt, pretzels, tortillas, peanut butter sandwiches, vegetarian burgers in buns, and, yes, soda and sour-tasting juices such as lemonade and grapefruit juice.

Box 9.4

Making Your Own Fluid Replacement Beverage

Use the following recipes to make a fluid replacement beverage based on fruit juice that provides 6 to 7 percent carbohydrate by volume, 600 to 700 milligrams of potassium, and 291 milligrams of sodium (if 1/8 tsp salt is used) or 581 milligrams sodium (if 1/4 tsp salt is used). The beverage will be a natural mixture of glucose, fructose, and sucrose. To add an interesting twist, experiment with adding fresh herbs such as mint, basil, or rosemary; a splash of flavored fruit vinegar; or a twist of citrus. These can also be added to plain or sparkling water to enhance drinkability.

Recipe 1

3/4 cup (177 ml) of apple juice (preferably filtered)

1-1/2 cups (354 ml) of tart cherry, pomegranate, or grape juice

Approximately 2 cups (472 ml) cold water to make 1 liter

1/8 to 1/4 tsp (0.75-1.5 g) table salt (not light, preferably iodized)

Recipe 2

2-1/4 cups (531 ml) of grape juice (preferably filtered)

Approximately 2 cups (472 ml) cold water to make 1 liter

1/8 to 1/4 tsp (0.75-1.5 g) table salt (not light, preferably iodized)

Note: 1 tsp (6 g) of table salt contains about 2,325 milligrams of sodium.

When it comes to drinking soda during an ultraendurance event, forget the carbonation rule. A bubbly, cold soda or the taste of sour juice may be just what you need in the middle or end of the event. Just remember to follow it with an equal amount of water. Finally, tuck in a few packets of salt. Salt may be what you are craving and can enhance the palatability of your carbohydrate-rich foods. This is the time you might want to put salt on your watermelon and even your peaches to help replenish sodium and possibly potassium lost during prolonged sweating.[36] Taking in sodium may also reduce the risk of hyponatremia, although this has not been completely backed up by research. A rough guideline is to strive for 230 to 460 milligrams of sodium and 119 to 195 milligrams of potassium per liter of fluids replaced.[36] If you prefer drinking plain water, the added sodium can come from salting your food or eating salty food. The important thing is to listen to your body. If you are craving salt during or after an event, consume it. There is a chance you might need it.

A Special Note for Team Sports

Team sports such as soccer, basketball, volleyball, and football also present a unique set of challenges. If you are on a team, whether or not you spend time on the bench, you need to be prepared to play at all times. Team athletes also must consume carbohydrate and fluids at times that are allowed by the rules of the game (e.g., half-time or time-outs). In many cases, team athletes are limited to specific sport drinks or products and may not be allowed to eat solid foods such as bananas or watermelon slices on the sideline. And you must remember that both your fluid and carbohydrate needs vary depending on how

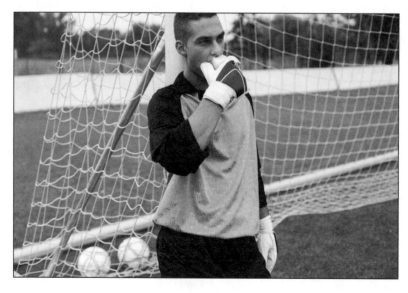

Aim for variety in your during-exercise snacks, and determine a method and schedule for intake that works for you.

Mosquidoo/fotolia.com

much of the actual game or match you play and then supplement accordingly. Going crazy on sport drinks and carbohydrate supplements when you have little playing time can result in unwanted weight gain (see chapter 13).

Keep a water bottle or two labeled with your name nearby at all times, and consider filling one with a sport drink for more-intense or prolonged practices. In a study of elite Australian basketball, netball, and soccer players, researchers found that the factors influencing fluid replacement during exercise included provision of individual water bottles, proximity to water during training sessions, encouragement to drink, and athlete awareness of his or her own sweat rate.[37] The duration and number of breaks or substitutions and the rules of the game are also influential, but you have no control over these influences. If you don't particularly like water—some athletes tell me they don't—try some of the suggestions proposed in box 9.4.

Prioritizing the Postexercise Meal

The meal after exercise or competition is critical for providing the nutrients necessary for recovery and training adaptation. This meal, however, is often the one most neglected by athletes, often because many do not have an appetite after grueling or long training sessions, particularly in the heat. Athletes also may not have immediate access to food or may have the desire to relax or celebrate—after all, they have just worked hard! Getting inadequate nutrition after exercise, however, can negate hard training efforts and also make training difficult in the following days.

It is recommended that athletes consume a mixed meal providing carbohydrate, protein, and fat soon after training, practice, or competition and also strive to replace fluid lost during the session.[1] To replace lost body fluids, aim to consume about 125 to 150 percent of your body mass lost during exercise or about 1.25 to 1.5 liters of fluid for every kilogram of body mass lost (3 cups for every pound lost), and include sodium and potassium in your recovery meals. This is important not only because both of these nutrients are lost through sweat and need to be replenished, but also because their replenishment helps restore fluid balance. Recent research from the United Kingdom found that fluid replacement beverages, orange juice, and milk may be more effective at promoting fluid retention than water, coffee, tea, or lager.[38] Although a mostly whole-foods, plant-based diet is likely to contain ample potassium, which is abundant in fruits and vegetables, it may lack sodium-containing foods. As previously noted, sodium intake can be a concern during periods of heavy training in athletes who avoid salt and processed foods. In fact, a more liberal intake of sodium is often appropriate for athletes, particularly those who are salty sweaters or find they have incredible cravings for salt. Remember also that ingestion of higher-sodium noodle soup in the pre-event meal promotes ad libitum fluid or water intake during exercise and can ensure good fluid balance during and after exercise.[42]

Vegan View: Finding Your Balance for Food Before and During Races

I have a strong stomach and can tolerate a high intake of fiber—sometimes reaching 100 grams on high-calorie-need days—but I'm still careful about what I eat before and during an event. I limit my fiber intake for three days before a big race by reducing my leafy greens, switching out my whole grains, and eating more refined foods. We can point to research and give guidelines, although nothing beats personalizing the approach that works best for you as you experiment during training and less-important events. For example, I found that I need less water than my body weight would predict and that an extra hour or so of sleep before a big event is more important than having a full breakfast. For Ironman-distance triathlons, instead of waking up at 3 a.m., my preference is to sleep as late as possible and consume a caffeinated beverage (usually coffee) immediately, to ensure I have a bowel movement. Then 10 minutes before the gun, I drink a carbohydrate-rich drink or eat a small banana. If I'm well trained and have eaten adequately the day before, this can get me through the swim and onto the bike, where I'll consume more carbohydrate drink.

Your specific postexercise nutrition priorities, however, depend on the intensity of your training that particular day and your (or your coach's) training plans for the following days. For example, if you performed a two-hour run and have a fast-paced tempo run on your schedule the next day, your goal to replace muscle glycogen is a higher priority than if you have a rest day scheduled. Similarly, if you play most of a grueling volleyball match in the early morning, you need to aggressively replace as much carbohydrate as soon as you can if you hope to play your best in a match that evening or the following morning. In contrast, if you complete a tough 45-minute weightlifting or plyometric workout, which is not likely to have depleted your glycogen stores, your focus will be on consuming protein along with carbohydrate to facilitate muscle growth and repair. In this case, neglecting postevent nutrition prevents you from optimizing the benefits of your resistance training.

Because muscle glycogen stores can be completely depleted at the end of a hard practice or workout, carbohydrate consumption should always be a priority on harder training days. Consumption of carbohydrate (0.7 g/kg) 20 to 30 minutes after exercise is essential for replenishing muscle glycogen stores and enhancing muscle recovery and muscle protein synthesis. Research has consistently shown that muscle glycogen can be replenished within 24 hours, providing the postevent intake and overall diet is high in carbohydrate. Again, this is particularly important if training is to be resumed the following day because low muscle glycogen stores can impair subsequent training and performance.

The current recommendation for replacing muscle glycogen and ensuring rapid recovery for events that will occur in less than eight hours is to consume 1.0 to 1.2 grams of carbohydrate per kilogram of body mass every hour for four to six hours after exercise.[1] Evidence also indicates that a postexercise meal containing both protein and carbohydrate may be more effective for rapidly replacing muscle glycogen than ingesting carbohydrate only.[39] Researchers have shown benefits using a ratio of both 3 grams of carbohydrate to 1 gram of protein and 4 grams of carbohydrate to 1 gram of protein, but there is probably no magic to these ratios. Again, because hard exercise and competition often suppress your appetite—particularly during running events—it may be easier to consume a carbohydrate and protein-containing beverage or snack immediately after exercise and then eat a mixed meal providing carbohydrate, protein, and fat a few hours later (see table 9.3 for snack suggestions that provide both carbohydrate and protein). This regimen allows you to begin replenishing muscle glycogen stores while you shower, travel home, or find a restaurant for a postcompetition meal.

Efforts to consume a mixed meal that provides a high-quality source of plant or dairy protein, such as soy, other legumes, eggs, milk, or Greek yogurt, are probably sufficient for most athletes who eat a plant-based diet. Consuming high-quality protein along with carbohydrate after endurance or resistance training supplies the needed amino acids to stimulate muscle protein synthesis. Recent thinking is that the amino acid leucine may serve as a signal to stimulate muscle protein synthesis but it needs to be ingested with a dose of about 8 to 10 grams of essential amino acids.[43,44] While some studies suggest the superiority of dairy protein on rapid accrual of muscle protein because of its content of well-absorbable leucine and branched-chain amino acids, a recent meta-analysis by Messina and colleagues found no differences in the effect of supplementing with soy compared to dairy or other animal proteins on strength and lean body mass gains over six or more weeks of training.[40] This suggests

TABLE 9.3 Vegetarian Postexercise Snacks That Provide Carbohydrate and Protein

Food	Carbohydrate-to-protein ratio (g)
Small apple and 1 cup milk	27:8 (3.4 to 1)
Small apple and 1 slice soy cheese	15:6 (2.5 to 1)
Large banana and 2 tbsp peanut butter	30:7 (4.3 to 1)
2 tbsp raisins and 2 tbsp almonds	15:7 (2.1 to 1)
4 graham cracker squares and 1 cup soy milk	34:10 (3.4 to 1)
1/2 large bagel with 1/4 cup cottage cheese	30:12 (2.5 to 1)
1/2 cup fruit with 1 cup plain yogurt	28:8 (3.5 to 1)
6-in. tortilla filled with 1/2 cup beans	30:7 (4.3 to 1)
1 cup low-fat chocolate milk	26:8 (3.2 to 1)

Note: Refer to appendix F for guidance on converting English units to metric.

that even if there is a short-term advantage of dairy immediately postexercise, it is not evident with long-term training. Research on other proteins, including combinations of vegetable proteins, is warranted.[1] To date, no studies have evaluated combinations of food-based vegetable proteins, many of which are rich in leucine.

Research also suggests that consuming protein along with carbohydrate after endurance or resistance training stimulates the building and repair of muscle and other tissue. As discussed in chapter 5, athletes who are trying to gain muscle should pay particular attention to their postexercise protein intake and aim to consume about 15 to 25 grams of protein or 0.25 to 0.3 grams of protein per kilogram body mass for a more exact target. As an example, the 198-pound (90 kg) male track athlete and the 132-pound (60-kg) female cyclist mentioned earlier would aim to consume 23 to 27 and 15 to 18 grams of protein, respectively, to promote adequate recovery under these guidelines. As a final point, including fat in a recovery meal may also be important for replacing muscle fat droplets following high-volume endurance training,[41] as discussed in chapter 4.

So there you have it! Consuming the right food and fluid before, during, and after exercise has great potential to improve—or at least optimize—your training and performance. In fact, prioritizing nutrition at these times has the potential to greatly affect your performance to a greater degree than any dietary supplement or ergogenic aid, the topic of the next chapter.

10 | Choosing Whether to Supplement

In the late 1990s, my colleagues and I conducted a study assessing the effect of creatine supplementation on off-season performance in female collegiate soccer players. My distinct memories from this study focus on one athlete, an extremely health-conscious semi-vegetarian player I had always enjoyed talking with. She worked hard, loved tofu, and had been raised by parents who I believed were a lot like me. When we approached her team about the creatine supplement study, she was reluctant and told me in private that she was not comfortable taking anything "artificial" into her body. I totally respected that! For some reason (probably related to peer pressure), however, she gave her consent to participate, which involved blindly receiving either creatine or a placebo mixed in a sport drink during the 13 weeks of spring training. Knowing what I knew, I was relieved to find out she had been randomized to the placebo rather than the creatine group. (Because I was the one in charge of dissolving the creatine or placebo in the sport drink and delivering it to the team after practice, I was privy to the randomization scheme.) What was interesting was that despite being given the placebo treatment (unbeknownst to her) she began experiencing side effects, which included nausea, headaches, shakiness, and weight gain. She dropped out of the study two weeks before it ended because she was convinced she was in the creatine group. She told me she couldn't take it any longer but did agree to let us have access to her final performance data. Later, when we broke the code, she was extremely embarrassed and apologetic. Given the background events, however, it was understandable. She was so against taking the supplement—or any nonherbal supplement for that matter—that her mind allowed her to experience many of its side effects. As a consolation, we presented her with a bag of dried cranberries—a natural, albeit not very concentrated, plant-based plant source of creatine.

– Enette

Although it is probably stereotyping, I believe that plant-based athletes as a whole think a little differently about sport supplements. Like most athletes we enjoy outrunning, outjumping, and outcompeting the competition, but as I see it, many of us tend to draw a different line between acceptable and unacceptable ways to gain a competitive edge. Plant-based athletes don't necessarily want to win at all costs. They want to win by training hard, eating properly, and taking care of their health, rather than by taking a magic performance-enhancing formula (with unknown health risks). This does not mean, of course, that we are not interested in herbal supplements to increase immune function, allay the discomforts of menopause, or promote longevity. Plant-based athletes may indeed be just as likely to use herbal or other botanical supplements as omnivorous athletes, but not as likely to swallow the latest, most popular artificially synthesized performance-enhancing formula.

Because athletes are constantly bombarded with media advertisements or advice from coaches or teammates promoting new supplements, this chapter aims to help you understand the various types of supplements, their current level of regulation, and when or if you may want to consider their use. Having had the honor of serving on the Medical and Scientific Commission of the International Olympic Committee's expert panel on the role of dietary supplements in the high-performance athlete, it is evident now more than ever that dietary supplements can be a legitimate part of the high-performance athlete's preparation.[1] When used appropriately, supplements can play a role in maintaining good health, supporting effective training, and optimizing performance in competition.[2] This likely goes for fitness buffs and recreational athletes who strive to push their limits.

Defining dietary supplements, however, is associated with challenges. The International Olympic Committee (IOC) Medical and Scientific Commission agreed that supplements would be defined as a food, food component, nutrient, or nonfood compound that is purposefully ingested in addition to the habitually consumed diet with the intention of achieving a specific health or performance advantage.[1] By this definition, dietary supplements include those used to prevent or treat nutrient deficiencies, provide a practical form of macronutrients, and directly or indirectly improve performance. Because dietary supplements (including iron and vitamin D supplements, sport bars, sport drinks, and gels) used to prevent or treat nutrient deficiencies and provide a practical form of macronutrients, respectively, have been covered throughout this book, this chapter focuses on supplements meant to improve performance (or ergogenic aids) and on specific herbal and botanical products that have purported health benefits. Supplements that affect inflammation will be discussed in the next chapter.

Because so many products are available in the marketplace, this chapter also provides information on how to evaluate each dietary supplement that appears on the shelf so you can make an informed choice to supplement or not supplement—either now or in the future. The chapter ends with a summary of several ergogenic aids that the IOC Medical Commission felt displayed robust evidence of enhancing sport performance when used according to established protocols[1,3] and a few others thought to be of interest to plant-based athletes.[4] A detailed discussion of all herbal and botanical products, however, are beyond the scope of this text. If you would like to know more, refer to the resources listed in table 10.1 or access the IOC special issue on dietary supplements at https://journals.humankinetics.com/toc/ijsnem/28/2. The papers by Maughan and colleagues,[1] Peeling and colleagues,[3] and Rawson and colleagues[5] may be of particular interest.

Supplement Primer

Athletes spend billions of dollars on dietary supplements each year for the purpose of improving performance or health. Athletes' attraction to supplements can probably be explained by their competitive instincts. History tells us that ancient warriors used various concoctions believed to possess magical properties to help them outfight their enemies just like ancient and current-day Olympians have used them to gain an edge over their opponents.

TABLE 10.1 Sources for Information About Dietary Supplements

Organization	Information
American Botanical Council (ABC) www.herbalgram.org	This online resource for herbal news and information is supported by the ABC, a leading independent, nonprofit, international member-based organization that provides education using science-based and traditional information to promote the responsible use of herbal medicine. It provides information on Commission E. Nonmembers have access to some of ABC's general resources and samples from the databases. Full access is available to members who pay a yearly fee.
American Herbal Pharmacopoeia (AHP) www.herbal-ahp.org/index.html	AHP's mission is to promote the responsible use of herbal medicines and ensure that they are used with the highest degree of safety and efficacy achievable. AHP has developed standards for identity, purity, and analysis for botanicals, as well as a set of qualitative monographs on specific herbal supplements, including many of the Ayurvedic, Chinese, and Western herbs most frequently used in the United States. Monographs are available on the website for a fee. Also check availability through your local library.
Dietary Supplement Quality Initiative (DSQI) www.supplementquality.com	This site provides information and a method for obtaining and sharing information on supplement quality and supplement manufacturers.

(continued)

TABLE 10.1   *(continued)*

Organization	Information
HerbMed www.herbmed.org	This interactive, electronic herbal database provides hyperlinked access to the scientific data underlying the use of herbs for health. It is an evidence-based information resource provided by the nonprofit Alternative Medicine Foundation. Information on 20 popular herbs is available for free, and information on more than 100 other herbs is available to subscribers. In addition to reports on clinical research, case studies, and descriptions of traditional use, listings also link to further information on contraindications, toxicity, adverse effects, and drug interactions, as well as an herb's chemical constituents and biochemical mechanisms of action.
National Institutes of Health Office of Dietary Supplements https://ods.od.nih.gov	This site provides a current overview of dietary supplements, including individual vitamins and minerals, and dietary supplements promoted for exercise, athletic performance, and for weight loss. It offers a fact sheet geared toward both consumers and health professionals and provides an A to Z index.
National Collegiate Athletic Association (NCAA) banned drug lists www.ncaa.org/2018-19-ncaa-banned-drugs-list	This site provides basic information on drugs and substances prohibited for use by NCAA athletes.
Natural Medicines database	Natural Medicines is an evidence-based database that seeks to answer questions about natural medicines by systematically identifying, evaluating, and applying scientific information along with clinically practical information for health professionals. Natural Medicines is continuously updated and requires an annual subscription. Check for access through your local library.
PubMed Central www.pubmedcentral.nih.gov	The U.S. National Institutes of Health offers a free digital archive of biomedical and life sciences journal literature. The user can search the site using text or key words to gain access to published research on supplements. All abstracts and some papers are available electronically.
U.S. Anti-Doping Agency Athlete Guide to the 2018 Prohibited List www.usada.org/substances/prohibited-list/athlete-guide-2018-prohibited-list	This site provides practical guidance on how the World Anti-Doping Agency (WADA) Prohibited List may affect an athlete. It includes a quick link to banned substances including anabolic agents, peptide growth factors, B-2 agonists, metabolic modulators, diuretics, and masking agents. Also see WADA for additional information: www.wada-ama.org.

Data from "Using Dietary Supplements Wisely," NIH National Center for Complementary and Integrative Health, accessed January 7, 2019, https://nccih.nih.gov/health/supplements/wiseuse.htm.

Supplements that promise even a small advantage are appealing in the athletic arena because events can be won or lost by the slimmest of margins: less than a second during a sprint to possess the ball or a sprint to the finish line. The breathtakingly close finish at the 2005 New York City Marathon is one example. After running 26 miles (41.8 km), Paul Tergat of Kenya and Hendrick Ramaala of South Africa ended up neck and neck for the final 385 yards (352 m), with Tergat eventually winning by just a step. Shorter events are often won by an even closer margin. In the 1996 Olympic Games in Atlanta, for example, the United States' Gail Devers won the women's 100-meter track event. Her time of 10.95 seconds was 0.01 seconds faster than the third-place finisher. Also, who can forget the finish of the men's 100-meter butterfly in the 2008 Beijing Olympics, where Michael Phelps beat Milorad Cavic by a mere 4.7 millimeters? No matter what your philosophy or level of competition, the temptation to take a supplement that may offer you a split-second advantage is always there, challenging your desire to perform better, feel better, or live longer. Believe me, as a mother of three athletic children, I have observed split-second differences deciding which athlete runs on the high school varsity team. It's not always just a matter of winning the race.

Before we continue, it is important to readdress the definitions of supplements and ergogenic aids, particularly because athletes and coaches often use these terms interchangeably. In the United States, the Dietary Supplement Health and Education Act of 1994 (DSHEA) defines a *dietary supplement* as a food product (other than tobacco) added to the total diet that contains at least one of the following ingredients: a vitamin, mineral, herb, botanical, or amino acid metabolite; it could also be a constituent, extract, or a combination of any of these ingredients.[6] An *ergogenic aid,* on the other hand, is typically defined as a substance or strategy that improves athletic performance by improving work production. The word's roots are *ergo,* which means work, and *genic,* which means generation.

Before DSHEA, botanicals and herbal supplements were considered neither food nor drugs. Now, all dietary supplements—including those that promote improved athletic performance—are considered a subcategory of food and are regulated by DSHEA,[7] whereas ergogenic aids that are not supplements, including high-altitude sleeping chambers, aerodynamic handlebars, and leg shaving, are not regulated by DSHEA.

Can Supplements Be Trusted?

Although the practice of medicine is, for the most part, grounded in science, the same cannot necessarily be said for supplements. For a medical treatment to become an accepted practice or standard of therapy, there must be evidence, supplied by human clinical trials, that the treatment is likely to benefit rather than harm the people who receive it.[8] If a treatment shows no benefit, it will not make it into the standards of care manual or to the shelves of your local pharmacy.

Before a pharmaceutical company can seek approval for a prescription or over-the-counter drug, the U.S. Food and Drug Administration (FDA) requires that the company conduct clinical trials in adults.[8] During these trials, the participants' response, side effects, and established doses are monitored and documented. The study results are then reported to the FDA and likely submitted for publication in peer-reviewed scientific journals. Although not perfect, this process, lasting approximately 15 years from discovery to consumer use, reduces the likelihood that ineffective and unsafe drugs reach the market. Once a drug is released, the FDA mandates that information pertaining to the drug's active ingredients, safety, dosage, and expected reactions be available and also expects physicians to report any ill effects experienced by patients taking the drugs. The drug may then later be removed from the market. For instance, this happened with the weight-loss drug sibutramine (Meridia) because of concern about its side effects.[9]

Supplements, on the other hand, require much less regulation before they are available to the consumer. Clinical trials documenting efficacy, safety, and dosage are not required and are exempted from FDA evaluation by the 1994 DSHEA act.[6] In fact, under DSHEA, manufacturers are exempt from providing premarket evidence of product safety and efficacy.[7] Similar regulations (or lack thereof) apply in most other countries where dietary supplements are not subject to stringent regulations applied to the pharmaceutical industry.[1] As a result, supplements are released on the market sooner than and without the same level of regulation as a pharmaceutical product.

Once a supplement reaches the shelves, the FDA can remove the product only if it can be proven unsafe when taken as directed. Furthermore, whereas the FDA has the authority to inspect the facilities of any drug manufacturer and to verify that the ingredients are pure, this safeguard does not apply to supplements. In the past, contaminated supplements have produced adverse reactions that were difficult to treat because the source of the contaminant was not easily identified. One serious example occurred a few years ago when an herbal "cleansing system" was found to be contaminated with the heart medication digitalis. This caused life-threatening cardiovascular reactions in two women.[8] The potential for inadvertent contamination does not seem to have improved. Numerous case reports link supplement use to adverse health outcomes or inadvertent anti-doping violations because the supplements are spiked with actual drugs and drug analogs.[7,10]

That said, however, it is also important to mention that the seemingly lax regulation of dietary supplements by the FDA does not mean that all supplements are unsafe or that their effects are poorly documented. Herbs are in fact regulated by Germany's Commission E, the equivalent of the FDA.[8] Any herb that is widely used in Germany or other parts of Europe, where herbal remedies are an accepted part of medical practice rather than being considered "alternative medicine," is likely to be accompanied by reports from studies concerning its effectiveness and safety. These reports are typically published in German medical journals, and summaries of specific herbs are available to the public (see table 10.1). Some are translated and available through scientific databases such as Medline or online resources such as the American Botanical Council. Additionally, evidence-based information is available to the public from the National Institutes of Health (NIH) Office of Dietary Supplements and through a subscription to the Natural Medicine database (see table 10.1). As a result of growing interest, it is becoming easier to find herbal remedies in the United States from reputable companies using standardized extracts that are equivalent to those used in Germany and to be reasonably certain of their effects. However, there is much less supporting evidence for nonherbal supplements and ergogenic aids, including enzymes, prohormones, hormones, and amino acids. This was part of the reason the Medical and Scientific Commission of the IOC assembled a panel of experts to evaluate dietary supplement use by high-performing athletes.

Evaluating a Supplement for Potential Benefits and Risks

To decide whether a dietary supplement is right for you, you must keep both an open mind and a watchful eye. Keeping an open mind, however, may be a bit easier for some athletes than for others. I must admit, I still struggle with the concept of using supplements, particularly ergogenic aids, even though I have read hundreds of scientific reports, served on the IOC dietary supplement committee, and even noted improvements in strength performance from using creatine, both in my studies[11] and in my own experience. What I have finally come to terms with—by keeping an open mind—is that some supplements have the potential to enhance the health and performance of athletes under certain conditions, particularly when used over the short term. But regular use of these supplements should be considered only after an athlete—plant-based or not—1) ensures that he or she is adequately training and following a good sport diet (see box 10.1) and 2) evaluates each supplement for its potential risks and benefits. The IOC dietary supplement committee recognizes similar points,[12] and stresses that performance supplements should not be considered until the athlete has reached an appropriate level of maturity and competitive readiness and has a nutrition plan in place[13,14] (see figure 10.1). Supplements are also not recommended for young athletes.

In my case, I tried creatine for several months as we prepared to conduct our supplementation study on female soccer players[11] and noted an amazing improvement in my bench press performance, which had not budged for years. I did not continue using creatine for very long, however, because I felt that as a recreational athlete who was planning to start a family, any small benefit to my already acceptable strength performance was not worth the unknown risks of long-term supplementation. Maybe I would have decided differently if I had been a close contender for the Olympic Trials. I also may think differently as I begin my journey as an aging plant-based athlete.

Keeping a watchful eye then becomes important for athletes at all levels who are interested in either performance- or health-enhancing dietary supplements. It involves carefully evaluating the supplement of interest, its research, safety, and cost so that you can decide whether the potential benefits outweigh the known and unknown risks and deciding whether taking the supplement fits into your personal value system. These steps are discussed in detail in the following sections and can be used to evaluate all types of dietary supplements.

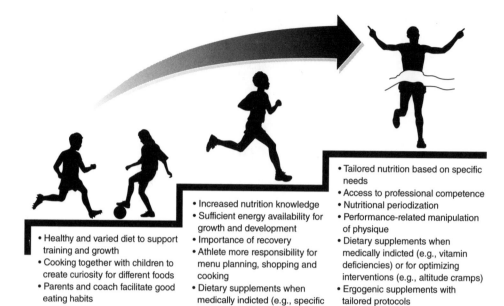

FIGURE 10.1   Stages in the athletic, educational, and nutrition development of the young athlete.

Reprinted by permission from R. Garthe and R.J. Maughan, "Athletes and Supplements: Prevalence and Perspectives," *International Journal of Sport Nutrition and Exercise Metabolism* 28, no. 2 (2018): 126-138.

Box 10.1

Do You Really Need to Supplement?

Before taking a supplement, ask yourself the following questions:

1. Do I eat breakfast regularly?
2. Do I eat at least three meals a day at regularly scheduled times?
3. Am I consuming enough but not too much energy to support my level of physical activity?
4. Do the bulk of my calories come from carbohydrate? Alternatively, am I taking in the recommended amount of carbohydrate for my sport and level of training?
5. Do I watch my fat intake, making sure my choices are smart and that I am getting enough but not too much of the right kinds of fat?
6. Do I eat a variety of foods from each of the major food groups?
7. Do I eat at least three servings of fruit a day?
8. Do I eat at least two servings of vegetables a day?
9. Do I consume adequate carbohydrate and fluids when training and during competition?
10. Do I drink enough water to maintain normal hydration?

If you cannot answer yes to each of these questions, why take a supplement? Don't expect supplements to replace a daily balanced diet.

Evaluate the Product and Its Claims

The first step in evaluating a supplement is to carefully evaluate the product and the claims being made. This includes taking a look at who is making the claims and whether the claims seem possible. Many times, products are sold by testimonials from other athletes, fitness buffs, self-proclaimed nutritionists, or medical doctors, all of whom can be convincing. If the product sounds too good to be true, it probably is. Also, consider whether the product claims that it contains secret ingredients or special formulas. Under an amendment to DSHEA, companies are now required to list all of the ingredients but are not required to tell which ones are likely to be beneficial. For example, creatine and caffeine have known chemical structures with known actions, but they are not heavily advertised by themselves. Instead, cocktails containing "magic," "proprietary," or "special" formulas of these and other ingredients are advertised. Although it is probably more profitable and exciting to offer a special concoction, such formulas require that you—the athlete—look up each ingredient to determine its possible effectiveness and safety. Furthermore, it is less likely that research supporting the benefit of a formula is available than research on a pure herb or compound. And it is more likely the formula could contain contaminants along with suspect ingredients.

Determine Whether Research Exists to Back Up the Claim

The next step is to determine whether adequate and scientifically sound research is available to back up the supplement's claims or support its effectiveness. The research should, of course, be done on humans, preferably athletes, and not on mice, rats, or chickens. Also, you don't need to have a PhD in nutrition to figure out whether the research is sound. This step entails checking the supplement company's website (which typically lists supporting studies), calling the company to get further details, and most importantly, searching for the product and published product research from reputable sources including the NIH Office of Dietary Supplements or PubMed Central if you are interested in looking for the research yourself (see table 10.1). In your search, remember that a compelling story or a single study does not signify research. Neither does an abstract or two from a meeting or an unpublished study described only on a supplement company's website. The studies conducted should also include controlled clinical trials.[15] Those that provide the strongest evidence are randomly assigned, placebo controlled, and double or single blinded. Randomly assigned, placebo controlled means that about half the athletes are randomly assigned to take the supplement and the other half are assigned to take the look-alike placebo that has no supplement.[1] Double blinded means that neither the athlete nor the investigators conducting the test know who is taking what. This helps eliminate bias on the part of the athlete and the investigator. Single blinded means that just one party, for example, the athlete, is unaware of who is taking what. Although not as scientifically sound, this protocol is used when it is impossible to "blind" a party. For example, it would be difficult to blind athletes randomly assigned to a plant-based compared to a mixed diet or a high-carbohydrate compared to a low-carbohydrate diet (although studies have successfully done the latter).

Studies should also, if possible, include a crossover design in which study participants are assigned to one treatment—supplement or placebo—and later cross over to the other treatment. Crossover studies, however, are difficult to use with athletes because of training influences and are almost impossible to conduct when supplements are stored in the body for longer than a week or so (as is true with creatine and carnitine). Studies in which all participants knowingly take a supplement are for the most part worthless because of the placebo effect. This well-documented phenomenon holds that about one-third of the people given a sugar pill, or placebo, will experience benefits or side effects simply because they are told that they will. With that said, the strongest evidence comes from meta-analyses and systematic reviews, which compile the evidence from multiple trials. Many clinical trials and meta-analyses are used as references throughout this book.

Determine Whether the Supplement Is Safe, Plant-Based, and Legal

If, after your research, the product still seems promising, the next steps are to determine whether safety or toxicity issues are associated with it, whether it is plant-based (or vegan), and whether it is indeed legal, and not necessarily in that order. A first step in this process may be to look up information on the noted and possible side effects from the published research or from one of the websites listed in table 10.1. The importance of this step is illustrated by the fact that in the United States in 2015, more than 23,000 emergency department visits were reported to be associated with dietary supplement use.[16] If the product seems relatively safe and you feel compelled to try it, the next step may be to seek a reputable brand. Although there are no guarantees, house brands from larger grocery or drug stores or pharmaceutical companies might be your safest bet. These brands—because of their visibility and economic clout—are more likely to impose high standards on their suppliers. Many may also be third-party tested, meaning that the dietary supplements are tested by an independent laboratory. Certification by NSF International is particularly important if you are a competitive college or national athlete who is subject to drug testing (see www.nsf.org for more information and to download the current NSF app). Certified for Sports by NSF is a program that ensures a product contains the nutrients listed on the label and is also free from contaminants and tested for banned substances.

Once you have selected a brand or two, search the website or call the company or manufacturer directly to obtain specifics on how the product is manufactured and whether animal derivatives are included as ingredients or in processing. This step is not necessary for an herbal supplement, which is of course vegan, or for collagen or bovine colostrums, which are not plant-based, no matter how you look at them. But it may be necessary for dietary supplements such as creatine, vitamin D_3, and melatonin. Commercially available melatonin preparations, for example, may be isolated from the pineal glands of beef cattle or chemically synthesized. Vitamin D_3 may be synthesized from sheep's lanolin or from lichen.

If you are an athlete who competes under anti-doping codes, a final step is to ensure that the supplement of interest is not banned or illegal. This can be done by checking directly with the national body governing your sport (if one exists) or competitive level. For example, the National College Athletic Association (NCAA) website lists all substances banned or restricted for athletes competing under the NCAA guidelines and includes anabolic agents such as dehydroepiandrosterone (DHEA) and androstenedione, and a list of popular stimulants including ephedra, Adderall, and bitter orange. Caffeine is also a limited substance. The World Anti-Doping Agency (WADA) also lists substances that are prohibited at all times, during competitions, and during participation in certain sports. If you are a collegiate or club athlete or compete at a national or international level, your coaches, trainers, and medical and nutrition support personnel should be aware of what supplements are banned in your particular sport. However, if you are unsure, it is best to err on the conservative side. All dietary supplements are taken at your own risk. And it is important that if you experience health problems of any sort or need to take a medication—any medication—tell your doctor what supplements you are taking and how long you have been taking them.

Determine the Potential Risks and Costs of Supplementing

The final step in this process is to determine whether supplementing is worth it. Taking a supplement—including an herbal one—has potential health, ethical, and financial risks. Remember that because the FDA does not strictly regulate the supplement industry, any given supplement may contain pesticides, banned substances, and other contaminants and may lead to long-term health complications or disqualification from an athletic event. Knowing how long people have been taking a certain substance may also help you determine its risks. Ginseng, for example, has been used as an herbal therapy for years (although not in the United States) and its safety, when not mixed with other products, is well documented. In contrast, creatine has been on the market for about 20 years. Although it appears to be safe over the shorter term, its long-term effects as well as those of many supplements are simply not known.

Also, as a plant-based athlete, you need to ensure that supplementation fits your value system and your budget. Do you define natural as what you get from food and herbs or does it also include an artificially synthesized ergogenic aid? If it is OK to supplement with a commercially produced carbohydrate–electrolyte beverage, is it also OK to mix in a little creatine or beta-alanine, or is that somehow cheating? Although your response may depend on your competitive level and whether your opponents are taking supplements, the question is one that only you can answer.

The final important question comes down to economics. Can you afford the cost of the supplement? You should consider this in the context of how much the supplement costs as well as how much healthy food you could purchase if you were not spending that money on supplements. For instance, if you believe that fresh blueberries or whole-grain sourdough bread from the local bakery is too expensive, you should think twice about buying supplements. Also consider how much benefit you are likely to gain from taking the supplement. In other words, what is its cost-to-benefit ratio? A final unfortunate fact is that you may be paying for a supplement that may not even contain the intended product. According to the Office of Dietary Supplements, analyses of dietary supplements sometimes find a discrepancy between quantity on the label as opposed to that in the product. For example, an herbal supplement may not contain the correct plant species, or the amounts of the ingredients may be lower or higher than the label states. That means you may be taking less (or possibly more) of the dietary supplement than you realize. There is nothing like paying money for something you are not even getting.

Supplements of Interest to the Plant-Based Athlete

Although a zillion supplements are out there, a handful may be of interest to athletes in general because ample evidence supports their claim of benefit[1] or to plant-based athletes specifically because they take in small amounts of these substances through their diet.[4] Discussion of these products is by no means an endorsement of their use, but it is an effort to provide information about their potential benefits and to expose hype, whichever the case may be, and the list is not exhaustive. However, if you decide to try a supplement, you should first ensure that you are eating well (see box 10.1). And remember, you should never substitute supplements for a good sport diet. If you would like to learn about other supplements, check out the 2018 IOC Expert Group Statement on Dietary Supplements in High-Performing Athletes or consult any of the sources listed in table 10.1.

Creatine

Most of the creatine in the body is found in skeletal muscle, where it exists primarily as creatine phosphate, which is an important storage form of energy that buffers ATP (see chapter 2). Many studies conducted since the early 1990s have found that oral creatine supplementation is effective at increasing muscle creatine stores (by as much as 30%), and performance during repeated high-intensity, short-duration exercise tasks such as those that occur in many team sports, and during high-intensity cycling or sprinting intervals and weight training.[3] Supplementation also enhances outcomes of resistance and interval training programs and can lead to greater gains in lean mass and muscular strength and power.[17] The IOC Expert Group on Dietary Supplements in Athletes felt there was sufficient evidence of the efficacy of creatine. Creatine supplementation, however, may be detrimental for endurance performance in events in which body mass must be moved against gravity (such as high jump or pole-vault) or when a specific body mass must be achieved.[2]

The average dietary intake of creatine is about 2 grams per day in meat eaters[18] and is negligible in vegetarian diets. This makes sense because creatine is found primarily in muscle tissue. Even though creatine can be made in the body from the amino acids glycine, arginine, and methionine, low concentrations of creatine in the blood[19-21] and skeletal muscle[22-24] are found in vegetarians, as well as nonvegetarians placed on a vegetarian diet. Several studies have also found that vegetarians respond better to oral creatine supplementation than nonvegetarians do.[20,24] In these studies, vegetarians were found to experience greater increases in skeletal muscle creatine phosphate, lean tissue mass, and work performance during weight training[24] and anaerobic bicycle exercises[20] than nonvegetarians did. One study, however, did not find these benefits.[25] Thus, it is often suggested that vegetarian athletes may benefit from regular or periodic supplementation with creatine.

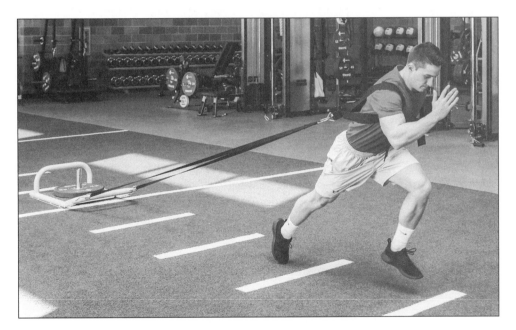

Creatine may help increase body mass and performance during high-intensity, short-duration activity. Because vegetarians often don't obtain much creatine from their diets, it's a supplement they could consider.

Tom Kimmell Photography

Creatine supplementation has not been associated with detrimental short-term or long-term (up to four years) health effects, if appropriate protocols are followed. Creatine comes in several forms. The pure powder form can be dissolved in warm water and mixed into smoothies or carbohydrate-containing beverages. Some evidence suggests taking creatine concurrently with about 50 grams of a carbohydrate or protein source enhances creatine uptake into muscle through an insulin response.[1] Several well-known manufacturers synthesize creatine without using animal derivatives. If you try creatine, take pure creatine monohydrate, not creatine mixed with a cocktail of other ingredients, and contact the manufacturer to verify that your brand is plant-based. The usual dose is 3 to 5 grams per day. Although many studies have used loading protocols of 20 grams per day (divided into four equal daily doses) for five to seven days followed by the lower maintenance dose, this loading phase is not necessary because a regular dose of 3 grams per day will achieve the same increase in muscle creatine over a slightly longer time frame.[26]

Carnitine

Carnitine (or L-carnosine) plays a central role in the metabolism of fat. Its role is to transport fatty acids into the body's energy-generating powerhouse—the mitochondria—to be burned for energy. Carnitine is found in meats and dairy products but not in plant foods. Like creatine, blood and muscle concentrations of carnitine have been found to be lower in vegetarians[19,27] despite the liver's ability to produce it from the amino acids lysine and methionine. In addition, blood carnitine concentrations are found to be lower in nonathletic people who are obese and following a diet that is very low in calories,[28] which suggests that carnitine levels could be low in anyone who restricts calories.

Not surprisingly, carnitine has been targeted as a potential "fat burner" and endurance-performance enhancer. Studies addressing the ergogenic potential of carnitine, however, have been ambiguous, with several suggesting a beneficial effect of carnitine supplementation and others indicating no effect at all.[3] It has also been noted that although carnitine concentration in blood goes up with supplementation, the enzyme system responsible for transporting fatty acids into the mitochondria is not increased. This suggests that supplementation is unlikely to enhance what capacity the body already has. Although carnitine supplements are generally not considered an effective ergogenic aid for athletes,[3] some sources[4] suggest that supplements be considered for vegetarians who may not consume adequate carnitine or its precursor amino acids in their diets. However, a study in male vegetarians and omnivores found that 12 weeks of supplementation with carnitine had no effect on muscle function or energy metabolism, despite an increase of about 13 percent in muscle carnitine concentration.[21] Research suggests that clearance of carnitine by the kidney is dampened in vegetarians compared to omnivores, which may suggest that vegetarians are able to preserve their carnitine stores.[21,27] Carnitine is available in pill and liquid forms and many companies offer a plant-based version. Adverse side effects have not been found from taking 2 to 6 grams per day for up to six months.

Caffeine

Caffeine is probably the most casually and widely used sport-enhancing supplement because of its availability and social acceptance. Caffeine and its sister derivatives theophylline or theobromine occur naturally in certain plant-based foods, including coffee, tea, and chocolate, and caffeine is also added to soda, sport bars and gels, and some medications (see table 10.2). Caffeine is thought to improve performance by both stimulating the central nervous system (CNS) and facilitating force production in the muscle.[3] As a CNS stimulant, caffeine specifically affects perception of effort, wards off drowsiness, and increases vigilance and alertness, which may offer performance benefits. Well-controlled laboratory studies have found that caffeine (3-6 mg/kg body mass) taken one hour before or during exercise improves endurance performance, most notably including improvement of about 3 percent in performance times in a race-like setting. Studies demonstrating a benefit of caffeine on shorter, more-intense

TABLE 10.2 Caffeine and Theobromine Content of Selected Beverages and Foods

Food or beverage	Portion	Caffeine (mg)	Theobromine (mg)
Coffee, breakfast blend, brewed from grounds	6 fl oz	70	—
Coffee, instant	1 tsp	31	—
Espresso, restaurant brewed	1 fl oz	63	—
Tea, green, brewed	6 fl oz	21	not reported
Tea, oolong, brewed	6 fl oz	39	4
Hot cocoa	12 fl oz	4	115
Cola	12 fl oz	29-99	—
Lemon-lime soda with caffeine	12 fl oz	55	—
Rockstar energy drink	8 fl oz	75	—
Red Bull energy drink	8 fl oz	80	—
Milk chocolate	1 bar (1.55 oz)	9	90
Clif Bar (cool mint chocolate and peanut toffee buzz)	1 bar	50	—

Note: Many energy bars and gels contain caffeine. Check the product information and website from your favorite coffee shop and for your favorite brands of sport supplements (caffeine content is not typically listed on the label). Use these values to convert English measurements to metric: 1 fl oz = 29.6 ml = 28.4 g; 1 tsp = 4.7 g.

Values obtained from USDA Food Composition Databases (https://ndb.nal.usda.gov/ndb/) and selected manufacturers.

events, such as a 1-kilometer (0.6 mile) cycling time trial, are less abundant but suggest an ergogenic potential. A growing body of research suggests that lower doses (<3 mg/kg/body mass) can have an ergogenic potential[29] and also reduce risk of negative side effects, including nausea, anxiousness, restlessness, and insomnia.

Plant-based athletes who enjoy coffee, tea, or other caffeinated beverages may find it beneficial to consume a large mug or two of strong coffee or tea about an hour before exercise, although some suggest that anhydrous caffeine from pills or supplements may be more effective.[1,30] Contrary to previous ideas about caffeine consumption,[30] habitual caffeine intake does not appear to diminish caffeine's ergogenic properties.[3] Nor does it lead to dehydration or electrolyte imbalance during exercise.[31] High levels of caffeine are banned by the NCAA, but at levels possible only from supplementation. For example, an athlete would have to drink approximately six cups (~ 1,400 ml) of strong coffee before exercise to exceed the urinary caffeine allowable level of 15 micrograms per milliliter. In the past, caffeine was prohibited by the International Olympic Committee, but in 2004 it was moved to its monitoring program.

Dietary Nitrates and Beetroot Juice

Both beetroot juice and dietary nitrate (NO_3^-) have become increasingly popular supplements that offer potential ergogenic and health benefits. Initial studies conducted nearly 10 years ago found that supplementation with beetroot juice has the potential to improve performance and lower blood pressure.[32,33] The performance benefits of beetroot juice are caused by the high concentration of nitrate in the beetroot, and attributed to its capacity to increase nitric oxide (NO).[34] NO is an important signaling molecule that modulates many physiological processes, including blood flow, muscle contractility, muscle cell differentiation, and vascular tone. Its most important performance-enhancing mechanism appears to be its ability to lower the energy (caloric) cost of submaximal exercise, which in essence enhances exercise efficiency. The improved efficiency is thought to occur through improved contractile function in fast-twitch (type II) muscle fibers or improved muscle oxygenation or some combination of both. Nitrate or beetroot supplementation has been associated with a 1 to 3 percent improvement in sport-specific time trials lasting more than 40 minutes and a 3 to 5 percent improvement of high-intensity intermittent, team-sport exercise lasting 12 to 40 minutes.[2,3] However, performance gains from dietary nitrate are harder to obtain in a well-trained athlete. Just ask my daughter Marlena; beetroot consumption did nothing for her performance during her sophomore high school cross country season (despite her intense belief it would).

Of importance to the plant-based athlete, drinking natural or concentrated beetroot juice seems to be more effective than nitrate supplementation in the form of sodium or potassium nitrate.[35] In fact, the availability of NO can be enhanced by consuming more leafy green and root vegetables, including spinach, arugula (rocket lettuce), beets, and beetroot juice.[36,37] Maybe this is another reason Marlena experienced no supplemental benefit. An optimal nitrate-loading regimen has not yet been established and is thought to vary among athletes and be generally higher in those who are well trained. Acute performance benefits are seen within two to three hours after consuming 310 to 560 milligrams.

Many studies, however, have tested the consumption of approximately 2 cups (472 ml) of beetroot juice for several days; these studies suggest that supplementation longer than 15 days may result in greater physiological benefit. Furthermore, the amount of nitrate thought to offer health and performance benefits (and which is found naturally in beetroots and green leafy vegetables) is significantly less than the amount that leads to toxicity.[38] Additionally for plant-based athletes, increasing the amount of nitrate-rich vegetables in the diet might serve as an easy strategy for optimizing performance.[39] And it offers another reason to eat your beets and arugula (which, by the way, grows like weeds—even in Wyoming).

Beta-Alanine and Sodium Bicarbonate

Beta-alanine and sodium bicarbonate augment the body's buffering capacity, which helps dampen the buildup of acid during high-intensity exercise. Beta-alanine is the rate-limiting precursor to an important muscle buffer, carnosine, which provides a defense against acid accumulation within muscle cells during exercise. A fairly good-sized body of research[3,40] has shown that daily supplementation increases muscle carnosine content and is associated with small but potentially meaningful performance improvements of 0.2 to 3 percent during continuous or intermittent bouts of high-intensity exercise lasting 30 seconds to 10 minutes.[1] Beta-alanine supplementation, however, seems to be less effective in well-trained athletes. The current supplementation protocol is 65 milligrams per kilogram of body weight, ingested in split doses (0.8-1.6 g every 3-4 hr) for 10 to 12 weeks. This dosing regimen is thought to reduce possible side effects, which include itching, skin rash, and transient paralysis.[3]

Sodium bicarbonate, on the other hand, augments the body's extracellular buffering capacity, which is the amount of buffering agents found in blood. Buffering the acid content in the blood helps "pull out" acid from the exercising muscle. Numerous studies conducted since the 1980s[41] have shown that supplementation has the potential to enhance performance by about 2 percent during high-intensity sprinting lasting about 60 seconds. Reduced effectiveness is observed as the exercise task exceeds 10 minutes.[1,3] The issue with bicarbonate supplementation, however, is that gastrointestinal (GI) distress is a well-established side effect. The standard supplementation protocol is 0.2 to 0.4 grams per kilogram of body mass taken 60 to 150 minutes before exercise. Alternative strategies such as split doses (smaller doses given over the same time period), coingestion with carbohydrate-containing meals, or supplementation with sodium citrate may reduce GI distress.

Herbal and Other Supplements

Depending on your objective, several herbal and other types of supplements may provide supplementary health benefits. Although Commission E and Natural Medicines databases may be the best sources of information about these supplements, table 10.3 lists a handful of herbal or phytochemical products that are generally considered safe and effective for their reported uses. If you are interested in these or other dietary supplements, evaluate each supplement—herbal or otherwise—using the tools discussed earlier, paying particular attention to data obtained from the websites listed in table 10.1. While you may find that many botanicals have supportive evidence for specific circumstances, you may also find that the effect is small. In the big picture, you may still get the biggest bang for your buck by following a plant-based diet.

TABLE 10.3   Selected Herbal and Other Supplements That May Offer Health Benefits

Supplement	Use	Reported value and effect
Echinacea	Stimulates immune system function. Prevents upper-respiratory-tract infections.	May be beneficial in reducing the severity and duration of symptoms associated with the common cold and flu; should not be viewed as a cure for the common cold.
Ginger	Thought to alleviate nausea associated with motion sickness, morning sickness, diarrhea, irritable bowel, chemotherapy, and so on.	Clinical studies suggest it may be effective for morning sickness, painful menstrual periods, osteoarthritis, vertigo, and postoperative nausea and vomiting, but not motion sickness.
Ginkgo biloba	Improves memory and mental sharpness. Acts as an antidepressant. Improves circulation. Thins blood. Acts as an antioxidant.	Research suggests it may be valuable for an array of health concerns related to problems with microcirculation in the brain, legs, and sex organs. Its neuroprotective effects are well established, and its benefits in improving mental function and memory in healthy subjects looks promising.
Ginseng	Relieves stress. Enhances athletic performance. Promotes well-being. Enhances immune system and reduces inflammation. Acts as a stimulant. Lowers blood sugar. Improves cognitive function.	Scientific evidence of the benefits is considered inconclusive. The adaptogenic role of ginseng has proven beneficial for many thousands of years, so ginseng may, therefore, prove valuable for normalizing substances during stressful conditions.
St. John's wort	Alleviates mild depression.	May be effective as a low-dose tricyclic antidepressant in treating mild depression. St. John's wort, however, should not be used to treat depression without consent of a medical doctor.

Supplement	Use	Reported value and effect
Melatonin	Promotes sleep. Reduces symptoms of jet lag. Slows the aging process. Increases secretion of sex hormones. Acts as an antioxidant.	Serves as a nonaddictive alternative to over-the-counter chemical sleep aids. Particularly useful as a short-term regulator of sleep–wake cycles (e.g., resetting your body clock after crossing several time zones). It can induce or deepen depression in susceptible people. Melatonin supplements may also be dangerous for people with cardiovascular risks.
Probiotics	Decreases severity and duration of GI problems. Decreases incidence, duration, and severity of upper-respiratory-tract infections.	Offers modest benefits to athletes prone to GI problems or traveling to regions where such problems are more likely. Supplementation needs to begin well ahead of competition.[5]
Quercetin (polyphenolic flavonol)	Provides anti-inflammatory effects. Acts as an antioxidant.	Results of research are equivocal; some studies note benefits and others see no effect.[42] Benefit of supplementation on performance and metabolic outcomes is likely to be trivial for both trained and untrained athletes.[43]
Turmeric (curcumin)	Provides anti-inflammatory effects. Reduces arthritis symptoms. Reduces symptoms of and enhances recovery from muscle-damaging exercise.	Benefits of supplementation (5 g/day) are noted after exercise that involves eccentric contractions (muscle lengthens under load, such as weight training and downhill running), but not after endurance exercise. Preliminary evidence shows it may reduce symptoms associated with inflammatory bowel diseases, osteoarthritis, and rheumatoid arthritis.

Note: Please refer to reputable websites for updates and information about safety concerns and recommended dosages. All supplements listed are thought to be safe for generally healthy people when supplemented at the suggested doses.

After reading the overview of dietary supplements in this chapter, you are now armed and ready to evaluate supplements and their place in your plant-based diet. The next chapter focuses on how diet and certain dietary supplements may influence two common athletic maladies: muscle cramps and inflammation.

11 | Reducing Muscle Cramps and Inflammation

As I've traveled around the country giving talks on sports nutrition, the most common reaction I hear from athletes who have recently adopted a plant-based diet is that eating this way significantly reduces their workout recovery time—no matter the sport. This is anecdotal, of course, and while there isn't much research that looks specifically at recovery time in athletes who eat plant-based diets, we do know there are mechanisms related to compounds and vitamins found in plant foods that theoretically reduce inflammation and therefore could reduce recovery time. There is strong evidence that plant-based nutrition can significantly reduce your risk for cardiovascular diseases and the same compounds and mechanisms involved in disease prevention may benefit the plant-based athlete. Phytochemicals, antioxidants, and nutrients such as potassium can increase blood flow, repair damaged cells, and protect arteries from future damage. More than 25,000 phytochemicals have been discovered in plant foods, and the unique benefits of most are still unknown. It is likely that many of these phytochemicals could be working to naturally enhance postexercise recovery in athletes who eat plant-based diets or helping to prevent overuse inflammatory injuries.

– Matt

Both muscle cramps and overuse inflammatory injuries are common, painful physiological disturbances that regularly frustrate athletes. Because both can be caused by a change in daily training routine—for example, you run faster or farther than you are accustomed to or pump more weight than usual—your diet can potentially assist in controlling or reducing these maladies. The latest thinking on muscle cramps is that they may be brought on by muscle fatigue, fluid and electrolyte imbalances or a combination of both. This suggests that dietary factors could be involved. Nagging overuse and inflammatory injuries could similarly be affected by diet. The dietary components implicated in muscle cramps commonly include fluids, electrolytes, and carbohydrate, whereas those involved in inflammation include mainly omega-3 fatty acids, vitamin D, and certain phytochemicals, such as polyphenols.

This chapter reviews the basics of both muscle cramps and inflammation and discusses the dietary factors that could potentially—but not necessarily—help prevent or control muscle cramps and musculoskeletal inflammation. Unlike the information in the other chapters, however, the information presented here is provocative and somewhat speculative.

Inside a Muscle Cramp

Most everyone has had a muscle cramp and understands that cramps are painful, involuntary contractions that seem to come out of the blue. Typically, they are of little medical consequence but can pose an inconvenience for athletes if they occur regularly. Muscle cramps tend to occur most frequently at night (nocturnal cramps) or during or after unusually prolonged exercise (exercise-associated cramps), but they can also occur during apparently typical exercise conditions, either early or late in the session. Unfortunately, despite their pervasiveness and interest from the sports medicine community,[1] their cause (or causes) is not well understood[2] and may in fact be caused by factors unique to each athlete.[3] This lack of understanding has resulted in a perpetuation of myths and anecdotes about the cause and treatment of cramps. This includes the belief by athletes, coaches, and trainers that eating bananas[4,5] or consuming mustard or pickle juice[6] are effective ways to prevent and treat muscle cramps.

Causes of Muscle Cramps

Sport scientists have recently begun investigating what makes a muscle cramp and when it does, what occurs during a cramp. In the past, muscle cramps were thought to be caused by extremely hot or cold environments, imbalances of fluids or electrolytes, or inherited abnormalities of carbohydrate or fat metabolism.[1] An imbalance of electrolytes—including sodium, potassium, calcium, and magnesium—was initially suspected because these electrolytes are involved in generating electrical currents in the body. These minerals can also be lost through moderate-to heavy-sweating, particularly in the heat.

More recent research suggests that muscles can cramp during a diverse range of conditions,[1,2] but the underlying cause—according to the bulk of the evidence—is due to neuromuscular cause. Specifically, muscles seem to cramp when the sensitivity of the reflex signals between the skeletal muscles and its tendons and the spinal cord are altered.[7,8] Researchers from the University of Cape Town Medical School in South Africa first reported in 1997 that muscles cramp because of both sustained firing of the nerves in the spinal cord to the muscle and limited protective reflex function by the Golgi tendon organ governor.[8] This enhanced excitability in the spinal cord results in increased discharge by the nerves of the muscle fibers (called the alpha motor neurons), resulting in localized muscle cramps.[2] Normally, excitatory signals from the spinal cord are fired in an intermittent rather than sustained pattern, and protective impulses from the Golgi tendon organ governor (communicating back through the spinal cord) cause muscles to relax under excess tension. These neuromuscular imbalances occur in association with fatigue and are particularly notable in the muscle groups that contract in a shortened position for prolonged periods, such as the quadriceps and hamstrings during cycling and running, the calf muscles during swimming or when sleeping, and the diaphragm muscles in most physical endeavors. Muscles that undergo frequent lengthening during exercise, in contrast, seem to be resistant to cramping because the stretching movement of muscle activates the protective stretch reflex via the Golgi tendon organ.

While it was previously thought that the underlying cause of the typical muscle cramps which occur during endurance and ultra-endurance events were due to fluid and electrolyte disturbances, an analysis of previously published findings found that few studies supported this thinking. [7] Instead, fatigue was the only consistent underlying cause. For instance, a study evaluating predictors of muscle cramps in male runners participating in a 35-mile (56 km) race found that going out too fast during the first portion of the race, beginning the race with already damaged or fatigued muscles, or a history of cramping predicted who developed muscle cramps during the race;[9] neither dehydration nor electrolyte imbalances were predictors in this or other studies. Additionally, it has consistently been observed that athletes prone to cramping are no more likely to be dehydrated or experience higher sweat rates or sodium or fluid losses than athletes who do not cramp.[2] With that said, however, it is important to note that this data does not suggest that fluid or electrolyte imbalances do not provoke cramps, but that the typical cause of muscle cramps is engaging in physical effort that is greater than the muscle is prepared for.

Moreover, determining whether electrolyte imbalances are involved in muscle cramping has proven to be elusive. This is because the body defends its concentrations of many electrolytes in the blood—including sodium, potassium, calcium, and magnesium[10]—and because the electrolyte concentrations in blood may not reflect those in the muscle during a cramp. That is, of course, if we could manage to collect a blood sample at the exact moment when the muscle cramps. Hence, it is possible that the concentration of certain electrolytes may be low within the muscle cell, but appear normal or just slightly lower in the blood when the sample is taken. As you can imagine, collecting this data is precluded for practical reasons because the only way to currently measure muscle electrolyte concentrations is by taking a muscle biopsy. Muscle biopsies can themselves also induce cramping. Tying this back to dietary intake, you can also imagine that obtaining accurate results is difficult when studies compare only electrolyte intake of athletes who cramp compared to those who do not.

Treatment of Muscle Cramps

Taking into account the neuromuscular theory, the accepted treatment for cramps is moderate static stretching of the affected muscle.[1,8] This type of stretching has proven to be effective for most muscle cramps, other than heat cramps[2] that may be brought on by fluid and electrolyte imbalances. Static stretching also reduces the electrical conductivity of the muscle, which in one study was found to be elevated in endurance athletes experiencing muscle cramping.[11] In contrast, fluid replacement does not seem to be a treatment or cure for muscle cramps. One study noted that exercise-associated muscle cramps still occurred in 69 percent of athletes when carbohydrate–electrolyte fluids were ingested at a rate that matched sweat loss.[12] Although no strategies have proven effective for preventing exercise-induced muscle cramping, research collectively supports that adequate sport-specific conditioning, correction of muscle imbalances and posture, and sport psychology therapy aimed at mental preparation for competition may be helpful.[2] Preliminary studies also suggest that ingestion of a transient receptor potential (TRP) channel agonist (available over the counter in sport products such as HotShot) reduces and may help prevent exercise-associated muscle cramps.[13] TRP channels are found on nerves throughout the body and are thought to respond to stimuli such as heat, cold, pain, and even pungent spices. The activation of these receptors at the mouth by ingredients in HotShot (as well as mustard, wasabi and even pickle juice) are hypothesized to calm hyperactive nerves that cause the muscles to cramp. Regular stretching—despite its benefit in the treatment of exercise-associated cramps—is not shown to be beneficial in the prevention of cramps.[2] The benefit of dietary factors, such as maintaining adequate carbohydrate reserves and ensuring adequate mineral electrolyte status through diet, which will be discussed in the next section, are still considered speculative.

Diet and Muscle Cramping

If you look at the information presented in most exercise physiology and sports nutrition books, you will notice the lack of discussions about muscle cramps. This is likely because little is known about the role that diet plays in the tendency for muscles to cramp. Nonetheless, I am a true believer that imbalances of fluid or the mineral electrolytes—sodium, potassium, calcium, and magnesium—in the diet should be ruled out as contributors to all nocturnal and exercise-associated cramps. Excess fatigue brought on by inadequate carbohydrate intake before or during prolonged or strenuous exercise should also be ruled out.

Fluid Imbalances and Dehydration

Whether fluid imbalances and mild dehydration can trigger muscle cramping is open to debate. Although we know that muscle cramps can and do occur with severe dehydration and heat injury, there is no conclusive evidence that consuming adequate fluid with or without electrolytes will prevent exercise-associated or nighttime cramping. In fact, studies have observed that athletes,[2] including runners, cyclists, triathletes and rugby players, who develop cramps during an endurance event are no more likely to be dehydrated or to have lost greater amounts of bodily water than are those who do not develop cramps during the same race.[14-17] However, exertional heat cramps are known to occur in football[18] and tennis[19,20] players in association with extensive sweating and appreciable sodium and chloride losses. In my practice, I have noted anecdotally that maintaining fluid balance indeed helps many endurance and team athletes avoid cramps, particularly those that occur after exercise or when sleeping at night. In one case, I worked with a male tennis player from Switzerland who had a history of severe cramping and fatigue after practice that was relieved by a regular and diligent fluid-consumption schedule. In her book, well-known sports nutritionist Nancy Clark tells a story about a runner who eliminated painful muscle cramps by following the simple postexercise advice to "first drink water for fluid replacement and then have a beer for social fun."[21] Thus, the importance of maintaining hydration and electrolyte balance as a prevention

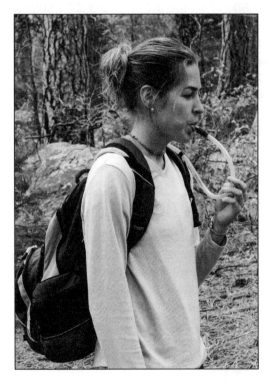

Readily available fluid sources such as hydration packs during prolonged activity are important for helping prevent dehydration, but they may not prevent painful muscle cramps. Also, use caution because overdrinking can lead to hyponatremia (see chapter 7).

strategy for athletes susceptible to exercise-associated muscle cramps should not be ignored,[2] no matter the underlying cause of the cramping.

Sodium

Sodium is one of the main positively charged mineral ions or electrolytes in body fluid. Sodium is needed to help maintain normal body-fluid balance and blood pressure, and is critical for nerve-impulse generation and muscle contraction. Sodium is distributed widely in nature but is found in rather small amounts in most unprocessed foods. In most developed countries, however, a significant amount of sodium is added by food manufacturers in processing (as listed on the food label) and to a lesser extent by use of the salt shaker (1 tsp [6 g] contains 2,325 mg of sodium). Sodium intake, however can vary; dietary intake for adults ages 19 to 50 averages about 3,744 milligrams per day for men and 3,090 for women.[22]

Because sodium plays an important role in regulating blood pressure, fluid, and electrolyte balance, the body has an effective mechanism to help regulate the levels of sodium in blood despite varied dietary sodium intakes. If the sodium concentration in the blood starts to drop, a series of complex events leads to the secretion of a hormone called aldosterone, which signals the kidneys to excrete less. If sodium levels are too high, aldosterone secretion is inhibited, which allows the kidneys to get rid of excess sodium through urination. Another hormone, called antidiuretic hormone (ADH), also helps maintain normal sodium levels in body fluids by signaling the kidneys to retain water along with sodium. Typically, levels of both aldosterone and ADH increase during exercise, which helps conserve the body's water and sodium stores.

Actual sodium-deficient states due to inadequate dietary sodium are not common because the body's regulatory mechanisms are typically quite effective. Additionally, humans have a natural appetite for salt. This helps assure that we consume enough sodium to maintain sodium balance. I have great memories of sprinkling table salt on already salty tortilla chips after long cycling races in the Arizona heat. Thankfully, these sodium-conserving mechanisms are typically activated in athletes who lose excessive sodium and other electrolytes during prolonged sweating (see box 11.1).

Although some reports suggest that muscle cramps occur during the sodium-deficient state, research does not suggest that alterations in sodium balance[11,15,24] are the underlying cause of exercise-associated cramps. This is despite the fact that significantly lower postexercise blood sodium concentrations were found in some athletes who experienced cramps during a race or competition compared to those who did not develop cramps. One reason this may be downplayed is because serum sodium concentrations are physiologically defended (as mentioned earlier) and still remain within the normal clinical range even in athletes who experience lower blood sodium

Box 11.1

Composition of Sweat

Sweat is about 99 percent water but does contain several major electrolytes and other nutrients. The major electrolytes found in sweat are sodium and chloride. Although it varies, an average of about 2.6 grams of salt, or 1.01 grams of sodium, are lost with each liter of sweat produced during exercise. A typical sweat rate is 800 to 1,500 milliliters per hour, but may be even higher during exercise in hot and humid environments, including the outdoors and non-air-conditioned gymnasiums. Additionally, some athletes are known as "salty sweaters" and lose more sodium through sweat than other athletes. Preliminary evidence suggests this may include athletes with tattoos over a significant amount of skin who may have over 60 percent higher concentrations of sodium in their sweat.[23] Other minerals lost in small amounts include potassium, calcium, magnesium, iron, copper, zinc, and iodine. Certain athletes—particularly those who sweat heavily—may need to increase their dietary intake of these nutrients to replace losses.

levels with muscle cramps.[24] In other words, statistically significant decreases in serum sodium noted in some studies[15,17, 24] result in low-normal sodium but are not found in all studies comparing athletes who cramp to those who do not. It is also important to note that whole-body sodium deficits are usually not detectable from measurements of serum sodium or other electrolytes.[25]

Nonetheless, it is important for athletes to consume enough sodium to replace what is lost through sweat[25] (see box 11.1). Despite the regulatory mechanisms discussed earlier, it is possible for athletes to be at risk for muscle cramps and other problems if their sodium and chloride losses through sweat are not offset promptly and sufficiently by dietary intake. Plant-based athletes may be at particular risk if they ignore their salt-craving cues and eat mostly unprocessed and unsalted foods. Athletes at greatest risk are those who are salty sweaters (and experience noticeable salt residue on black clothing after exercise.). The recommendation set by the USDA's Dietary Guidelines for Americans to keep sodium intake to 2,300 milligrams or less per day and the more conservative guidelines of 1,500 milligrams suggested by the American Heart Association to help lower blood pressure are not appropriate for most athletes because of their higher sodium losses. Thus, while it is not likely that low sodium intake is the cause of cramps in most athletes, it is certainly possible that a vegetarian athlete prudently following a low-sodium diet for health reasons might experience muscle cramps that would be relieved with more liberal use of the salt shaker. A documented case of a 17-year-old nationally ranked tennis player with extensive sodium losses nicely illustrates this point.[19] The athlete was able to eliminate heat cramps during competition and training by increasing daily intake of sodium.[19] With that said, there is no magic to pickle juice—one of the currently hot treatments—to prevent or treat muscle cramps. Research suggests that despite its high sodium concentration, pickle juice consumption does not increase blood sodium levels,[6,26] and its use in the prevention of muscle cramps has not been studied. Pickle juice, however, may be tastier to ingest than salt water. One tablespoon contains approximately 230 milligrams of sodium.

Potassium

Potassium is the major electrolyte found inside all body cells, including muscle and nerve cells. Potassium works in close association with sodium and chloride in the generation of electrical impulses in the nerves and the muscles, including the heart muscle. Potassium is found in most foods, but is especially abundant in fresh vegetables, potatoes, certain fruits (melon, bananas, berries, citrus fruit), milk, meat, and fish. Table 11.1 lists the 20 best plant-based sources of potassium.

Potassium balance, like sodium balance, is regulated by the hormone aldosterone. A high serum potassium level stimulates the release of the hormone aldosterone, which leads to increased potassium excretion by the kidneys into the urine. A decrease in serum potassium concentration elicits a drop in aldosterone secretion and therefore less potassium loss in the urine. As with sodium and calcium, potassium is typically precisely regulated, and deficiencies or excessive accumulation is rare in healthy individuals. Potassium deficiencies, however, can occur during conditions such as fasting, diarrhea, and regular diuretic use. In such cases, low blood potassium concentrations, called *hypokalemia,* can lead to muscle cramps and weakness, and even cardiac arrest caused by impairment in the generation of nerve impulses. Similarly, high blood potassium concentrations, or *hyperkalemia,* are not common but can occur in people who take potassium supplements far exceeding the recommended daily allowance. High blood potassium concentrations can also disturb electrical impulses and induce cardiac arrhythmia, although they are not provoked by high potassium intake in the diet.

Even though little evidence is available to support a link between potassium intake and muscle cramps, it is interesting that most athletes—and nonathletes alike—think that the banana is the first line of defense in preventing muscle cramps.[5] If only it were that simple. One study of nine active men found that consuming up to three medium-sized bananas resulted in only a marginal increase in blood potassium levels that took 30 to 60 minutes to occur.[4] Thus it is difficult to argue that bananas be considered effective treatment for exercise-associated muscle cramps.[4] Furthermore, even if potassium or "banana" deficit were the cause of muscle cramps (it's not), athletes following vegetarian diets would not be at risk because plant foods provide an abundance of potassium. An athlete who is recovering from an intestinal illness, restricting calories, or taking diuretics or laxatives should, nevertheless, make an effort to consume potassium-rich foods (see table 11.1), not just bananas, particularly if he or she

TABLE 11.1   Top 20 Plant-Based Sources of Potassium

Food	Portion	Value (mg)
Beet greens	1 cup cooked	1,309
White beans, canned	1 cup	1,189
Baked potato, flesh and skin	1 medium	1,081
Green soybeans	1 cup cooked	970
Lima beans	1 cup cooked	955
Marinara sauce, commercially prepared	1 cup	940
Hash browned potatoes, home prepared	1 cup cooked	899
Winter squash, all types	1 cup cooked	896
Soybeans, cooked	1 cup cooked	886
Spinach, cooked	1 cup cooked	839
Tomato sauce	1 cup	811
Plums, dried or stewed	1 cup	796
Sweet potatoes, canned	1 cup cooked	796
Pinto beans	1 cup cooked	746
Lentils	1 cup cooked	731
Plantains	1 cup cooked	716
Kidney beans	1 cup cooked	713
Split peas	1 cup cooked	710
Navy beans	1 cup cooked	708
Prune juice	1 cup	707

Note: The recommended daily intake for potassium is 4,700 milligrams per day for adults. Refer to appendix F for guidance on converting English units to metric.

Data from report by single nutrient for potassium, USDA Food Composition Databases (https://ndb.nal.usda.gov/ndb/nutrients/index).

is experiencing muscle cramping. Note also that the banana is not even on the top 20 list (one medium banana contains 422 milligrams of potassium) of high-potassium foods, but its cousin, the plantain, is. Because of the dangers of hyperkalemia, potassium supplements are not recommended unless closely monitored by a physician.

Calcium

As discussed in chapter 6, the vast majority of calcium found in the body is in the skeleton where it lends strength to bone. Calcium, however, is involved in

Vegan View: The Plant-Based Potassium Advantage

In 2015, the Dietary Guidelines Advisory Committee prepared a report for the U.S. Departments of Health and Human Services (HHS) and Agriculture (USDA). In it, potassium was called a "nutrient of public health concern" because national intake was far below recommendations; only 3 percent of adults met the adequate intake of 4,700 milligrams per day.[27] Potassium is critical for athletes, and eating a plant-based diet is an easy way to significantly bump up intake to cover your needs (see table 1.1).

And an increased intake of potassium is not just beneficial for athletes. A small study published in 2014 showed an inverse relationship between potassium intake and arterial stiffness in young, healthy adults.[28] The researchers didn't test endothelial function, but did state that it is already well established that potassium increases nitric oxide production, which protects the endothelium and increases blood flow. Dietary potassium can lower blood pressure and reduce the likelihood of developing hypertension, the "silent killer."

Additionally, potassium in fruits and vegetables is associated with citrate and other bicarbonate precursors that are beneficial for bone strength because these precursors reduce calcium losses in urine. Meats, dairy products, and cereals are also sources of potassium, but they have fewer bicarbonate precursors and are less effective.[29]

muscle contractions, including that of the heart, skeletal muscle, and smooth muscle found in blood vessels and intestines, as well as the generation of nerve impulses. Blood calcium is tightly controlled and regulated by several hormones, including parathyroid hormone and vitamin D.

Although impaired muscle contraction and muscle cramps are commonly listed as symptoms of calcium deficiency, many exercise scientists feel that low calcium intake is not likely to play a role in most muscle cramps. This is because if dietary calcium intake were low, calcium would be released from the bones to maintain blood concentrations and theoretically provide what would be needed for muscle contraction. This thinking, however, does not completely rule out the possibility that muscle cramping could be caused by a temporary imbalance of calcium in the muscle during exercise. Certainly, we know that people with inborn errors in calcium metabolism in skeletal muscle (which will be discussed later) are prone to muscle cramping.

Despite so little being known about low calcium intake and muscle cramps, calcium is one of the nutritional factors people most associate with muscle cramp relief, second only to the potassium-rich banana. Although studies have not assessed whether dietary or supplemental calcium affects exercise-associated cramping in athletes, a recent report found that calcium supplementation was ineffective for treating pregnancy-associated leg cramps (despite evidence that women experience fewer leg cramps after treatment with calcium supplementation).[30] On the other hand, anecdotal reports from athletes are common. Nancy Clark tells of a hiker who resolved muscle cramps by taking calcium-rich Tums and of a ballet dancer whose cramping disappeared after adding milk and yogurt to her diet.[21] Because calcium intake can be low in the diet of some vegans and vegetarians, inadequate calcium should also be ruled out in vegetarians experiencing muscle cramps.

Magnesium

In addition to its role in bone health, magnesium plays an important role in stabilizing adenosine triphosphate (ATP), the energy source for muscle contraction, and also serves as an electrolyte in body fluids. Muscle weakness, muscle twitching, and muscle cramps are common symptoms of magnesium deficiency.

Limited data have suggested that magnesium status is indirectly related to the incidence of muscle cramps in endurance athletes. In these studies, blood magnesium concentrations were found to be significantly lower in cyclists who cramped during a 100-mile (160 km) bike ride[17] and significantly higher in runners who cramped during an ultradistance race.[15] In both studies, serum magnesium remained within the normal range for athletes who cramped, but was low-normal in the cyclists and high-normal in the runners. Studies in pregnant women have found that, like calcium, magnesium supplementation taken orally for two to four weeks did not consistently reduce the frequency of leg cramps compared with placebo or no treatment.[30] Research has not yet addressed whether dietary or supplemental magnesium can prevent or reduce muscle cramps in athletes.

Vegetarian athletes are not likely to experience muscle cramping as a result of low magnesium intake because the typical vegetarian diet is abundant in magnesium. Low magnesium intake, however, is possible in athletes who restrict calories or eat a diet low in whole foods and high in processed foods. Thus, low magnesium intake should still be ruled out in athletes prone to muscle cramping. Table 11.2 lists the 20 best vegetarian sources of magnesium. A more extensive list is found in table 6.1 on page 88.

Carbohydrate

Inadequate carbohydrate stores have also been implicated as a potential cause of muscle cramps. Although it makes some sense that hard-working muscles might experience cramping in association with the depletion of the power source—carbohydrate—little evidence to date supports a benefit of consuming carbohydrate for the prevention of muscle cramps. For example, a controlled hydration study in men with a history of exercise-associated muscle cramps found that a carbohydrate–electrolyte beverage did not prevent cramps when participants performed calf-fatiguing exercises in the heat.[12] Nevertheless, while all athletes should consider the recommendations presented earlier to optimize performance, athletes with a history of cramping during prolonged exercise should ensure that they consume adequate carbohydrate during exer-

TABLE 11.2   Top 20 Plant-Based Sources of Magnesium

Food	Portion	Value (mg)
Spinach, frozen	1 cup cooked	156
Pumpkin seeds	1 oz	151
Soybeans	1 cup cooked	148
White beans	1 cup cooked	134
All-Bran cereal (Kellogg's)	1/2 cup	109
Green soybeans	1 cup cooked	108
Brazil nuts	1 cup cooked	107
Lima beans, frozen	1 cup cooked	101
Beet greens	1 cup cooked	98
Navy beans	1 cup cooked	96
Okra, sliced	1 cup cooked	94
Baking chocolate, unsweetened	1 square (28 g)	93
Southern peas, black-eyed and crowder	1 cup cooked	91
Oat bran muffin	1 medium (57 g)	89
Pinto and great northern beans	1 cup cooked	86
Buckwheat groats, toasted	1 cup cooked	86
Brown rice	1 cup cooked	84
Raisin Bran cereal (Kellogg's)	1 cup	80
Kidney beans	1 cup cooked	80
Almonds and cashews	1 oz	78-79

Note: Refer to appendix F for guidance on converting English units to metric.

Data from report by single nutrient for magnesium, USDA Food Composition Databases (https://ndb.nal.usda.gov/ndb/nutrients/index).

cise and in the days before and days following an endurance event because carbohydrate consumption provides other benefits (see chapter 3 for a review).

Checking Your Diet

If you have a history of muscle cramps—either nocturnal or exercise induced—a first step may be a nutrition check to ensure that your diet is not contributing to the cramps (see box 11.2). While the latest evidence suggests that cramps most commonly occur in athletes who work their muscles to exhaustion, they can also occur in association with hypohydration and electrolyte imbalances,[31]

Box 11.2

Ruling Out Nutritional Causes of Cramps

Nutrition may be involved in nocturnal or exercise-associated muscle cramps. Although the following nutrition tips are not guaranteed to resolve this malady, they should help ensure that a poor diet does not contribute to the underlying cause of cramping. Keep in mind that dietary change may not immediately resolve cramps.

- Follow the guidelines for fluid intake before, during, and after exercise (see chapter 9). Both too little and too much fluid can potentially induce muscle cramps.

- Consume enough sodium in your diet to replace what is lost through sweat. Vegetarian athletes eating mostly whole and unprocessed foods and who do not salt their food may risk low sodium intake. Salt intake during exercise may be beneficial for salty sweaters or when undergoing prolonged exercise in the heat. The American College of Sports Medicine suggests that sodium ingestion be considered during exercise in athletes with high sweat rates (>1.2 L/hr), salty sweat, or exercise sessions exceeding two hours.[31]

- Eat an abundant amount of fresh fruits and vegetables—not just bananas. The plant-based diet is typically rich in potassium, but people who eat poorly or who take laxatives or diuretics may have poor potassium status.

- Obtain calcium from a variety of plant sources and, if appropriate, dairy sources. Plant foods that are rich in easily absorbed calcium include low-oxalate, green, leafy vegetables (collard, mustard, and turnip greens), tofu set with calcium, fortified soy and rice milks, textured vegetable protein, tahini, certain legumes, fortified orange juice, almonds, and blackstrap molasses. (Refer to chapter 6 for more information.)

- Eat a diet packed with whole grains, nuts, seeds, and legumes. Although vegetarian athletes may be at an advantage when it comes to dietary magnesium intake, athletes who eat diets high in refined foods should watch their intake of magnesium. Plant foods that are rich in magnesium include seeds, nuts, legumes, unmilled cereal grains, dark-green vegetables, and dark chocolate. Refined foods and dairy products tend to be low in magnesium.

- Consume ample carbohydrate both in your overall diet and in association with exercise (as discussed in chapters 3 and 9). Muscles depleted of their carbohydrate stores may be more likely to cramp.

- Consume adequate energy. Insufficient energy consumption can compromise your intake of important electrolytes, including potassium, calcium, and magnesium.

- If you experience cramps regularly, keep a cramping journal. Document food and fluid intake as well as training status. This journal may help a sports dietitian or physician determine the cause of and treatment for your cramping. Ingesting sport products with TRP channel agonists[13] such as HotShot may also be worth a try.

affecting athletes who experience heavy sodium losses through sweating,[19] and well-conditioned athletes for no apparent reason. Paying attention to the timing and pattern of cramping can be helpful. Cramps associated with dehydration typically occur in the latter parts of prolonged exercise or at the beginning of an event if the athlete begins exercise partially dehydrated. Dehydration-induced cramps often begin with small spasms and tend to occur on both sides of the body.[25] In contrast, muscle cramps that are associated with fatigue or overexertion usually come on more suddenly, with consistent cramping of a specific muscle on one side of the body (e.g., solely the right calf). Technically, cramps caused by a deficiency of sodium, calcium, or magnesium could occur any time and not necessarily during exercise.

Although making improvements in your diet will never hurt—and may in the long run help you improve your overall health and performance—making these improvements is not guaranteed to prevent muscle cramping. I worked with a former training partner who began to experience severe calf cramps during running but not cycling. The cramps started suddenly sometime in her early 30s and did not appear to be related to poor conditioning or a change in her training. Despite trying everything imaginable—nutritionally and otherwise—she finally gave up running only to find herself placing in master's cycling events. Oddly, she never experienced a cramp during cycling.

My colleagues and I also worked with an indoor-fitness enthusiast who taught the toughest spinning class I have ever taken. Despite being in awesome shape, he could not exercise outdoors without his quadriceps locking up. Many times he had to hobble home because his cramps would not let up. After assessing him in the lab, we came to the conclusion that his cramping was related to malignant hyperthermia (MH), a rare genetic condition characterized by an abnormal release of calcium from its storage site in muscle, the sarcoplasmic reticulum. Although his sister had been diagnosed with MH, discovering that the condition was the cause of his cramping was beneficial because people with MH can experience severe reactions during anesthesia, including muscle rigidity, increased body temperature, metabolic acidosis, and even death.[32] Nothing could be done to his diet to improve his condition. In addition to MH, other genetic and metabolic disorders that can result in exercise-associated cramping in seemingly fit athletes include a deficiency of muscle carnitine palmitoyltransferase[33] (the enzyme that helps escort fat into the mitochondria for oxidation) and myotonia.[34]

Inflammation and Injury 101

Inflammation is something every athlete has experienced. We know it as redness, swelling, and pain, but it is technically an immune response that helps our bodies repair injuries, get rid of irritants, and fight off diseases. Without the inflammatory response, the body would not be able to protect itself from infection, repair damaged tissue, and begin healing. During an inflammatory response, the immune system quickly responds to signs of injury or infection—

which could include broken cell parts and spilled cell constituents—by sending out its special immune cell army; this results in the accumulation of fluid along with a variety of immune cells.

Tissue damage that results from a sport injury typically involves local and short-lived inflammation, which in some cases can become long term or chronic. Tissue damaged in response to injury recruits white blood cells traveling through blood to the scene of the injury (see figure 11.1). The immune system then activates other types of immune cells. Many of these cells contain and secrete tissue-remodeling agents that play a role in healing, while others stimulate blood clotting to halt bleeding or gently pry open the tissue so it can begin to sew itself back together and close up a wounded area. Acute inflammatory reactions can be painful because swollen tissue compresses nerves and because chemical messengers activate nerve cells and communicate to the brain that the injury hurts. The purpose of pain, of course, is to get you to pamper your injured area a bit so it can heal, but we all know how well that works in athletes. Once the cause is resolved, the inflammation usually subsides. In cases such as joint stress in osteoarthritis or the autoimmune response with rheumatoid arthritis, the inflammation reaction continues out of control and can cause tissue damage rather than repair.

Chronic inflammation can develop if the irritation (such as overuse or overtraining) is ignored or not resolved. For example, think about how many times athletes run through shin splints or continue to throw with a sore shoulder. These injuries are often termed overuse injuries and typically result from continued athletic activities despite the presence of symptoms associated with previous injury or inadequate rehabilitation.[35] They also may appear following alterations in the athlete's equipment or clothing (including shoes) or an abrupt increase in training volume or intensity. The immune system is also involved in chronic inflammation, but in this case it is more low-grade and chronic and can break down tissues and result in a weakening of cartilage, tendon, muscle, and bone.

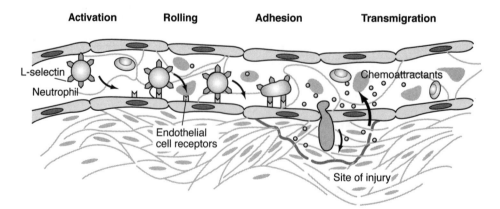

FIGURE 11.1   Tissue damaged in response to any type of injury (including a sport-related injury) recruits white blood cells traveling through blood to the scene of the injury. Illustrated here is the activation of a type of white blood cell called neutrophils that then move into the injured tissue in response to chemical signals. This process is important for tissue healing.

Overall, chronic, unchecked inflammation from any cause is not desired. On the whole-body level, it is a common underlying factor in many chronic diseases, including arthritis, Alzheimer's disease, diabetes, heart disease, and cancer.[36-38]

Diet and Inflammation

Given what we know about inflammation, an important question is whether diet can influence how your body reacts to acute inflammation from a sport injury or more chronic inflammation from an overuse injury. Although no one would expect good nutrition to prevent an ankle sprain or a contact contusion, it is possible that the type of foods you consume could potentially help control the inflammatory response that occurs after the ankle is sprained or the body bruised from contact, perhaps allowing injured tissues to heal faster or more completely. It also might help control the reaction to more chronic overuse injury. Nutrients that might be involved—and therefore deserve a nutrition check—include the omega-3 fatty acids (or the ratio of omega-6 to omega-3 fatty acids), vitamin D, and the anti-inflammatory phytochemicals found in plant foods and seasonings (see box 11.3). Interestingly, since the publication of the first edition of this book, the concept of the anti-inflammatory diet was born.[39] This diet encourages careful selection of foods that are anti-inflammatory in nature while avoiding foods that are proinflammatory. This diet focuses on whole, plant-based foods that are rich in healthy fats and phytonutrients, along with increased plant proteins, small amounts of natural meats if desired, decreased processed carbohydrate, and the avoidance of overconsumption of calories.[39] Sounds just like the focus of this book doesn't it?

Omega-3 Fatty Acids

As discussed in chapter 4, both omega-3 and omega-6 fatty acids are used to create a family of signaling molecules called *eicosanoids* (and include the prostaglandins). The eicosanoids are important and potent controllers of many body functions, including inflammation and immune function.[39] The signaling molecules created from omega-3 fatty acids, however, behave differently than those created from the omega-6 fatty acids. Those created from the omega-3s direct blood vessels to dilate, encourage blood to stay fluid, and reduce the inflammation response, whereas those created from the omega-6s (particularly arachidonic acid found in eggs, meat, and dairy) promote blood clotting, constrict blood vessels, and encourage inflammation. Overall, the type of inflammatory response is determined by the type of fat consumed in the diet. Research has shown that increasing the omega-3 fatty acids in the diet, particularly the longer-chain eicosapentaenoic and docosahexaenoic acids, reduces the production of and tissue response to aggressive inflammatory-response cellular signals, called cytokines.[43] These cytokines control the wide range of symptoms associated with trauma and infection and are thought to promote the inflammation associated with a variety of ailments including arthritis, inflammatory bowel disease, and asthma.

Although omega-3s are thought to reduce inflammation and lower the risk for many age-related diseases, it is not known whether they affect nagging athletic injuries. A recent study of exercise-trained men found that supplementation with about 4 grams of omega-3s (as EPA and DHA) for six weeks decreased inflammation biomarkers at rest, but not following an intense treadmill climb.[44] Studies in individuals with rheumatoid arthritis have also shown that regularly consuming 2 to 3 grams of omega-3 fats helps decrease joint tenderness and swelling;[45,46] the effect seemed to be improved by including olive oil and limiting arachidonic acid found in animal products. Thus, at the moment, the benefit of incorporating more omega-3s in the diet or as supplements for exercise-associated inflammation is limited. Nonetheless, if you are prone to inflammatory injuries, it may not hurt to give it a try for a month or two. Even if bumping up the omega-3s in your diet at the expense of the omega-6s has no effect on your nagging injuries, it may provide other health benefits. It is hard to predict where you might feel the effects of increased omega-3 intake, but it could have an impact anywhere you experience inflammation, including your joints, muscles, or tendons.

Practically speaking, the easiest way to improve your ratio of omega-6 to omega-3 fatty acids is to strive to include two or more servings every day of foods that supply omega-3 fats and limiting—as much as possible—foods high in omega-6 fats: oils made from corn, safflower, sunflower, and cottonseed and dairy products, eggs, and meats (if you are consuming even small amounts), which are high in arachidonic acid. A serving of omega-3 fats is one teaspoon of flaxseed oil, two teaspoons of canola oil or soybean oil, one tablespoon of ground flaxseed, or a quarter-cup of walnuts.[47] Other good sources of omega-3 fatty acids can be found in table 11.3 (also see figure 4.5 on page 63). If you decide to bump up those omega-3s at the expense of the omega-6s, keep in mind that dietary changes may not produce immediate results because it takes time to significantly alter the fatty-acid composition of your cell membranes through diet, which is the fat storage source used to make inflammatory markers.

Vitamin D

In addition to its major influence on bone, vitamin D also plays a role in modulating the body's inflammatory and immune responses.[48] Vitamin D exerts its anti-inflammatory effect by blocking production of inflammatory cytokines (at the gene level) and regulating the function of certain inflammatory cells.[49] Because of this, vitamin D may be important in maintaining healthy muscles and joints over the long haul and aiding in controlling chronic joint inflammation. As with the case of the omega-3s, few studies have addressed the importance of vitamin D in inflammation during acute or chronic sport injuries in athletes. While some[50] but not all studies[51,52] in athletes have found associations between decreased vitamin D status and increased markers of inflammation, only a few provide evidence that either maintaining adequate vitamin D status or vitamin D supplementation is beneficial for injury prevention in a variety of sports, including swimming, football, and ballet dancing.[52,53,54] To date, however, the

TABLE 11.3 Plant Sources Rich in Omega-3 Fatty Acids

Food	Portion	Total fat (g)	Omega-6 (g)	Omega-3 (g)
Canola oil	1 tbsp	14	2.8	1.3
Camelina oil	NA	—	—	—
Chia seeds	2 tbsp	9.2	1.7	5.3
Flaxseed	2 tbsp	8.2	1.0	4.3
Flaxseed oil	1 tbsp	13.6	1.7	7.3
Hemp seed oil[a]	1 tbsp	14	2.5	7.0
Soybean oil	1 tbsp	13.6	6.9	0.9
Walnuts, English[b]	7 halves (14 g)	9.2	5.4	1.3
Walnut oil[b]	1 tbsp	13.6	7.2	1.4
COMMERCIAL PRODUCTS[c]				
Flax Plus Multibran Flakes (Nature's Path)	3/4 cup	1.5	N/A	0.5
Flax Plus Waffle (Nature's Path)	2 waffles (78 g)	9	—	1.0
Flax and soy granola cereal, (Zoe's)	1/2 cup	5	N/A	2.2

Note: Use these values to convert English measurements to metric: 1 tbsp = 14.2 g; 1 cup = about 230 g (see appendix F).

[a]Obtained from product label; information not contained on USDA nutrient database.

[b]English walnuts, but not black walnuts, are a good source of omega-3 fatty acids.

[c]Commercial products with added flax or hemp are becoming available in local, national, and international markets.

Data from reports by single nutrient, USDA Food Composition Databases (https://ndb.nal.usda.gov/ndb/nutrients/index).

best evidence supporting a beneficial effect of vitamin D on inflammation in athletes comes from a clinical trial, which intentionally induced muscular injury in a randomly selected leg of seven young men with sufficient vitamin D status and six men with insufficient status.[55] The most interesting finding was that sufficient vitamin D status increased the anti-inflammatory response to the muscle injury. While additional research is needed, these results suggest that maintaining vitamin D status may be important in healing and rehabilitation after an injury by increasing the body's anti-inflammatory responses.

It is not known how much vitamin D is needed to help keep the body's inflammatory system in check. The Vitamin D Council recommends that blood concentrations of 25-hydroxyvitamin D be maintained above 80 nanomoles per liter (approximately 30 ng/ml), which can be accomplished by sensible sun exposure (usually 5-30 min of exposure to the torso, arms, and legs two or three times a week depending on skin tone)[56] or regular intake of foods fortified with vitamin D or supplements[48] (see chapter 6). Vitamin D supplementation at the level of 1,500 to 2,000 international units per day[57] might be worth trying if you are experiencing muscle inflammation or bone, joint, or tendon problems, including swelling and stiffness. (See chapter 6 for additional information on vitamin D.)

Anti-Inflammatory Agents

Many plant products—including fruits, vegetables, plant oils, and herbs—contain specific nutrients or phytochemicals that may have antioxidant as well as anti-inflammatory properties. Antioxidants—including vitamins C and E—protect body tissues, which include muscles and joints, against free radical

---

Box 11.3

Nutrition Tips for Reducing Inflammation

- Strive to improve the ratio of omega-6 to omega-3 fatty acids in your diet by consuming at least two servings of foods that supply omega-3 fats every day and limiting your intake of omega-6-rich corn, safflower, sunflower, and cottonseed oils as well as arachidonic-rich animal products including industrial-raised eggs and meat products. Omega-3-rich foods are listed in table 11.3 and include walnuts and flax, chia, camelina, canola, and hemp seeds and their oils, as well as commercially available products with added flax. If omega-3 supplements are desired (at least temporarily), look for vegan versions derived from microalgae.[40]

- Maintain adequate levels of vitamin D, either by spending time outside in the sun or through supplementation (see box 6.1 on page 100). Vitamin D supplementation of 2,000 international units per day might be worth trying if you experience bone, joint, or tendon problems, including swelling and stiffness.

- Consume a diet rich in fruits, vegetables, fresh herbs, and spices[39,41] (see box 11.4). One source suggests that about two-thirds of the volume of the diet should come from vegetables and fruits.[42] When experiencing inflammation from a nagging sport injury, try green or white tea, ginger tea, turmeric-rich East Asian food, basil pesto, dark-cherry and pomegranate juices, and other foods naturally high in anti-inflammatory compounds, including polyphenols (which give fruits and vegetables their vibrant colors).

- Drink tea instead of coffee. Although there is nothing wrong with coffee, tea contains antioxidants and polyphenols that may contribute to reducing inflammation. Although black, green, and white teas all contain phytonutrients, green and white teas have the highest levels. Tea should be made with near-boiling (not boiling) water.

- Select whole-grain carbohydrates that contain all their original parts (bran, germ, and endosperm) and limit their refined counterparts. Fiber-containing, whole grains induce a lower insulin response and reduce inflammatory markers in the blood.

- Avoid excess alcohol consumption. While a little wine or microbrew may provide some health benefits, excess alcohol consumption can increase inflammatory markers in the blood.[39]

- Stay tuned for more research!

damage and possibly also age-related degeneration (see chapter 8 for review). Anti-inflammatory agents, on the other hand, block or reduce the inflammatory response, acting in a manner that is either similar to or different from the action of nonsteroidal anti-inflammatory agents, aspirin, and ibuprofen[64] (see box 11.4). While many identified and yet to be identified components of plants may exhibit these properties, mounting evidence suggests that polyphenols—which are prevalent in fruits, vegetables, and teas—play an important role in reducing inflammation.[39] Polyphenols neutralize free radicals and also activate gene-transcription factors that inhibit activation of a signaling molecule called *NF-kB* that activates inflammation.

It is not yet known whether dietary antioxidants or anti-inflammatory agents can help prevent or reduce symptoms associated with sport or overuse injuries. A recent study found that mice fed an anti-inflammatory diet recovered faster from an inflammatory injury than did mice fed a standard American diet.[60] The anti-inflammatory diet contained a variety of plant-based components, including epigallocatechin gallate, sulforaphane, resveratrol, curcumin and ginseng, which have been shown to have anti-inflammatory properties. Epigallocatechin gallate is found mainly in tea, whereas resveratrol is found in red grape skins, grape juice, and red wine, and curcumin is found in the spice turmeric. Recent studies of athletes also support the possible effectiveness of curcumin supplementation (at a dose of ~ 5 g per day) to reduce inflammation, muscle damage, and delayed-onset muscle soreness.[61] Similarly, tart cherry juice has been shown to decrease muscle damage and inflammatory markers following intense resistance and endurance exercise.[62,63] Studies in patients with inflammatory conditions such as diabetes, metabolic syndrome, and arthritis, also suggest benefits from a variety of other plant foods including pomegranate juice, ginger, garlic, green tea, cayenne, oregano, and cat's claw.[41,64,65] Because

---

Vegan View: Beets and Chocolate for the Win!

Beets are a unique source of betanin and vulgaxanthin, two examples of the phytochemical group betalains, which have anti-inflammatory and antioxidant properties. They are why beets are such a beautiful, dark-red color. Beets also supply naturally occurring, nonsynthetic nitrates that are converted to nitric oxide, which increases vasodilation. With wider blood vessels, more oxygen-rich blood flows through the body and reaches muscles sooner, allowing them to work at a high intensity for longer periods. Increased blood flow also helps to dissipate the heat created during physical activity.

Chocolate is made from the cacao bean, a plant food exceptionally rich in phytochemicals. According to a Harvard study, cacao increases blood flow because of the positive effect of flavanols, a subgroup of phytochemicals, on the nitric oxide system.[58] The theobromine in cacao may also increase vasodilation. Dark chocolate may increase physical performance through this mechanism.[59] Dark chocolate is also an excellent source of magnesium; yet another reason for athletes to love it.

learning about each of these plant foods can be daunting, your best bet is to ensure that your diet is rich in a variety of fruits and vegetables, including tomato products[66,] and contains olive oil[67] and fresh herbs and spices. Giving green tea, ginger tea, tart cherry juice, and dishes with turmeric, basil, and olive oil a try may not hurt. Beyond that, stay tuned for the research to evolve. It may be that following a plant-based diet rich in colorful fruits and vegetables accompanied by a variety of herbs is already an anti-inflammatory diet. (See table 3.4 on page 42 for a list of phytochemicals found in fruits and vegetables of a variety of colors).

If you are prone to muscle cramps or muscle or joint inflammation, you can use the information in this chapter to make diet choices that may help prevent or alleviate them. The next chapter discusses how you can incorporate all the information covered so far into a healthy plant-based meal plan.

Box 11.4

Herbs and Plant Products Considered to Have Anti-Inflammatory Properties

- Basil
- Oregano
- Olive oil, which contains oleocanthal in newly pressed extra-virgin versions
- Willow bark, which contains salicin, the chemical in aspirin
- Pomegranate fruit
- Tart cherry juice (Montmorency cherries)
- Green tea (epigallocatechin-3-gallate)
- Cat's claw
- Hot peppers, including cayenne (capsaicin)
- Thunder god vine
- Turmeric (curcumin)
- Ginseng
- Grape skins (including certain grape products such as wine)
- Ginger
- Tomatoes and tomato-based drinks
- Red onion, kale, chokeberry, cranberry, apples (quercetin)

This list of plant and herb products that may have anti-inflammatory properties is not meant to be inclusive nor be an endorsement for product use. It was compiled from various sources.[60-69]

12 | **Creating a Customized Meal Plan**

The women's athletic trainer asked me to see a 22-year-old tennis player to determine whether her weakness, fatigue, and history of frequent infections were related to her diet. Like several of the vegetarian athletes I had worked with, she was from Germany. She had a hearty appetite and reported eating a diet that consisted mostly of bagels with European cheese, potatoes, rice, pasta, cereal, dense crusty bread (when she could get it), and lots of vegetables. She said she consumed at least two servings of dairy products a day but typically ate fruit only in the morning. She was also a coffee drinker and admitted to recently adding a little fish to her diet to see if it would help her fatigue. She had no interest in taking a multivitamin (as recommended by her coach). Despite her fatigue and regular infections, she denied any real detriment to her playing record.

Although her eating habits were not too bad, her meal plan needed revising. Without a doubt she was getting ample carbohydrate, but I was a little concerned about her protein, iron, and zinc intake. Because results from a routine blood analysis were pending—and would have provided only a basic screening for anemia—I could not directly pinpoint whether her diet was the cause of her frequent infections. I could, however, work with her to customize a meal plan that would better provide all of the essential nutrients. In her case this meant improving the overall nutritional quality of her diet by incorporating legumes, nuts, fruit, and powerhouse vegetables, such as leafy greens and orange and red vegetables, and limiting coffee to one or two cups (236-472 ml) daily. In my nutrition note, I documented that we had reviewed a vegetarian eating plan emphasizing easy ways to add fruit and plant-protein foods to her current plan.

–Enette

The task of eating well can be daunting for many athletes. There are too many nutrients to consider—or at least it often seems that way—along with the additional nutrition guidelines for athletes. You need enough carbohydrate to fuel high-intensity activity, enough protein to build body tissue, including muscle, and enough but not too much energy in the form of calories. You also need the right balance of dietary fat and an adequate intake of calcium, iron, iodine, zinc, riboflavin, vitamin C, vitamin K, and many other vitamins and trace minerals. On top of that you need to think about all those phytochemicals. Or do you?

Quite honestly, what you need is a game plan: a meal plan upon which to build a healthy diet to ensure that you get enough of the right kinds of macronutrients (carbohydrate, fat, and protein), micronutrients (vitamins and minerals), and phytochemicals. The meal plan should be the framework for establishing a healthy eating pattern for a busy vegetarian athlete and then set you free to eventually eat well intuitively. Indeed, the purpose of this chapter is to help you put together all the pieces discussed in this book to come up with a customized eating plan for yourself. The remaining step, which will be covered in chapters 14 and 15, is learning how to whip up simple meals and snacks that fit into your customized game plan.

Pieces of a Healthy Diet

Various eating plans have been developed to teach people how to meet nutrient needs through good food choices. These food guidance systems have been available in the United States since before the 1930s and have included the basic seven food groups (the basic seven has three fruit and vegetable groups classified by color: green/yellow, orange/red and all other), the basic four food groups, the USDA Food Guide Pyramids, and now USDA's MyPlate.[1] Although most food guidance systems developed by the government or private entities were designed for an average citizen, not an athlete, we can borrow and easily customize a plan for vegetarian athletes from any of the available food guidance systems designed for the general population (such as MyPlate), athletes, or vegetarians (see figures 12.1 and 12.2 and appendix B). The design of the USDA's MyPlate in particular emphasizes that one size does not fit all.[2] Before we begin, however, it is important to first understand the pieces that contribute to a healthy diet: food groups and variety.

Why Food Groups?

In my earlier days as a nutritionist, I failed to recognize the importance of food groups. I was disturbed by some of the categories: the meat group for obvious reasons and the fruit and vegetable groups, which incorrectly categorize many fruits—including tomatoes, squash, and pumpkin—as vegetables. It was not until I taught my first college-level sports nutrition course to exercise science and health promotion students that it hit me—during my own lecture—just how ingenious this system is. Maybe you are a faster learner than I was, but foods grouped within each category contain similar key nutrients (see table

12.1). Although some variability exists among the different foods in each category, this system *guides* people to select a variety of foods from each group to meet their nutrient needs so that they can enjoy eating rather than trying to remember which foods provide B vitamins, protein, or iron, for instance.

The estimated number of servings from each category was initially determined based on how much food from each food group people need to consume to meet daily nutrient needs, and more recently to reduce risk of many chronic diseases. Taking fruit and vegetables as an example, consuming the recommended number of servings of fruits and vegetables daily helps ensure the needs for vitamins A and C and fiber are met. It also helps reduce risk for chronic diseases such as heart disease and certain cancers. If fruits and vegetables alone made up the bulk of your diet (or your calories) instead of grains, you might lack B vitamins, iron, and zinc even though you would get ample carbohydrate, fiber, and vitamins C and A. Therefore, you need to choose foods from each food group and use them to build and create individual meals and snacks.

Admittedly, I am not enthralled with the category names and mandatory inclusion of the dairy group—because they are somewhat limited for vegans and vegetarians—but I do find that the food categories in general make considerable sense. Basically, the grain group includes cereals, bread, pasta, rice, and all other whole or milled grain or grass products (quinoa, wild rice, kamut), which provide carbohydrate, some protein, iron, potassium, zinc, copper, thiamin, niacin, riboflavin, folate, vitamin B_6, biotin, and vitamin E. The protein group (also

---

Vegan View: Are All Vegan Foods Healthy?

There's an incredible movement afoot to replace foods that are traditionally from animals, like burgers, mayo, milk, and yogurt, with plant-based versions. Just 10 years ago, it would have been hard to imagine that pizza shops would carry vegan cheese or you could order a tasty, meatlike burger at a pub or bar. This is good news in terms of using fewer animals for food, but the impact these foods could have on our collective health is unknown. Does replacing a regular cheesesteak with a vegan version improve health outcomes? No research has looked closely at this just yet, but Harvard researchers, using a cohort of 200,000 health professionals, found that a healthier plant-based diet had a greater reduction in risk for type 2 diabetes, than a less-healthy one. Even a small reduction of animal food intake reduced risk, but those who ate a diet with a higher healthy index eating score (meaning more whole grains, fruits, and vegetables), had the biggest reduction.[15] This suggests that just because something is vegan, such as a burger or pizza, doesn't mean it's healthy. Despite originating from plants, most of these products are not whole foods and have lost many of the compounds associated with the benefits of whole plant foods. That doesn't mean that vegan comfort foods can't be part of a healthy diet. They can! But if eating a nutrient and phytochemical dense diet for good health and longevity is your goal, the emphasis must still be on whole foods. It's important to know the fat, calorie, and salt content of these new products, so be sure to check the nutrition label and adjust your choices as needed. And think of comfort foods as complements to, not the focus of, your overall eating plan.

TABLE 12.1   Key Nutrients Provided by the Food Categories Used in Most Food Guidance Systems

Category	Nutrients provided by group	Food and typical servings
Grains	Carbohydrate Protein (some) Minerals: iron, potassium, zinc, copper, selenium,* iodine* Vitamins: thiamin, niacin, riboflavin, folate, B_6, biotin, E Phytonutrients Whole grains also provide fiber, magnesium, chromium, vitamin E.	**1 equivalent =** 1 slice (1 oz) bread 1/2 cup cooked grain, rice, or pasta 1 oz ready-to-eat cereal 1 biscuit, small pancake, or minibagel
Vegetables	Carbohydrate (starchy vegetables) Fiber Minerals: iron, potassium, zinc, selenium,* iodine* Vitamins: A and carotenoids, C, folate, K Phytonutrients Dark-green leafy vegetables also provide riboflavin, vitamin B_6, magnesium.	**By MyPlate** 1 cup vegetables = 1 cup raw or cooked vegetable or juice 2 cups raw leafy greens **By other food guides** 1/2 cup cooked = 1 cup raw
Fruits	Carbohydrate fiber Vitamins: A and carotenoids, B_6, C, folate (selected fruits) Phytonutrients	**1/2 cup fruit =** 1 small to medium-sized fruit 1/2 cup cut fruit or fruit juice 1/4 cup dried fruit
Milk	Protein Minerals: calcium, iodine, potassium Vitamins: riboflavin, B_{12}, biotin, A, D (fortified)	1 cup milk, yogurt, or soy milk 1-1/2 oz natural cheese 2 oz processed cheese 1-1/2 cup ice cream
Meat (for comparison)	Protein Minerals: iron, zinc Vitamins: thiamin, niacin, B_6, B_{12}	1 oz any type of meat
Beans (legumes) and meat analogues	Protein Minerals: calcium, iron, magnesium, potassium, zinc, copper, molybdenum Vitamins: folate, thiamin, niacin, riboflavin, B_6, biotin	**1 protein equivalent =** 1/2 cup cooked legumes (MyPlate uses 1/4 cup) 1/2 cup tofu or tempeh (MyPlate uses 1/4 cup [2 oz] tofu or 1 oz tempeh) 1 oz meat analogue 1 egg 1 oz cheese
Nuts	Protein fiber (some) Minerals: iron, calcium, magnesium, zinc, copper, chromium, selenium* Vitamins: folic acid, E, other tocopherols Essential fatty acids: linoleic acid, linolenic acid	**1 protein equivalent =** 1 oz nuts or seeds (~ 2 tbsp) or 2 tbsp nut or seed butter (MyPlate uses 1/2 ounce nuts and seeds and 1 tbsp nut or seed butters)
Healthy oils	Essential fatty acids: linoleic acid, linolenic acid, Vitamin E	1 tsp

Note: Refer to appendix F for guidance on converting English units to metric.

*Content of selenium and iodine varies significantly depending on the content of the soil.

Serving sizes obtained from MyPlate (2), the Vegetarian Food Guide Pyramid (3), and the national nutrient database as outlined in previous tables in this book.

called the meat and bean group in some guidance systems) provides protein, along with iron, zinc, thiamin, niacin, and vitamins B_6 and B_{12}. The fruit group is divided from the vegetable group based on their carbohydrate and general nutrient profile, which are slightly different. The only group whose inclusion is arguable is the dairy group because certain foods from each of the other categories, with the exception of fruit and oil, can contribute significantly to calcium intake (see figure 12.1). Additionally, calcium-rich foods include fortified soy milk and other nondairy alternatives. Dairy foods do however provide a source of riboflavin and vitamin B_{12} for vegetarians. The final group is the leftover group, or discretionary calorie group, which includes sweets, fats, and even sport supplements. MyPlate largely ignores discussing these, which we commonly think of as junk foods. MyPlate also does not officially have an oil group, but it does outline the whole foods that contain oil—including nuts, vegetables, olives, and avocado.

Why Variety?

Although the concept of variety has been discussed in other parts of this book, it is mentioned here briefly to emphasize that the additional piece of a plan for healthy eating includes the selection of a variety of foods from each major food category. Because there are no perfect foods, the variety of components increases an athlete's chance of taking in adequate vitamins, minerals, and phytochemicals. For example, although walnuts are the only nuts high in omega-3 fatty acids, the other nuts provide different oils and alpha and gamma tocopherols (vitamin E derivatives) that also contribute to a healthy diet. Spinach—which is not an absorbable source of calcium—is one of the top sources of folate, vitamin B_6, beta-carotene, lutein, vitamin E, and magnesium. In addition, fruits and vegetables lacking in one type of anti-inflammatory phytochemical may be high in another phytochemical that enhances the body's ability to detoxify cancer-causing agents. Thus, the more variety, the better!

Helpful Models for Vegetarian Athletes

Teaching vegetarian athletes what their meal plan should look like can be a bit more challenging than educating nonvegetarian athletes. First, for vegetarians in general, the framework of what makes up a nutritious meal is not always there—particularly for those who grew up in a meat-centered household where the response to "What's for dinner?" was answered based on the meat being served. Chicken was for dinner rather than chicken, rice pilaf, garden salad, and whole-grain bread. This way of thinking often leaves new vegetarians with the idea that they need to have a meat analogue for dinner and that rice pilaf with almonds and leafy greens cannot stand alone as a meal. My husband is still known to say, "We did not have any protein tonight," and then have to listen as I recall the content of all the protein-rich plant foods in the meal along with the nuts and occasional egg and cheese in the seemingly "no-protein" dishes.

Second and third, no food guidance systems exist specifically for vegetarian athletes, and those that offer options for vegetarian eating can be misleading for athletes who consume little or no dairy. For example, a vegetarian version of a food plan for endurance athletes developed in the 1990s recommends that vegetarian athletes consume 5 to 10 1-cup (236 ml) servings of milk products per day, depending on their energy intake.[4] Yes, this is quite a bit more milk than most vegetarian athletes desire or tolerate. More recent food plate models —whether designed for vegetarians, vegans, or the general population—struggle with where to place the calcium-rich foods and dairy, incorporating them as a circle silhouette at the top right of the plate, where a glass of milk might go (see MyPlate[2] in appendix B) or placing them on the plate itself (see the Athlete's Plate in appendix B). This presents a challenge when educating athletes about calcium, which is found both on the plate as dark-green leafy vegetables such as kale, calcium-set tofu, and yogurt, and in a glass such as soy milk or cows' milk. The Athlete's Plate[6] (see appendix B), developed by the U.S. Olympic Committee (USOC) dietitians and the University of Colorado at Colorado Springs (UCCS) Sports Nutrition Program, lumps low-fat dairy with legumes, nuts, and soy foods as an option on the plate and also includes it as a beverage option at the top of the plate. Although this is a good way to illustrate how calcium-rich foods might be incorporated into the diet, it can be confusing to some athletes.

Food guidance systems designed for vegans[3,5] (see appendix B) or the vegetarian tips offered by MyPlate[7] may model insufficient calories for athletes and also lack flexibility in recognizing that appetite and energy needs can vary according training volume, intensity, and training phase. The USOC and UCCS Athlete's Plate[6] guides provide plate options for easy, moderate, and hard training or game days to help tailor intake of carbohydrate, protein, and fat to training requirements (and they are can be adapted for vegetarians). This might seem like a minor point to the nonathlete, but having the tools to help understand how eating patterns may change according to different stages of training is important. As an example, a 121-pound (55 kg) female endurance athlete in a heavy training phase may have calorie needs similar to those of a 190-pound (86 kg) softball player during her strength-building season. Although they both require 2,800 to 3,000 calories per day, the endurance athlete might need more carbohydrate, which would dictate the servings of carbohydrate-rich grains and fruits and starchy vegetables, and the softball player might need a bit more protein. The Athlete's Plate model allows the endurance athlete to choose the plate for hard training and the softball player the plate for easy training and weight management.

With that said, however, I have successfully used many of the food guidance systems—including the USDA Food Guide Pyramid (food guidance system before MyPlate), USDA's MyPlate, Great Britain's Eatwell Plate (see appendix B), the Vegetarian Resource Group's My Vegan Plate,[5] the USOC and UCCS Athlete's Plates,[2] and the Vegetarian Food Guide Pyramid published in 2003 by Messina, Melina, and Mangels[3] (see figure 12.1) to help vegetar-

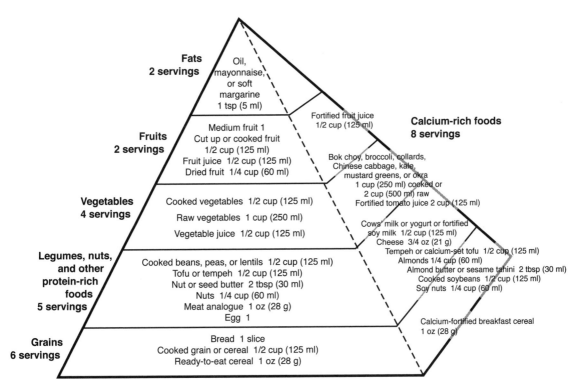

FIGURE 12.1 Vegetarian Food Guide Pyramid.

Reprinted from *Journal of the American Dietetic Association,* vol. 103, Messina et al., "A New Food Guide for North American Vegetarians," pp. 771-775, Copyright 2003, with permission of The Academy of Nutrition and Dietetics.

ian athletes develop a custom plan or to simply fine-tune their current eating plan. Although my current favorites are the USOC and UCCS Athlete's Plates models—which I can easily flip to vegan or vegetarian—I often use MyPlate initially with some athletes because personal plans are readily available online (www.choosemyplate.gov/MyPlatePlan), and I still find myself using the Vegetarian Food Guide Pyramid. MyPlate can be useful for athletes who initially need structure, whereas the three-dimensional aspect of the Vegetarian Food Guide Pyramid is particularly nice for athletes who need specific education on plant-based sources of calcium. Remember that the goal for using a food plate, food pyramid, or even spinning top (see appendix B for international food guidance models including Japan's spinning top) is to provide a framework or set of guidelines to help establish a pattern of healthy eating and learn to eat instinctively. In my experience, one model simply does not fit all.

Customizing Your Meal Plan

Although the various food-plate models and the Vegetarian Food Guide Pyramid each present limitations to vegetarian athletes, they can guide you in customizing your meal plan and learning to eat intuitively. This section discusses how you can use MyPlate, the Vegetarian Food Guide Pyramid, or your favorite food guidance system to put together a custom meal plan. We explain how to adapt the food-plate model for a more intuitive eating approach. If you feel you already have a healthy eating pattern, read on or jump ahead. Toward the end of the chapter, we discuss learning to eat intuitively and how food models such the Athlete's Plates can serve as a visual reminder for making food choices according to your hard and easy training phases or days (and appetite of course). Again, the food guidance systems simply provide a foundational framework for healthy eating—one to help educate yourself about healthy eating or one to come back to if eating habits stray.

Your first step in customizing a meal plan is to estimate your energy needs using one of the methods discussed in chapter 2 and to round your estimate to the nearest 200 calories. It is also helpful to estimate your carbohydrate and protein needs as discussed in chapters 3 and 5. If your training varies drastically from day to day or across the weeks, months, or year, you may also want to estimate calories, carbohydrate, and protein for each of your training phases. The next step is to consult table 12.2 to obtain the recommended number of servings you need to consume from each of the major food groups if using MyPlate (top of table) or the Vegetarian Food Guide Pyramid (bottom of table) as your food model. The daily allowance for the oils, however, is suggested and should not be a concern unless you make high-fat choices for all your food options or completely avoid fat. Remember that oils enhance the flavor of foods, and that fat is an important nutrient (see chapter 4). If your energy needs are greater than 3,000 calories per day, you can use the 3,000-calorie recommendations as a starting point because, as we will discuss later, these servings are an estimate of the *minimum* number of servings needed in each group for a healthy diet. Thus, you will simply follow a 3,000-calorie diet but eat larger portions at each meal or increase your intake of protein-rich or carbohydrate-rich plant foods or healthy oils depending on your training phase and goals. You can also consult table 12.3 if you need ideas for which food groups could be added to extend calories.

In deciding which guidance system to consult, use MyPlate if you regularly consume two to three servings of milk, yogurt, or cheese daily, and the Vegetarian Food Guide Pyramid if you are vegan or consume few milk products. The Athlete's Plate can be your visual model to help understand how your food choices may change with your different training days or phases, as appropriate. Again, one advantage to using MyPlate is that it has an interactive online version that allows you to print out custom worksheets. In fact, if you decide to use MyPlate as your framework, using the downloadable worksheets for a few weeks may be all you need to get on track for intuitive eating. On the other hand, if you prefer another food guidance system in appendix B, use what works best for you.

Once you have an idea of your estimated daily servings from each category, the next step is to begin customizing your plan on paper. An example of a 3,000-calorie diet based on MyPlate is shown in table 12.4, and table 12.5 shows a 3,000-calorie diet based on the Vegetarian Food Guide Pyramid. The

TABLE 12.2 Creating a Meal Plan Using USDA's MyPlate or the Vegetarian Food Guide Pyramid

AMOUNT OF FOOD FROM EACH MAJOR FOOD GROUP, BASED ON MYPLATE, REQUIRED TO SATISFY VARIOUS CALORIC NEEDS FOR ACTIVE VEGETARIANS							
Calories per day	1,800	2,000	2,200	2,400	2,600	2,800	3,000
Grains[b]	6 eq	6 eq	7 eq	8 eq	9 eq	10 eq	10 eq
Vegetables	2-1/2 cups	2-1/2 cups	3 cups	3 cups	3-1/2 cups	3-1/2 cups	4 cups
Fruits	1-1/2 cups	2 cups	2 cups	2 cups	2 cups	2-1/2 cups	2-1/2 cups
Milk	3 cups	3 cups	3 cups	3 cups	3 cups	3 cups	3 cups
Beans and analogues[c]	5 eq	5-1/2 eq	6 eq	6-1/2 eq	6-1/2 eq	7 eq	7 eq
Oils (general)	5-6 tsp	5-6 tsp	5-7 tsp	5-7 tsp	5-7 tsp	5-7 tsp	5-7 tsp
Added sugars (maximum, g)	45	50	55	60	65	70	75
TABULATION							
Carbohydrate range (g)[b]	256	271	288	311	332	352	386
Protein range (g)[c]	78-97	81.5-101	87-108	92.5-115	98.5-124	104-131	106-134
Discretionary calories	195-290	265-310	265-310	265-310	360-510	360-510	360-510

AMOUNT OF FOOD FROM EACH MAJOR FOOD GROUP, BASED ON VEGETARIAN FOOD GUIDE PYRAMID, REQUIRED TO SATISFY VARIOUS CALORIC NEEDS FOR ACTIVE VEGETARIANS							
Grains[b]	6 eq [a]	6 eq	7 eq	8 eq	9 eq	10 eq	10 eq
Vegetables	2 cups	2-1/2 cups	3 cups	3 cups	3-1/2 cups	3-1/2 cups	4 cups
Fruits	2 cups	2 cups	2 cups	2 cups	2 cups	2-1/2 cups	2-1/2 cups
Beans, nuts, and analogues	5 eq	6 eq	6 eq	7 eq	7 eq	8 eq	8 eq
Fat[a]	2	2	2	2	2	2	2
TABULATION							
Carbohydrate range (g)[b]	227.5	247.5	270	292.5	318	355	365
Protein range (g)[c]	63-82	70-90	74-96	83-107	87-113	96-124	99-127

Servings sizes for MyPlate from USDA MyPlate (https://www.choosemyplate.gov/MyPlatePlan).

Note: Serving sizes for the Vegetarian Food Guide Pyramid were modified from the original source by V. Messina, V. Melina, and A. Mangels[3] (see figure 12.1) by adding additional servings of various food groups as energy needs increase and correspond with the serving sizes presented in Table 12.1 for grain equivalents and bean and protein equivalents. Refer to appendix F for guidance on converting English units to metric.

[a]Values in this row for each group are the minimum amounts, according to the Vegetarian Food Guide Pyramid, necessary to meet nutrient needs for nonathlete vegetarians. Vegetarian Food Guide Pyramid fat servings do not increase as calories increase because it is a minimum requirement.

[b]Carbohydrate content is estimated using the methods described in chapter 3, assuming half of the vegetable servings are starchy and half are not, half of the protein servings are from legumes, and half the milk (if appropriate) is from carbohydrate-rich milk or plain yogurt (rather than from cheese). Carbohydrate content under each energy level can be increased by selecting mostly starchy (carbohydrate-rich) vegetables and adding discretionary carbohydrate sources, including simple sugars and sport drinks, bars, and gels.

[c]Protein content is estimated using the methods described in chapter 5, where each protein and milk equivalent provides 7 to 8 grams of protein and each grain and starchy vegetable provides 2 to 3 grams of protein.

TABLE 12.3   Food Combinations That Provide 250 Additional Calories

Combination	Suggested serving	Example	Actual nutrients in example
Bean (protein)	1 equivalent (eq)	1/2 cup black beans	228 kcal
Fruit	1 cup	1 cup pineapple	8 g protein, 5 g fat, 40 g carbohydrate
Healthy oil	1 tsp	1 tsp hemp seed oil	
Bean (protein)	1 eq	1 cup pinto beans	165 kcal
Healthy oil	1/2 tsp	1/2 tsp canola oil	15 g protein, 2.5 g fat, 44 g carbohydrate
Grain	2 eq	1 cup white rice	287 kcal
Nuts	1 oz	1 oz walnuts	6 g protein, 18 g fat, 26 g carbohydrate
Grain	2 eq	2 slices whole-grain bread	222 kcal
Healthy oil	1 tsp	2 tsp trans-fat-free margarine	6 g protein, 11 g fat, 26 g carbohydrate
Starchy vegetable	1 cup	1 large sweet potato	222 kcal
Healthy oil	1 tsp	1 tsp hazelnut oil	9 g protein, 9 g fat, 37 g carbohydrate
Fruit	1 cup	1 cup peaches in own juice	250 kcal
Dairy or soy milk	1 cup	1 cup yogurt	11 g protein, 5 g fat, 40 g carbohydrate
Healthy oil	1 tsp	1 tsp flaxseed oil	
Healthy oil	2 tbsp	1 tbsp olive, flaxseed, or coconut oil	230 kcal
		1 tbsp ground flax seeds	23 g fat

Note: The energy and macronutrient values are approximate and will vary depending on actual food choices. They will also vary depending on the accuracy of portion sizes. Refer to appendix F for guidance on converting English units to metric.

easiest way to start customizing your plan is to start with each group, such as the grain group, and divide the suggested number of servings into meals and snacks. Remember to include the nutrition you'll take in during exercise, if appropriate. Keep in mind that there will be room for added fats and discretionary calories depending on your energy needs. In the sample plan in table 12.4, 3 of the 10 grain equivalents were placed in the breakfast meal, 3 in the lunch meal, and 4 in the dinner meal. If a during- or postexercise carbohydrate-rich snack were needed, another option (not shown) would be to have one less grain at breakfast and dinner, and incorporate two grains as a 30-gram carbohydrate-containing snack. As discussed in chapter 3, each serving of grain provides about 15 grams of carbohydrate.

Once you have placed all of the groups, list several ideas for foods and mixed dishes for each group. This is easier to do when lunch consists of a cheese sandwich made with two slices of bread and either 1.5 ounces (42 g) of cheese and a half-cup tofu (mixed with mustard and onion) instead of vegetable and cheese pizza, minestrone soup, or stir-fry. Because combinations of foods

TABLE 12.4 3,000-Calorie Vegetarian Meal Plan Using MyPlate

Meal	Categories	Suggested serving	Sample plan 1	Sample plan 2
Breakfast	Grain Fruit Milk	3 equivalents (eq) 1/2 cup 1 serving	2 slices whole-wheat toast 1 tbsp no-trans-fat margarine* 1 oz cornflakes 1 medium orange 1 cup skim milk	3 (5-inch) pancakes 1 tbsp no-trans-fat margarine* 2 tbsp maple syrup* 1/2 cup blueberries 1 cup vanilla nonfat yogurt
Morning snack	Fruit Protein	1 cup 1 eq	1/2 cup raisins 1 oz almonds	1 large apple 2 tbsp peanut butter
Lunch	Protein Grain Milk Vegetable	2 eq 3 eq 1 serving 1 cup	Vegetarian burger (60 g) on a large poppy seed bagel 1/2 oz cheddar cheese 2 cups mixed greens 1 tbsp Italian dressing*	1 cup marinated and baked tofu with 1 tsp sesame oil* 1-1/2 cups wild rice 8 oz skim or soy milk 1 cup steamed yellow squash
Afternoon snack	Vegetable	1 cup	1 cup baby carrots 1 tbsp ranch dressing*	1 baked potato topped with 2 tbsp light sour cream*
Dinner	Protein Grain Milk Vegetable	3 eq 4 eq 1 serving 2 cups	1-1/2 cups black beans with 1/2 cup onions 2 cups long-grain rice with 1 tbsp olive oil* and topped with 1/2 cup tomato 1 cup skim milk 1 cup steamed spinach	1-1/2 cup lentil taco mix with 1/2 cup onion 4 (6-inch) tortillas 1 oz cheddar cheese 1/2 cup each tomato, red bell pepper, green bell pepper, and lettuce
Evening snack	Fruit Protein	1 cup 1 eq	1 cup sliced bananas 1 oz walnuts 1/2 cup frozen yogurt*	Large baked pear 1 oz pecans Brown sugar*

Note: Refer to appendix F for guidance on converting English units to metric. Sample meal plan 1 provides about 3,066 kcal (56% carbohydrate, 30% fat, 14% protein), 442 g carbohydrate, 114 g protein, 105 g fat (7% saturated), 4.6 grams omega-3 fats, 1,348 mcg folate, 141 mg vitamin C, 27 IU vitamin E, 1,728 mg calcium, 32 mg iron, 15 mg zinc, and 797 mg magnesium. It also provides more than the RDA for male and female athletes for riboflavin (3.7 mg), vitamin B$_6$ (3.9 mg), and vitamin K (119%) and adequate levels of other trace minerals. Sample meal plan 2 provides about 3,065 kcal (55% carbohydrate, 29% fat, 16% protein), 442 g carbohydrate, 125 g protein, 110 g fat (7% saturated), 2.4 grams omega-3 fats, 1,062 mcg folate, 299 mg vitamin C, 12 IU vitamin E, 2,118 mg calcium, 31 mg iron, 18 mg zinc, 624 mg magnesium and vitamin K (94.7%). It also provides more than the RDA for male and female athletes for riboflavin (2.5 mg), and vitamin B$_6$ (2.9 mg) (94.7%) and adequate levels of other trace minerals.

*Discretionary calorie items

from two or more food groups are common in many diets, you will need to estimate how much of each of the different food types is in the dish to determine how it fits into the food-plate model. We say estimate because it is important to remember that the purpose of this exercise is to learn to eat healthy, not to become obsessed with mixed food items. For example, a slice of vegetable and cheese pizza contains a serving of grain in the crust, a half to a full serving of protein in the cheese, and an eighth-cup or so of vegetables, depending on

TABLE 12.5 3,000-Calorie Vegan Meal Plan Using the Vegetarian Food Guide Pyramid

Meal	Categories	Suggested serving	Sample plan 1	Sample plan 2
Breakfast	Grain Protein Fruit	3 equivalents (eq) 1 eq 1/2 cup	2 slices whole-wheat toast 1 tbsp no-trans-fat margarine* 1 oz cornflakes 1 cup fortified soy milk 1 medium orange	3 (5-inch) pancakes 1 tbsp no-trans-fat margarine* 2 tbsp maple syrup* 1 oz vegetarian sausage 1/2 cup calcium-fortified orange juice
Morning snack	Fruit Protein	1 cup 1 eq	1/2 cup raisins 1 oz almonds	1 large apple 2 tbsp peanut butter
Lunch	Protein Grain Vegetable	2 eq 3 eq 1 cup	Vegetarian burger (60 g) on a large poppy seed bagel 2 cups mixed greens 2 tbsp Italian dressing*	1 cup marinated and baked tofu with 1 tsp sesame oil* 1-1/2 cups wild rice 1 cup steamed yellow squash
Afternoon snack	Vegetable	1 cup	1 cup baby carrots 2 tbsp tofu-based dip*	1 baked potato topped with 2 tbsp soy sour cream*
Dinner	Protein Grain Vegetable	3 eq 4 eq 2 cups	1-1/2 cups black beans 2 cups long-grain rice with 1/2 cup onions and 1 tbsp olive oil* and topped with 1/2 cup tomato 1 cup collard greens	1-1/2 cups lentil taco mix with 1/2 cup onion 4 (6-inch) tortillas 1/2 cup each tomato, red bell pepper, green bell pepper, and lettuce
Evening snack	Fruit Protein	1 cup 1 eq	1 cup sliced bananas 1 oz walnuts 1/2 cup Soy Dream dessert*	Large baked pear 1 oz pecans 1 tbsp brown sugar*
Training snack	Other	—	2 cups fluid-replacement beverage*	1 cup fluid-replacement beverage*

Note: Refer to appendix F for guidance on converting English units to metric.

Sample menu 1 provides about 2,972 kcal (60% carbohydrate, 28% fat, 12% protein), 461 g carbohydrate, 91 g protein, 98.9 g fat (4% saturated), 4.2 g omega-3 fats, 1,258 mcg folate, 151 mg vitamin C, 29 IU vitamin E, 1,125 mg calcium, 29 mg iron, 12 mg zinc, and 630 mg magnesium. It also provides more than the RDA for male and female athletes for riboflavin (1.9 mg), vitamin B_6 (3.1 mg), and vitamin K (114%) and adequate levels of other trace minerals.

Sample menu 2 provides about 3,055 kcal (55% carbohydrate, 31% fat, 13% protein), 434 g carbohydrate, 104 g protein, 112 g fat (5.5% saturated), 3.6 grams omega-3 fats, 991 mcg folate, 320 mg vitamin C, 16.5 IU vitamin E, 1,630 mg calcium, 30 mg iron, 14 mg zinc, and 516 mg magnesium. It also provides more than the RDA for male and female athletes for riboflavin (2.9 mg), vitamin B_6 (3.8 mg), and vitamin K (114%) and adequate levels of other trace minerals.

*Discretionary calorie items

how loaded with vegetables it is. It is also likely to be fairly high in fat and thus contain some discretionary calories.

Learning to properly count mixed foods is easiest if you prepare the foods yourself so you know what went into the recipe and how much of that recipe you had for dinner. And while making your estimates, it is hoped that you will also recognize, based on your individual plan, that if you have pizza, several pieces are best served as a part of a meal consisting of a huge green salad on lighter training days and additional sources of carbohydrate, such as French bread, fruit, or fruit juice on higher training days. If not, count it as one of those treat days and don't be tempted to top off the whole pizza with a soda, multiple beers, and ice cream. Even if these items are vegetarian and you can afford the calories, the meal is not well balanced, even if the pizza includes a variety of vegetables.

In coming up with sample menu ideas, you should also evaluate whether the plan seems reasonable for you (based on your preferences and training schedule) and whether it is too structured. Although most plans specify a greater number of servings of vegetables than fruits because of the lower sugar content and presumed higher nutrient density and phytochemical content of vegetables compared with fruit,[3] the sample 3,000-calorie plans have too many vegetables and not enough fruit for my lifestyle. I have always found it easier to grab several colorful pieces of fruit than to prepare and eat the recommended vegetable servings. I also feel that the argument in favor of more vegetables than fruit is a moot point if you regularly include legumes in your diet. So I typically lump them together and aim to eat a combined total of 5 to 5.5 cups (1,000-1,180 g) of fruits and vegetables daily.

Furthermore, if this sample plan calls for more dairy products than you would like, you could drop one or two and include calcium-rich greens—as part of your vegetables—on the days you don't consume much dairy, or focus on including soy milk or another calcium-fortified veggie milk regularly. And if this plan appears too restrictive—because, for example, you don't want to be stuck with a vegetable every day for a snack—you can either grin and bear it for a few weeks or try the checklist approach (see figure 12.2). If you are just learning to adopt a more healthy eating pattern, you may want to stick with the sample plan for several weeks or months until you learn how to incorporate this healthy eating pattern into your lifestyle. Over the weeks, you will learn to intuitively select a variety of foods at meals and throughout the day. You can then drop the plan and move to more intuitive eating. Believe me, I am not introducing this plan as a forever plan, but one you follow just long enough to establish healthy (or healthier) eating habits.

The checklist approach, on the other hand, is a more flexible method of ensuring that you get adequate servings from each group. I have recommended many athletes, including my oldest daughter, use this checklist. I most distinctly remember counseling both a female collegiate volleyball player and a male mountain bike police officer who found the daily checklists were all they needed to maintain healthier eating patterns. Although both of these athletes were checking off foods to ensure that they made good choices and did not overeat, all athletes can use the checklist to ensure that they eat foods that will meet their nutrient needs. The checklist is something you use for a short time and reinstate later if your eating habits begin to stray off track. Within a short period, you will most likely find—as I do—that you can keep the checklist in your head to help you make healthy choices throughout the day. You may also find that some days you don't make it, and that is OK every once in a while.

Daily Target

Grains   _____ servings (1 oz, 1 slice, 1/2 cup)

Vegetables   _____ cups (raw or cooked)*

Fruit   _____ cups (1/2 cup + 1 medium fruit)

Milk and dairy   _____ 1 cup milk or 1-1/2 oz cheese

Omega-3 fats   _____ g

DAY OF WEEK _____					
Grains					
Vegetables					
Fruit					
Milk and dairy					
Protein					
Healthy oils					

Instructions: Carry in pocket or purse or post on refrigerator. Check box after eating a snack or meal. Strive to meet daily target (at a minimum). Refer to appendix F for guidance on converting English units to metric.

*1 cup leafy greens = 1/2 cup vegetables

FIGURE 12.2 Sample checklist for recording food intake.

From D.E. Larson-Meyer and M. Ruscigno, *Plant-Based Sports Nutrition* (Champaign, IL: Human Kinetics, 2020).

The last piece of the plan is to pencil in how you will meet specific personal nutritional goals that are not always obvious in MyPlate or other plans (see box 12.1). Examples include meeting your vitamin D needs by spending a little time in the sun, increasing your intake of omega-3 fatty acids, or remembering to use iodized table salt. Kudos to My Vegan Plate[5] for the reminders about vitamin D, vitamin B$_{12}$, and iodine.

Going With The Flow

At the risk of repeating myself, it is important to reemphasize that the plan is just a plan. It estimates what you need, and around this framework you will strive to make good food choices that will include mixed dishes and possibly also alcohol (see box 12.2). You will add or subtract foods and servings based on your training and your hunger level. As an athlete, your energy needs likely fluctuate daily with your training schedule and your nonsport activities. Attempting to follow a rigid meal plan would be crazy. That's what makes the various Athlete's Plates so useful. They provide a visual framework for healthy eating based on your training days and phases.

Day-to-day variability in the energy needs of athletes is also difficult for researchers conducting controlled clinical trials on this population. I understood this firsthand when I used myself as a research subject for a study requiring a three-day controlled diet when I was at the University of Alabama at Birmingham. I placed myself on a 2,800-calorie diet that met my needs the first two days—when I was sitting at my desk—but ended up being insufficient in calories on the third day, when I spent a little time gardening. By 5 p.m. I had consumed all of the food in my research bag and was starved the rest of the evening. If you ever run into my husband, you can bet he also has some memory of having to spend the evening with a calorie-deprived wife.

This presents the opportunity to state that the final step in the planning process is to begin following your custom meal plan while remembering that this plan provides a framework and does not list everything you are supposed to eat. At times you will likely want to supplement your diet with healthy oils and additional carbohydrate-rich foods, including sport products and healthy desserts to meet your training needs. Additional or larger servings of the foods listed are, of course, also appropriate. Again, this may be one advantage of using the Athlete's Plate models, which provide different food plates according to training phase, easy training vs. hard training, and game days.

The tabulation of the estimated carbohydrate and protein content provided for each calorie level (table 12.2) should help you determine whether you need to add more carbohydrate, protein, or fat. For the sample 3,000-calorie plans shown in tables 12.4 and 12.5, healthy oils, healthy desserts, and fluid replacement beverages were added to increase calories and carbohydrate. It is interesting to note, however, how much more room there is for these foods when milk is eliminated from the diet and that you can eliminate milk and still meet or exceed calcium recommendations. The addition of milk and dairy, however, help increase the protein content of the vegetarian meal.

Tips for Meal Planning

- See table 12.2 for a list of the estimated number of servings from each major food group required to satisfy various calorie needs for active vegetarians. Choose additional foods from any of the groups or from the discretionary calorie group as needed to meet energy needs.

- Choose a variety of foods from the major food groups.

- If you do not consume dairy products, choose five to six servings per day of calcium-rich foods. Those conveniently listed in the third dimension of the Vegetarian Food Guide Pyramid provide approximately 10 percent of an adult's daily requirements. A more extensive list of calcium-containing plant foods is found in chapter 6.

- To meet iron needs, follow MyPlate or another food-plate plan and select a variety of iron-rich grains and legumes. Aim to consume a fruit or vegetable that contains vitamin C along with most meals to boost absorption. See chapter 7 for more information.

- Incorporate healthy fats in cooking and in dressing up foods, and limit foods that are high in saturated and processed fat (as suggested in chapter 4).

- Include foods rich in omega-3 fatty acids as discussed in chapter 4 and shown in figure 4.5 on page 63.

- Although not mandatory, a daily serving or two of nuts or seeds is a good idea. Focus on seeds if you have a peanut or tree nut allergy. Nuts and seeds add energy, healthy fats, and an abundance of other nutrients (see table 12.1). Servings of nuts and seeds can also serve as a source of protein and be used in place of servings from the fats group for people limiting energy requirements.

- If you are vegan, include at least three good sources of vitamin B_{12} in your diet every day. These include 1 tablespoon (15 ml) of Red Star T6635 nutritional yeast, 1 cup (236 ml) of fortified soy milk, 1 ounce (28 g) of fortified cereal, and 1.5 ounces (42 g) of fortified meat analogue. Servings for vegetarians include half a cup (118 ml) of cows' milk, 0.75 cup (172 g) yogurt, and one egg.

- Use iodized salt when cooking and in salting foods, particularly if you live in an area where the concentration of iodine in the soil is low.

- Get adequate vitamin D from daily sun exposure or through fortified foods or supplements. Use of vegetarian vitamin D is controversial (see chapter 6).

- Get most of your daily calories from the whole-food choices. Limit consumption of overly processed foods, which contain added sugars, high-fructose corn syrup, and unhealthy fats.

This brings us to a final question of whether athletes should develop customized meal plans for rest days. The answer is to play it by ear. Many athletes with high energy needs actually eat more, not less, on their regularly scheduled rest days. A rest day allows them to catch up because it can be a struggle to maintain neutral energy and carbohydrate balance on vigorous training days. Athletes with varied training or work schedules, and therefore varied energy needs, might

Box 12.2

How Do Coffee, Tea, and Alcohol Fit In?

There is nothing wrong with a little coffee, tea, wine, or beer. Consumed in moderation, all can be included in a healthy sport diet and may even provide health benefits. Although many people are aware of the abundance of antioxidants found in both green and black tea,[8] some people may not yet know that several healthful phytochemicals have also been isolated from coffee, which in moderation may be associated with health benefits, including the prevention of type 2 diabetes and liver and neurological diseases.[9,10] I suppose we should not be surprised, because most plant foods seem to deliver their own set of unique phytochemicals. Similarly, although most people know about the health benefits of red wine, which are at least partially linked to polyphenolic compounds found in grapes and grape skins, others may not yet know that beer (particularly higher-quality microbrews or European-style beer is also chock full of nutrients and polyphenols originally found in the malted barley and hops.[11] In fact, both epidemiological and clinical studies have pointed out that moderate wine consumption (one to two glasses a day) is associated with decreased incidence of cardiovascular disease, high blood pressure, diabetes, and certain types of cancer, including colon, basal cell, ovarian, and prostate cancers, whereas moderate beer consumption likely has these same effects, but to a lesser degree.[12] The lower effect noted for beer, however, may be due to variety because different beer styles present different polyphenols in the end product as does fermenting or macerating grapes in the skins in the production of red versus white wines—allowing for a tenfold higher content of polyphenols in red wine. Overall, the health benefits of wine and beer are thought to be caused by the overall mix of polyphenolic compounds, not just one component. Sound familiar?

So how should these fit into your meal plan? Quite simply, they provide mostly discretionary calories. Although coffee and tea are basically calorie free, the sugar or cream added should be included in the discretionary group. For the latte or cappuccino fan, the amount of milk or soy milk mixed with your espresso may be nearly equal to one milk serving. Wine and beer offer calories from alcohol (7 kcal/g) as well as some carbohydrate. While I am often tempted to count a hearty microbrew as a grain or a glass of red wine as a fruit, I am not sure this would be legal with the food police.

When you should consume these beverages is another story. Because many of the components in tea and coffee potently inhibit iron absorption, they should not accompany a meal. Wine and beer do not appear to interfere with nutrient absorption, but you should limit them as suggested by the *Dietary Guidelines for Americans:* up to one drink per day for women and up to two drinks per day for men. Typically, 12 ounces (348 ml) of regular beer, 5 ounces (145 ml) of wine, or 1.5 ounces (43.5 ml) of 80-proof distilled spirits count as a drink. Although there are no hard-and-fast guidelines for tea and coffee, limiting intake to one or two cups (236-472 ml) per day is also a good idea. Athletes should also recognize that the postexercise period is not the best time to consume alcohol or caffeine-containing beverages because the body needs to rehydrate. Remember from chapter 7 that fluid replacement beverages, milk, and orange juice were found to be the most efficient beverages for rehydrating, not tea, lager, coffee, or diet cola.[13] Coffee and tea, however, may provide an ergogenic benefit when consumed before an event (see chapter 10).

develop a maintenance plan based on an energy level that includes regular physical activities (but not training) and then simply increase portions or add sport supplements and healthy desserts according to their hunger on training days.

Learning to Eat Intuitively

If you feel that what we have discussed so far takes too much planning or is simply not your style, you might find that simply thinking about the food-plate model as a reminder of what your plate should look like is all it takes to learn to eat well intuitively. What I have always liked about the food-plate models in general is that they seem less burdensome and more intuitive than other models—like the food pyramid, Japan's spinning top or a number of other international models like France's stair steps or Hungary's food house (not shown)—and some athletes seem to take to it more readily. Even before the launching of MyPlate, I frequently used the United Kingdom's food plate with many football players and cyclists because they related to it more easily. After all, they were eating on a plate. Unless they had specific concerns, I simply had them visualize their lunch or dinner plate or cereal bowl divided in quarters. One quarter contained protein, one or two quarters contained grains, and the remaining one or two quarters were made up of vegetables (depending on their training phase and calorie needs). The problem, of course, is that this still takes visual imagination and does not provide a perfect foundation for including calcium-rich foods or healthy oils, to name a few. Nevertheless, I have found that visualizing a healthy plate or cereal bowl helps many athletes pack healthier lunches, cook healthy dinners, and make better selections at restaurants or buffet meals. As a quick example, if I were serving black-bean chili for dinner, which is a source of protein and is also a vegetable, visualizing the plate might remind me to serve the chili over rice or with cornbread to add grains and with a leafy green salad or fruit salad or a healthy dessert.

Further Assistance With Meal Planning and Healthy Eating

You are lucky to live in a day and age where most of the foods you select at the grocery store "wear" nutrition labels and where accurate nutrition information is at your fingertips. Although the exact information that appears on food labels changes over time, these resources can help you figure out how specific foods—particularly mixed and unusual foods—fit into your meal plans.

Using Food Labels

Food labels—as you are aware—provide information on the nutrient content as well as the ingredients in most food products available in supermarkets. Most consumers are familiar with the nutrition facts label that lists the serving size by household portion and weight or volume; the number of servings in the container; the calorie content and grams of protein, carbohydrate, sugar (including amount of added sugars), fiber, fat and saturated fat and milligrams of sodium in a serving along with nutrients including vitamin D, calcium, iron and potassium. Although the nutrition facts are somewhat intuitive, it is important for athletes to remember to check serving sizes because the size of a serving is often small and to keep in mind that many of the percentages given are for a reference individual on a 2,000-calorie diet. You can, however, use the grams of carbohydrate, protein, saturated fat, and total fat to help determine how the product fits in with the rest of your daily requirements and whether the food is a good source of a selected nutrients including vitamin D, calcium and iron. As an example, the cereal in figure 12.3 provides 17%DV for calcium. Because the DV for calcium is 1,000 milligrams, the cereal provides 170 milligrams of calcium (0.17 × 1,000 mg = 170 mg). Also, without performing calculations, you can tell from the %DV that this product is a decent source of calcium. A good nutrient source provides 10%DV to 19%DV, and a high source provides more than 20%DV.

The ingredient list is the other important component of a food label. It lists the ingredients in the food product in descending order by weight. Hence, ingredients listed first are present in the largest amounts in the food, and those listed last in the smallest amounts. The labels, however, do not indicate how much of any ingredient is included in the food. Although the average consumer often ignores the ingredients list, it can be helpful in many instances. For example, the ingredients list can help vegetarian athletes get an idea of how much of a multigrain product contains whole grains, determine how much sugar in a product is from added sugars (versus those naturally found in foods such as fruit, vegetables, or dairy), and see whether a food product contains animal products. If you are interested in learning more about the vegetarian purity of specific common ingredients, the Vegetarian Resource Group offers a *Guide to Food Ingredients*.[14] Food ingredient lists are also important for athletes with allergies or intolerances to food products or preservatives such as monosodium glutamate.

Using the USDA or Other Nutrient Databases

The USDA Food Composition Databases are one of the best sources for looking up accurate information on food products. They are available free online (https:// ndb.nal.usda.gov/ndb) and allow athletes to quickly look up the nutrient profile for specific foods. The databases are a great source for looking up produce or for checking the nutrient profile of a common oil (before you buy it). For example, if you wonder whether it is worth it to give up your iceberg lettuce and switch to darker greens, you could do a quick comparison of iceberg and see that among other things, iceberg has 10 times less vitamin A per serving than red-leaf or other darker greens. The databases, however, are not perfect. They are missing several common vegetarian foods (or have them listed in unusual ways) as well as international foods such as vegemite and insect pro-

Nutrition Facts

Serving Size 1 oz (about 3/4 cup)
Servings Per Container about 12

Amount Per Serving		Cereal	with 1/2 cup skim milk
Calories		100	140
Calories from Fat		15	20
		% Daily Value**	
Total Fat 1.5g*		2%	2%
Saturated Fat 0g		0%	0%
Trans Fat 0g		0%	0%
Polyunsaturated Fat 1.1g			
Monounsaturated Fat 0.5g			
Cholesterol 0mg		0%	0%
Sodium 190mg		8%	11%
Total Carbohydrate 22g		7%	9%
Dietary Fiber 7g		28%	28%
Sugars 6g			
Protein 4g			
Vitamin A		0%	6%
Vitamin C		0%	0%
Vitamin D		0%	12%
Calcium		2%	17%
Iron		15%	15%
Potassium		3%	8%

*Amount in cereal. One-half cup of skim milk contributes an additional 40 calories, 65mg sodium, 6g total carbohydrate (6g sugar), and 4g protein.

**Percent Daily Values are based on a 2,000 calorie diet. Your daily values may be higher or lower depending on your calorie needs:

	Calories	2,000	2,500
Total Fat	Less than	65g	80g
Sat Fat	Less than	20g	25g
Cholesterol	Less than	300mg	300mg
Sodium	Less than	2400mg	2400mg
Total Carbohydrate		300g	275g
Dietary Fat		25g	30g

Calories per gram

Fat 9   Carbohydrate 4   Protein 4

Ingredients: Organic whole-wheat flour, organic corn, organic wheat bran, organic evaporated cane juice, organic flaxseed, organic oat bran, organic barley malt extract, rice extract, sea salt, tocopherols (natural vitamin E).

FIGURE 12.3   Sample nutrition facts label and ingredient list.

teins. Information on the nutrition content of many products can also be found on food company websites or by contacting the company.

After finishing this chapter, you should feel equipped to customize a vegetarian meal plan to support your current training. The remaining step—discussed in chapter 14—is learning how to whip up quick meals and snacks, with recipe options in chapter 15. You, however, should first consult chapter 13 if you struggle to maintain a healthy weight or feel you have to constantly restrict calories as part of your athletic training. If not, forge ahead to the fun.

13 | Adapting the Plan to Manage Weight

A division I collegiate volleyball player came to see me for weight loss in early January of her freshman year. She had gained a little more than 30 pounds (14 kg) during the fall season, and it was difficult to hide even on her 5-foot, 11-inch (180 cm) frame. She was under the impression—based on something her parents had said over the holiday break—that her weight gain was "caused by the carbohydrate." Because I had worked closely with the team in the preseason and during the season, I had an idea that there was more to the story. I knew it was not because of carbohydrate, unless there had been an abundance of the nutrient.

As we spoke further about her first semester on the volleyball team, it came out that she—like the majority of freshman players—traveled frequently with the team but spent more time sitting on the bench than playing. When the team went for their postgame meal, she feasted as much, if not more, than her older teammates who had played most of the game. And yes, even though her choices had been fairly healthy, she simply ate more calories than she was expending. Part of it, she admitted, was that she ate because everyone else was eating. The other part, however, was eating out of frustration and boredom. It is never easy sitting on the sidelines when you really want to play. She was a great player. Unfortunately, if she did not get her weight under control, she risked playing time in subsequent seasons.

– Enette

Athletes are not immune to struggles with body weight. Nearly three-fourths of the athletes I saw as a nutritionist for a National Collegiate Athletic Association (NCAA) Division I team came to me for concerns about weight loss or weight gain. Of course, this is a biased sample because I did not see all athletes, but it illustrates that many athletes, despite hours of hard training, are not immune to weight-related issues. Vegetarian athletes are no exception. Although some athletes struggle with real issues that may be caused by poor eating habits or a particular genetic makeup different than that dictated by their sport, other athletes struggle with issues related to unrealistic expectations—either their own or those of their coaches or parents. While it is true that excess weight can hinder performance in some athletic activities, athletes do not and should not feel that they need to fit a specific mold or body type in order to be a good athlete. They also should not be driven to unhealthy eating practices for aesthetics or to make a certain weight.

This section focuses on how a plant-based meal plan can be adapted when necessary to promote weight loss or weight gain and ultimately assist in life-long weight management. It also briefly addresses the relationship between body weight and performance and discusses conditions in which weight-loss or weight-gain efforts may not be appropriate.

Physics of Weight Management

Simply put, weight maintenance is a matter of balancing the energy consumed with the energy spent. Body weight is altered, up or down, when there is a long-term imbalance between energy consumed from foods, beverages, and some supplements, and calories expended during training and the activities of daily living. Theoretically, losing 1 pound (0.45 kg) of body fat requires an energy, or caloric, deficit of 3,500 calories—something called "Wishnofsky Rule." To lose this much in one week, there must be a negative balance of 500 calories each day for one week.[1] This is accomplished by eating less, being more active, or a combination of the two. To gain this much as body fat, there must be a positive balance of at least 3,500 calories.

That said, however, some individuals can overeat a bit on occasion and manage to avoid gaining weight, whereas others seem to gain weight every time they eat an excess calorie. This is because energy balance is not as simple as energy in equals energy out because changing one factor on the energy intake side can affect factors on the energy expenditure side and vice versa.[1,2] In other words, numerous factors work together to influence both sides of the energy balance equation. Thus, the difference in the aforementioned individuals is partially related to their ability to waste (or burn off) some of the excess energy consumed or unconsciously alter desire to eat following a bout of caloric excess.[3] The person who is prone to weight gain is not able to defend against caloric excess by compensating with either an increase in energy expenditure or a decrease in appetite at that body weight. The resistant gainer may—without even thinking about it—increase physical activity or fidgeting after overeating, thereby spontaneously increasing energy expenditure or decreasing his or her desire to eat. The average person wastes about 12 percent of the excess energy consumed and thus banks about 78 percent of the excess calories.[4,5] Easy gainers, however, put nearly every excess calorie into their body fat stores, and resistant gainers seem to be able to increase metabolism enough that a smaller proportion of the excess calories is stored as body fat. The opposite is true to some extent during active weight loss. The resistant reducer loses a bit less than predicted because metabolism slows somewhat to fend off weight loss, and he or she may even subconsciously decrease physical activity levels or experience an intense desire to eat or both. These reactions do not occur to the same degree in the person who loses weight easily. What causes these differences in metabolism and appetite regulation in response to overeating or calorie restriction is not yet understood.[3] Despite extensive research, we still have a lot to learn—particularly in the athlete who struggles with weight issues!

It should be stressed, nevertheless, that although differences in metabolism and appetite regulation exist, they are small relative to the big picture and do not support the contention that an athlete can cut calories by 3,500 calories per week with no effect to his or her weight. Instead, these differences in metabolism explain why two college athletes with similar energy needs who splurge on 500-calorie ice cream sundaes every night for two weeks (in excess of their energy requirements, of course) gain different amounts of weight, or why a person who eats 500 calories less than needed every day for a week loses three-quarters of a pound instead of the predicted pound. And if you are wondering whether your sex makes a difference—it might. Women are more likely to gain weight easily and have a difficult time losing it. But that is a generality. Some men have what we call a conservative metabolism that makes it easier for them to gain weight, and some women have a wasteful metabolism

---

Vegan View: Benefits of High-Volume Plant Foods for Weight Loss

Several books and research papers show that eating a plant-based diet can aid in weight loss, and the principle benefit can be explained rather simply: whole plant foods have more volume and fewer calories. Imagine, for example, a large plate of steamed broccoli. The space taken up by the broccoli is equivalent to a typical meal, but for a fraction of the calories. An entire stalk of broccoli is a mere 100 calories, but the same amount of gravy by volume, for example, would contain thousands of calories. Now, most people are not eating giant plates of broccoli (or gravy!), but the space vegetables take up in meals means fewer calories eaten. It expands the meal both visually and in the time it takes to consume; both aid in weight loss. This concept is called *caloric density*, and it is a key component in weight loss—so much so that athletes new to plant-based eating need to keep this principle in mind to make sure they are eating enough. For people trying to lose weight, adding whole plant foods each day crowds out more calorically dense foods and can help make weight loss a little easier to achieve.

that makes it easier for them to lose it. If truth be told, I have worked with male athletes who struggle to keep weight off and female athletes who are able to eat *everything* they want but cannot gain an ounce. Indeed, in our weight-conscious, food-abundant society, these women are considered lucky; however, during a famine, their faster metabolisms wouldn't serve them so well.

Overweight Issues for Vegetarian Athletes

Beyond the basic concept of energy balance, the prevention of weight gain and the promotion of weight loss are not simple issues, even for vegetarian athletes. Although athletes typically expend a lot of energy, they are still subject to both overeating and a sedentary lifestyle when they are not training. One or a combination of both can promote a positive energy balance that either leads to weight gain or prohibits body-fat reduction. Again, some athletes are more destined to weight gain because of their genetic makeup, which can include the tendency to overeat, move less, or efficiently bank excess energy.[2] Some have slightly lower metabolism at rest for their given lean mass, fat mass, age and sex or are genetically less fat burners than carbohydrate burners. Following a vegetarian diet may help dampen overeating, but it is certainly still possible to overeat vegan and vegetarian foods. As a group, athletes appear to be particularly prone to weight gain during their first year of college and after experiencing a major injury, undergoing surgery, taking a new job, getting married, having children, or going through menopause. While the reasons for weight gain are different for each athlete, typically stress, boredom, and the habit of eating a lot are somehow involved. My father, a former football player, for example, is overweight because he still eats as if he were training for the Fiesta Bowl. By the way, he is not vegetarian and enjoys typical American foods that are not nutritious.

Although it is also true that a very small percentage of athletes may experience problems with their thyroid—the gland that produces the important energy-regulating hormone[6]—most people gain weight simply because they eat more than they move. For example, collegiate athletes may gain weight during their first year because they play less during games or matches yet eat as much as their junior and senior teammates. They also may make poor food choices. Adult athletes often gain weight because real-life responsibilities either decrease the time they have to exercise or provide an environment that encourages overeating. From personal experience, I can testify that vegetarian athletes are also destined to gain weight if they shift uninformed to a vegetarian eating pattern. As you can imagine, weight gain is inevitable when you sprinkle sunflower seeds and cheese on everything just to ensure that you get enough protein.

Deciding Whether You Need a Weight-Loss Plan

Weight reduction is a different ballgame for athletes than it is for nonathletes. If you or your coach believe that you need to lose weight, it is important that you first seriously consider whether your weight-loss goals are necessary and realistic. I have worked with too many athletes who believe that they need to weigh a little less to run faster or look better in their team uniform. These athletes are not really candidates for a weight-loss diet, but for one that directs their focus toward better eating habits. Yes, some studies of physically fit subjects have found negative associations between body fat and athletic performance that requires the body to be propelled quickly in space, but the associations are actually weak, explaining less than 10 percent to as high as 50 percent of the variation in performance during various running and jumping activities. Also, because studies were typically conducted in cross-sectional groups of active people, not top-level competitive athletes, the results should not be taken to mean that you will perform better if you go on a "diet" to lose a few pounds of fat. You may instead lose lean tissue along with fat tissue. And loss of lean mass, if it is muscle that is important to acceleration, power, or other aspects of sport performance, could decrease performance. Loss of body fat can also be detrimental. Body fat serves as padding in contact sports and loss of too much fat may increase risk of injury and, in combination with a negative energy balance, alter the circulatory pattern of hormones, including estrogen, testosterone, and thyroid hormone.

Thus, the bottom line is that you should consider reducing your weight only if you have recently gained weight (not associated with puberty) and you are not performing as you did before. You may also consider modifying your diet according to a weight-loss plan if you have been slightly overweight your whole life, providing you are persistent in your efforts to improve your eating habits so that you can achieve a healthy body weight over the long haul. In that case, you are probably someone who gains easily and has a difficult time losing, so you will need to overcome your body's desire to overeat or store excessive calories by learning to eat just what you need. If you are an athlete with a stable body weight within the normal range and you perform decently, however, you should not embark on weight-loss efforts with the idea that you will perform or look better if you just drop a little weight. Part of being a strong and successful athlete is learning to accept your body for what it is and making the most of it through participation in athletics. Athletes come in all sizes and shapes!

Pieces of the Weight-Reduction Plan

The meal plan for an athlete trying to lose weight is similar to the meal plan for any athlete, but it contains slightly fewer calories than are necessary to maintain weight. Exactly how much fewer depends on your body size or total energy requirements and training and performance goals.[2,7] If you are a teen athlete, it also depends on your stage of development. I firmly believe that athletes should not restrict calories during the regular season or peak season, unless of course they have been benched, are redshirted, or are not expecting a peak performance that season. Restricting calories is a goal for the preseason, base-season, and off-season or as far from the competitive season as possible.[8] During this time, athletes on a weight-reduction plan should strive to eat 250 to 500 calories per day less than their required energy needs,[7,8] which would promote a weight loss of about 0.5 to 1 pound (0.22-0.45 kg) per week. Athletes weighing over 200 to 250 pounds (90-112 kg) or so can get by restricting up to—but no more than—1,000 calories a day, which should promote a reduction of 1 to no more than 2 pounds (0.45-0.9 kg) per week. In support, a study of a mixed group of elite male and female Norwegian athletes found that a slow weight reduction of 0.7 percent of body weight per week had more positive effects on lean body mass, strength, and performance than a faster reduction of 1.44 percent per week.[9] An athlete wanting to cut weight or body fat during the season should strive to improve his or her eating habits and then embark on weight-loss efforts during the off-season. Although it is common for athletes in

Weight loss does not necessarily ensure improved performance. Many factors go into the decision to try to lose or gain weight.

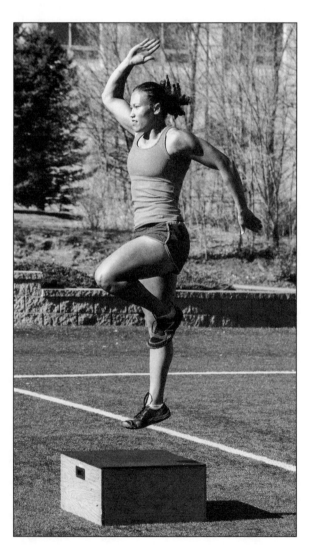

certain sports to restrict calories to make weight or cut body fat, this practice is not healthy[8] and may result in poorer-than-expected performance.

The biggest mistake an athlete can make during his or her efforts to reduce body weight or body fat is to choose a diet that excludes one or more of these vital nutrients: carbohydrate, protein, vitamins, minerals, and, yes, even fat. Another mistake is to follow a diet that excessively restricts calories and results in rapid weight loss. The next sections discuss why a balanced diet is vital to your performance and why weight loss should occur slowly.

Get Your Carbs   Carbohydrate is the only fuel that can sustain the moderate to high level of activity that is required in most sport and athletic endeavors and is the one preferred by the brain and central nervous system. (See chapter 3 for further information.) Excessively restricting carbohydrate diminishes your ability to train long and hard, which most likely will cause problems later. For example, if you go out for an hour run with low glycogen reserves caused by a low-carbohydrate weight-loss plan, chances are you will run at a lower percent effort and cover fewer miles. This, of course, will burn fewer calories and, unless it is your easy day, induce less of a training effect. If you have enough energy to make it through the run, you most likely will finish the workout more tired than usual and seek the comforts of your couch or cozy office chair and be less likely to expend effort (calories) getting out of the chair to walk down the hall, up the stairs, or into the kitchen. If you somehow make it into the kitchen, your carbohydrate-craving liver and muscles will most likely strain your willpower and, well, you get the idea—suddenly you may be eating ravenously. If you don't, you may experience fatigue.

How much carbohydrate you need on your weight-loss plan depends on your body weight and level and type of training, but a good general rule is to eat about 1 or maybe 2 grams of carbohydrate per kilogram of body weight *less* than you should be striving for (see table 3.1 on page 35). Another way to think of this is to strive for the lower end of the recommended range based on training needs. For example, a 242-pound (110 kg) baseball player would most likely require 5 to 7 grams of carbohydrate per kilogram of body weight (550-770 g of carbohydrate) during preseason training. If this athlete wants to reduce his body weight, he should aim for the lower range or about 5 grams of carbohydrate per kilogram of body weight (~ 550 g of carbohydrate). Reducing carbohydrate intake by just 1 gram of carbohydrate per kilogram would result in 440 fewer calories consumed (4 kcal per g × 110 g of carbohydrate) and be close to the 500-calorie deficit recommended to lose about a pound (0.45 kg) a week. You will know you have restricted carbohydrate intake too much if you experience early fatigue during your training or note a rapid change in your body weight. Typically, losing a pound or two over the course of a day or two can be attributed to the lost water weight that occurs when glycogen stores in the liver and muscle are low. This happens because every gram of glycogen in the muscle and liver is stored along with 3 to 4 grams of water. So if you reduced your body's glycogen stores by 500 grams, you would notice a 3.3- to 4.4-pound (1.5-2 kg) weight loss almost overnight. Although there is some indication that low-carbohydrate or very low carbohydrate diets, which induce ketosis (high blood levels of ketones as a result of increased fatty acid breakdown) may be used with some success for rapid weight loss,[10] these extreme diets may result in lean tissue loss[11] and poor performance.[12] They do not promote healthy plant-based eating over the long haul.

Get Your Protein   The obvious goal of a weight-reduction plan is to restrict intake of energy and energy-producing nutrients; however, this does not hold true for protein. During active weight loss, when your energy balance is negative, you may need to increase your protein intake to help reduce the loss of lean tissue and to prevent your resting metabolic rate from slowing. The current recommendation for protein intake in competitive athletes (and really any athlete undergoing intense training with performance goals in mind) is 1.6 to 2.4 grams of protein per kilogram of body weight per day.[13] One reason is because more dietary protein is "burned" for energy when the body has a negative energy balance, resulting in less protein available for building and repairing lean body tissue. Higher protein intake during active weight loss may dampen or prevent tissue loss and allow for a maintenance or improvement in athletic performance.[13] For instance, one study in resistance-trained male athletes found that energy-restricted diets containing 2.3 grams of protein per kilogram of body weight were significantly superior for maintenance of lean body mass than similarly restricted diets containing about 1 gram of protein per kilogram of body weight.[14] In addition, research suggests that protein, compared to fat and carbohydrate, promotes satiety and requires that your body expend more energy to digest and metabolize a meal (something called the thermic effect of food, see chapter 2). [15] Interestingly, there may also be something about legumes that has a similar effect—whether it be the plant protein or the soluble fiber. A recent meta-analysis by de Souza and colleagues found that adding a 3/4 cup (130 g) serving daily of beans, peas, lentils resulted in a modest spontaneous weight loss of just over half a pound (0.34 kg).[49] Hence, a little extra protein—perhaps in the form of legumes—may be advantageous during weight loss.

Although most experts agree that there may be an advantage to including more protein in an energy-restricted diet, it is not known just how much protein within the suggested range is beneficial for each athlete. A recent review by Hector and Phillips[13] found that higher protein requirements (in the upper recommendation range) are needed when weight loss is more rapid, whereas lower protein seems to be appropriate when resistance training is simultaneously undertaken. The quality of the protein consumed also seems to be important, with less total protein required when high-quality protein is consumed. This implies that vegetarian athletes may want to consider eating complementary proteins at most meals during active weight loss. Although this is not necessary when energy is balanced because the limiting amino acids consumed from a single plant source are buffered by the body's amino acid pools, it may be beneficial during weight loss when these amino acid pools are not as plentiful because of the lower energy intake combined with the body's increased use of protein for energy. No research currently supports this suggestion in vegetarians, but it does not take much effort to complement or eat higher-quality proteins because these foods are a natural part of our culture (see chapter 5 for further detail).

Include Fat Judiciously   Yes, although it is true that we should reduce dietary fat during weight loss, particularly to ensure that we get enough carbohydrate and protein, athletes should by no means attempt to follow a diet that is nearly fat free. The main reason is because humans like fat. It tastes good and allows us to enjoy the flavors of our foods even when we are trying to drop a few pounds. If we deprive ourselves of fat by eating the bread without the margarine or olive oil, or having the raisins without the walnuts, we may be setting ourselves up for an "I can't stand the deprivation any longer" binge. Athletes also need to recognize that a substantial amount of research suggests that it is easier to overeat fat-containing foods.[16] On the other hand, diets extremely high in fat, such as those recommended as part of the ketogenic diet (see chapter 4) may promote weight loss because the foods are not terribly palatable. Try eating only creamed onions, cheese, and salad with heavy dressing, and you will understand this comment.

Therefore, you should continue to include small amounts of smart fat choices—nuts, seeds, flavorful oils, full-fat soy products, and strongly flavored cheeses—in your daily diet, but cut back on fat-containing foods such as chips, crackers, fried tofu, or any food that triggers the "I have to eat the whole thing" effect. In fact, if you have a binge food, such as ice cream, chocolate, or cashews, avoid bringing them into your house or keeping them in your desk drawer, or purchase them only in small packages.

Include Fruits, Vegetables, Vitamins, Minerals, and Energy-Dense Foods
When you restrict your energy intake, you increase your chance of taking in inadequate amounts of vitamins, minerals, and phytochemicals. You can negate or even avoid the low-vitamin-and-mineral trap if you continue to eat nutrient-dense fresh and frozen fruits and vegetables—without limits. These foods are also high in soluble and insoluble fibers, which may promote satiety. Athletes who struggle in their decision about which foods to eliminate or reduce to create a calorie deficit may want to emphasize low-sugar, low-starch vegetables such as carrots, cooked and fresh leafy greens, onions, tomatoes, and parsnips and cut back on fruit juice and starchier vegetables. This is especially true if those vegetables are easy to overeat or overloaded with fat calories (e.g., potatoes, sweetened winter squash). In a recent clinical trial in overweight nonathletes, a low-fat, low-glycemic vegan diet (which did not necessarily emphasize calorie restriction) promoted greater weight loss over a six-month period than a pesco vegetarian, semivegetarian, or omnivorous diet.[17] Athletes who restrict energy may also want to consider taking a multivitamin and mineral supplement even though it is typically recommended when consuming less than 1,200 calories a day.

Drink Plenty of Water and Cut Back on Supplements   As mentioned in chapter 9, it is important to drink enough fluids daily to keep well hydrated. This is additionally important during weight loss because the body's need for fluid is often misinterpreted as a desire to eat. During weight reduction, drink plenty of water throughout the day and avoid high-calorie fluids,[2] such as regular soda, sweetened tea, and full-fat milk. Also drink fluid replacement beverages only when needed, for example, during a long training session. These and other sport supplements add calories and may even suppress fat oxidation during and after exercise. When you are actively seeking weight loss, it is better to drink water and snack on carbohydrate and protein-rich foods such as a banana with peanut butter and dairy or soy yogurt with fresh fruit. Save the sport foods and supplements for when you need them.

Watch Portion Sizes   As mentioned earlier, an eating plan that promotes healthy weight loss should look like the meal plan in chapter 12 but contain slightly fewer calories than required to maintain weight. Thus, if you already eat well, you may simply want to watch your portion sizes and avoid foods you tend to overeat without thinking about. If you don't eat well, you should take the time to create a meal plan for weight reduction. It is interesting to note that the amount of food considered to be a normal portion has escalated over the past 20 to 30 years. Research from the Department of Nutrition, Food Studies, and Public Health at New York University found that portion sizes in eating establishments are two to eight times greater than recommended serving sizes.[18] This has also influenced what we consider to be normal at home. Because you consume more calories when more food is on your plate, you can reduce energy intake simply by putting less on your plate and focusing on smaller portions. Although this may be difficult in certain social situations, for example, when eating with your running buddies or when celebrating with the team at the postgame meal, remember that everyone has a different metabolism. Either find a vegetarian buddy to split a healthy meal with or take half of it home for the next day. Another option is to choose a healthy soup and salad or a small entree with steamed vegetables. And by all means, avoid all-you-can-eat buffets. Buffets promote overeating even if the options for vegetarians are limited.

Go Slowly   If you are an overweight athlete, losing slowly is not necessarily the message you want to hear. College athletes and students in my sports nutrition course have often asked me why an athlete shouldn't simply go on a more extreme low-calorie diet for six to eight weeks during the off-season and be done with it. Why prolong this "dieting thing"? Although there are a multitude of reasons to go slowly, the first and most important reason not to rush things is that these extreme diets do not typically contain real foods and thus do not teach athletes how to make the appropriate changes to their eating and lifestyle habits that are necessary for long-term success. Second, rapid weight loss tends to promote greater loss of valuable lean tissue or muscle than does slower weight loss (discussed earlier) and also does not allow for much training apart from moderate walking or weight training. No athlete wants to lose muscle and experience a six-to-eight-week detraining effect. Chances are they may never perform the same again. Third, athletes are typically overachievers. If you place an athlete on a 1,000-calorie diet, he or she would likely strive for a 500-calorie diet, which would increase risk of adverse health issues. I saw an extreme case in which a football player placed himself on an extremely low calorie diet after being called "fatty" by his coach. By the time the team physician referred him to me, he had been consuming just a 6-inch (15 cm) sub sandwich and a liter of diet soda daily for eight weeks. He had dangerously elevated concentrations of creatine phosphate, an enzyme that dwells in skeletal and cardiac tissue and is released when tissue is damage. Indeed, he dropped 30 pounds (14 kg), but he had been experiencing such an amazing breakdown of muscle tissue that he could have ended up with acute renal failure. The final reason is simply that extremely low energy diets do not always bring about the best weight-loss results because they reduce lean mass, resting energy needs, and spontaneous physical activity. They are rarely successful.

Creating or Modifying a Plan for Weight Loss

A meal plan customized for weight reduction helps athletes determine an energy level that promotes healthy weight loss (see box 13.1). To customize your meal plan for weight reduction, estimate your energy needs using one of the methods discussed in chapter 2, subtract 500 to 1,000 calories (as will be reviewed in box 13.1), and round your estimate to the nearest 200 calories. Use this target energy level to obtain the recommended number of servings you need to consume from each of the major food groups as shown in table 12.2 on page 211 and to develop a meal plan designed specifically for weight loss. For example, if the estimated daily energy needs of a female synchronized swimmer were approximately 2,550 calories per day during her off-season, she would subtract 500 calories from her daily needs to promote weight loss and then round 2,050 to the nearest 200 calories to come up with a 2,000-calorie target. Her plan should contain six grain equivalents, 2.5 cups (575 g) of vegetables, 2 cups (460 g) of fruit, 3 cups (708 ml) of milk, and 5.5 to 6 servings of protein (if using MyPlate). A sample menu showing both a vegetarian and vegan 2,000-calorie-per-day weight-loss plan is shown in table 13.1.

Remember that with any plan, you may need to adjust the carbohydrate or protein foods a bit to meet your training needs and may also add servings of leafy greens and other nonstarchy vegetables, which contain only 10 to 20 calories per half cup (115 g) serving. The "Easy" or "Weight Maintenance" Athlete's Plate may be a helpful visual in this situation. If you find you are starving on the plan, feeling fatigued, or dropping weight too quickly, you may have underestimated your daily energy needs and should adjust up by adding an additional serving or two of carbohydrate or protein depending on your training needs.

TABLE 13.1   2,000-Calorie Vegetarian Meal Plan for Weight Loss

Meal	Categories	Suggested servings	Vegetarian meal (using MyPlate)	Vegan meal (using the Vegetarian Food Guide Pyramid)
Breakfast	Grain Milk Fruit	2 equivalents (eq) 1 serving 1/2 cup	1 slice (1 oz) whole-wheat toast 1 cup (1 oz) shredded wheat, 1 tsp no-trans-fat margarine*, 1 cup skim milk 1/2 cup sliced strawberries	1 multigrain English muffin (2 oz) 1 tsp no-trans-fat margarine* 1 tbsp apricot preserves*, 1/2 cup fortified orange juice
Morning snack	Fruit Protein	1/2 cup 1 eq	1/4 cup raisins 1 oz almonds	1 small apple 1 tbsp peanut butter
Lunch	Protein Grain Milk Vegetable	2 eq 2 eq 1 serving 1/2 cup	Vegetarian burger (60 g) on a French roll (2 oz) 1 cup milk 1 cup mixed greens 1 tbsp red-wine vinegar and 1 tbsp olive oil*	Tofu-salad sandwich made with 1 cup firm tofu, 1 tbsp soy mayonnaise, 1 tbsp mustard* 2 slices whole-wheat bread 1/2 cup baby carrots
Afternoon snack	Fruit	1/2 cup	1 medium orange	1/2 cup unsweetened apple sauce 1 cup hot tea
Dinner	Protein Grain Vegetable	2 eq 2 eq 1-1/2 cups	1 cup vegetable soup 1 cup black beans with 1/4 cup onions 1 cup long-grain rice with 1 tsp canola oil* and topped with 1/2 cup tomato 1/2 cup steamed spinach drizzled with red-wine vinegar	1 cup black-eyed peas topped with 1/2 cup green onions 1 cup brown rice 1 piece homemade cornbread made with canola oil* 1 cup steamed collard greens
Evening snack	Fruit Milk	1/2 cup 1 serving	1/2 cup sliced bananas 1 cup nonfat yogurt 1 tbsp honey*	1 small Asian pear 1 cup fortified soy milk* 1 oz walnuts*

Note: Refer to appendix F for guidance on converting English units to metric.

*Discretionary calorie items.

Other Tricks to Promote Weight Loss or Maintenance

In addition to understanding the basic principles of weight loss and following a meal plan, a handful of other "tricks" or ideas may aid in weight loss or in weight maintenance following weight reduction. These are briefly reviewed in the following sections.

Don't Skip Breakfast   You have been told this before, but now there is research to support it. Successful dieters who have lost weight and maintained

Box 13.1

Tips for Adopting a Plan to Promote Weight Loss

To promote a weight loss of about 0.5 to 1 pound (0.22-0.45 kg) per week, eat a well-balanced vegetarian diet that contains 250 to 500 calories per day less than you need. Larger athletes with higher energy expenditures can eat about 500 to no more than 1,000 calories per day less than needed. This should promote a reduction of about 1 to 2 pounds (0.45-0.9 kg) per week. Customize the meal plan for weight reduction by estimating energy needs (using one of the methods discussed in chapter 2), subtracting 500 to 1,000 calories, and rounding to the nearest 200 calories. This calorie target can then be used to develop a meal plan as discussed in chapter 12. Remember that you may need to reassess your energy needs and adjust your calorie needs downward as you lose weight. Use the following tips to reach your calorie target:

- Eat plenty of fresh fruits and vegetables, which are packed with water, fiber, vitamins, minerals, and much more. You can add as many nonstarchy vegetables to the plan as you want because they add few calories.
- Learn to take smaller portions of food.
- Avoid the all-you-care-to-eat buffets.
- Drink plenty of water and other low-calorie beverages.
- Limit your intake of alcohol and sugar-containing beverages, including sport drinks. For some athletes, just omitting the high-calorie beverages such as soda, fruit juice, energy drinks, flavored coffees and teas, or alcohol could help achieve weight-loss goals without making other changes.[2] While a glass of wine or beer may help you to relax at the end of the day, the calories in several beers or glasses of wine can add up quickly.
- Spread food intake throughout the day and don't skip breakfast—or for that matter, lunch or dinner. Three meals and three snacks as shown in the sample meal plans may be appropriate for spreading out food intake. This approach may help athletes from becoming too hungry and consuming foods not on their weight-loss plan.[2]
- Keep a food log recording when and why you eat. The worksheets downloaded from the MyPlate website (www.choosemyplate.gov) may be useful for logging your daily progress in relation to your plan.
- Assess your nontraining physical activity. If needed, get off the couch! Consider taking a walk after dinner.
- Watch emotional eating. If you feel like snacking, take a walk or have a cup of unsweetened tea or coffee instead.
- Fix an enjoyable vegetarian meal, and splash on the flavored vinegar if desired.
- Learn lifelong healthy habits that will help you maintain a healthy body weight. You will have greater success if you think you are following a healthy meal plan rather than a "diet".
- Go slowly and don't look for magic.
- If you need professional assistance, search out a registered dietitian specializing in vegetarian nutrition.

the weight loss report eating breakfast every day.[19] Eating a morning meal helps reduce later consumption of fat and minimizes impulsive snacking during the day. It is common for people who don't eat breakfast to make up the missed calories later in the day and even consume more calories than they would have if they had eaten breakfast. And as an athlete, you need the additional energy and carbohydrate to help you perform your best—even in the off-season. Be sure to include breakfast in your custom meal plan.

Start With a Low-Calorie, High-Volume Appetizer   Interesting research by Barbara Rolls—who has spent her career studying eating behavior and weight management—at Pennsylvania State University has found that consuming food or meals with a low energy density (measured in calories per gram of food), aids in weight control.[20,21] Our bodies, it seems, do not have calorie meters but rather volume meters, meaning that our hunger is satisfied by a certain volume of food, not a certain number of calories. Consuming foods with low energy density, such as certain fresh fruits and vegetables, whole-milled cereals and grains, legumes, and broth-based soups, helps us feel more satisfied with fewer calories than if we had eaten more dense foods, such as meats, cheese, pizza, ice cream, and candy. To incorporate this plan, try eating broth-based soup, yogurt, a leafy salad, or vegetable soup before or at the start of each meal and make it a point to select more foods with a low energy density. Choosing foods with fewer calories per volume allows more satisfying food portions and—if you make good choices—more vitamins, minerals, and phytochemicals per gram of food. Note, however, that drinking a calorie-free beverage such as water or diet soda with a meal does not count toward the volume of food it takes to satisfy the appetite, as some still believe.[22] And consuming a calorie-containing beverage adds to the total calories of the meal. It seems our bodies are simply unaware of the volume that comes from a beverage.

Limit Alcohol   Conventional wisdom states that the cause of a "beer belly" may be just that: the alcohol in beer. Advertisements for low-carbohydrate beer,[22] however, would like us to believe it is really the calories from carbohydrate and not the alcohol that increases our girth. It is true that excess calories cause weight gain—no matter what type of calories—but it is also true that alcohol intake can slow fat metabolism. In the early 1990s, a group of well-known energy metabolism researchers from Switzerland found that when alcohol was either added to the diet or substituted for other foods, 24-hour fat use decreased by nearly 33 percent in both cases.[23] Carbohydrate and protein metabolism were not affected. Energy expenditure was slightly increased (by 7 and 4%) but was not elevated enough to offset the effect of alcohol on fat balance. Although the researchers concluded that habitual consumption of ethanol in excess of energy needs favors fat storage and weight gain, the amount of alcohol used in the study (96 g) was quite a bit higher than one would consume in a 5-ounce (145 ml) glass of wine with dinner (16 g). The effects of just one glass of wine or a microbrew, however, are not known. Nonetheless, other reasons to limit alcohol are that it may promote snacking[24] and reduce your body's ability to store muscle glycogen.[25]

Try Vinegar   Research is preliminary, but given that vinegar can enhance the flavor of many vegetables and vegetarian dishes, adding it regularly in salad dressing or as a condiment may be worth a try. A few years back, Swedish researchers found that consuming vinegar as part of a meal reduces the body's insulin response to carbohydrate and increases feelings of satiety following that meal.[26,27] Researchers had volunteers consume three different amounts of vinegar on different days in random order, the highest amount being 2 to 3 tablespoons (30-45 ml) along with 50 grams of high-glycemic carbohydrate from white bread. The researchers found that the higher the vinegar intake, the greater the effects on dose response. Recent research is mostly in support, suggesting that vinegar may promote satiety, delay gastric emptying, suppress the activity of enzymes that break down disaccharides (such as sucrose), and aid in stabilization of blood sugar. While longer-term clinical studies are needed, current results suggest that adding vinegar to your meals may help you eat less and reduce cravings brought on by sugar peaks after meals.[28] Try a vinegar and olive oil dressing on fresh greens. Drizzle it on top of cooked greens, legumes, or legume-based soups, or use it in pasta salads and rice dishes. Even if it amounts to little weight loss, the acetic acid in the vinegar may enhance absorption of minerals such as zinc, calcium, and iron. Also, create a beverage by mixing a few tablespoons of a flavorful vinegar, such as raspberry or pomegranate, with plain or seltzer water. Vinegar-based drinks have taken off in Japan, owing to belief in their medicinal properties. Although vinegar is not likely to be the essential element for promoting weight loss, adding a bit to your meals may keep you on track.

Wear a Pedometer   Sure, you spend a lot of energy training for your sport, but what do you do when you are not training? Wearing a pedometer to get an idea of how physically active you are during your nontraining time may benefit your weight-loss program. I have found in working with athletes that many are sedentary when not training. Quite a few drive everywhere, circle the parking lot to get the closest spot, and spend a lot of time sitting at a desk or on the couch. If you exert little physical effort except during training, a pedometer may help you learn to be more physically active. Your goal? First, measure what you do now and then increase the value by 10 to 15 percent each week until you approach 10,000 steps. In addition to helping you control your weight, increasing your movement, particularly through walking, may also assist with active recovery because it increases blood flow to your hard-worked muscles. This helps provide a fresh supply of oxygen and other nutrients and removes lingering postexercise metabolites. Emerging research also finds that excessive sitting may be a serious health hazard even in people who are otherwise active.[29] As an athlete, however, keep in mind that you should increase your daily steps by walking more in your daily activities, including around your house and to and from practice, and not by engaging in racewalking. I also would not yet recommend a standing desk. Static standing thwarts blood flow and may not be the best for recovery. If you are injured, discuss this advice with your doctor as it may not be appropriate.

Write It Down, but Don't Tweet It   Research shows that monitoring the type of food you eat plays an important role in successful weight loss and maintenance. Writing down all the drinks and food you consume in a day, at least for a while, helps make you aware of the food you consume and why you consume it. Many weight-conscious people also feel that keeping food records keeps them accountable and helps them avoid binge foods because they don't want to have to write it down. As an athlete, writing it down also allows you to check the adequacy of your carbohydrate and protein intake. If you feel that tweeting it to the world might also make you accountable, however, consider your followers. Many may celebrate in your success, but most don't care about your day-to-day meal plans.

Don't Count on the Calcium   While the dairy industry wants you to believe that drinking milk or eating yogurt is important for wellness and weight management, limited evidence supports their marketing. A recent meta-analysis found that neither increasing calcium intake by 900 milligrams per day as supplements or increasing dairy intake to approximately three servings daily (approximately 1,300 mg of calcium per day) was an effective overall weight-reduction strategy in adults.[30] However, the meta-analysis found that consuming three servings of dairy products daily markedly accelerated body-fat loss during short-term caloric restriction in people who were overweight or obese, whereas calcium supplementation had no effect. Dairy products are thought to have this effect because of their assistance with appetite control, not because of the calcium, and potentially because of other components such as their protein. While casein in dairy in particular is thought to have satiety effects, it is possible that higher-fiber, plant-rich proteins could offer a similar effect during calorie restriction. Remember, as mentioned earlier, that adding a 3/4 cup serving daily of beans, peas, or lentils was shown to produce a spontaneous weight loss of just over half a pound (0.3 kg) in non-athletes.[49] If you created your customized meal plan from MyPlate, you have the dairy servings already built in. If not, this is another reason to ensure protein-rich options at each meal and snack.

Don't Think About the D Word   Believe it or not, one of the best ways you can achieve success is to forget the D word—diet, that is. Many people are done in by their "diets." They are overzealous, restrict too much, including their favorite foods, and suddenly begin cheating and maybe binging, and soon they are off the diet. Instead, stick to a healthy plan as suggested in this chapter that realistically restricts energy by about 500 to no more than 1,000 calories per day. This promotes a slow weight loss and allows you to incorporate some of your favorite foods. If you crave ice cream, have a small dish, but don't overindulge. In the big picture, you are trying to improve your eating habits over the long term, which includes learning to make better choices more often and overeat less often—if ever.

Don't Buy or Order Trigger Foods   Most of us have those foods we can easily overeat. For some it is ice cream; other people can't control themselves around cookies, flavored crackers, or chips. For me it is those darn Pringles. I don't even like them, but if I see a can in my cupboard after a swim or long run I start snacking, taking a few and another few. My solution is to just not buy them. If you have a craving for something sweet or savory, find a healthier, less-processed alternative like a frozen fruit smoothie, fresh-cut veggies with spicy yogurt, nut or tofu dip, or popcorn sprinkled with a pinch of flavored salt. Ever notice that the foods we can easily overeat are not carrots, apples, or oranges?

Don't Look for Magic   Every week, we hear about something new that is thought to aid in weight loss or help achieve a healthy body weight. Take oolong tea,[31] green tea, coffee,[32] or hop extract for example. In a study of rodents, researchers found that supplementing the diet with isomerized hop extract (containing isohumulones)—normally found in Indian and American-style pale ales and other styles of beer—prevented weight gain in rodents,[33] and may even have promise in humans.[34] Concerning caffeine,[34] a study conducted in the Netherlands found that people who consumed large amounts of caffeine (more than 300 mg) had greater success at reducing body weight, fat mass, and waist circumference (as well as maintaining resting energy expenditure) than did those who consumed little or no caffeine.[32] Certainly, if you already enjoy a glass of hoppy beer or cup of tea or coffee, relax and know it may help just a wee bit. If you don't, consider that the evidence is not strong enough for you to start taking hop extract, green tea, or caffeine pills.

Furthermore, always use caution when considering new weight-loss information (just as you do with ergogenic aids and herbal supplements). Although some of these aids are harmless foods or products you may already be using, others have the potential to be costly or dangerous, even if they are natural. A few years back, bitter orange peel—a seemingly innocent weight-loss aid—made the news. This product, which was touted as an ephedra-free weight-loss agent, can elevate heart rate and blood pressure in generally healthy individuals, especially when taken with caffeine, and may be no safer than ephedra. (See WebMD for additional information.) It is also considered a banned substance by the NCAA. The bottom line is to simply eat a well-balanced plant-based diet and know that there may be a bit of magic simply in some of what you're already doing. Also, remember that natural and plant-based items are not always safe. Bitter orange is obtained from the peels of Seville oranges, used to make real marmalade. Sure, it is safe in small concentrations, but maybe not when concentrated as a medicinal weight-loss agent.

Remember That a Calorie Is a Calorie   A recent scientific statement from the Endocrine Society addressing the development of obesity still highlights that a calorie is a calorie.[3] It is not fat or carbohydrate that contributes to weight gain, just overeating. Yes, athletes needing to reduce a few pounds are advised to limit alcohol, high-fat foods, and simple sugars, but overall overconsuming these macronutrients is the problem, not the nutrients themselves.

Physics of Weight Gain

Scientists know a lot less about the energy demands of muscle gain than they do about fat loss. We know that if you were to overeat 3,500 calories you should gain close to a pound (0.45 kg) of body fat, but most athletes are not looking to gain body fat. Furthermore, as mentioned earlier, the amount of weight that would be gained by consuming the extra 3,500 calories varies considerably. Some would gain almost exactly 1 pound (0.45 kg), and others, because they can "waste" a higher percent of the excess energy they consume, would gain a bit less. Gaining muscle, however, is more complex. One pound of muscle contains less energy than a pound of fat—about 2,500 calories compared to 3,500 calories—but additional energy costs are required to "build" lean tissue. These include the cost to run the body's protein-making machinery, to arrange the amino acids consumed in the diet into the proper sequence, and to perform the resistance training that stimulates muscle gain. Thus, as much as I hate to say it, the caloric recommendations for weight gain are not based on a lot of hard science. Typically, to keep things simple and allow leeway, most practitioners use a figure of 3,500 calories to represent the cost of gaining 1 pound of muscle tissue.

We do, however, know quite a bit about the potent stimuli for promoting muscle growth or *anabolism,* which includes feeding (as compared to fasting) and resistance training. Although feeding alone is not sufficient to induce muscle growth—otherwise most people in the Western world would look like professional bodybuilders—it supplies the amino acid building blocks, elevates many anabolic hormones, including insulin, and serves as a trigger for muscle protein synthesis.[35] Insulin is important because it helps muscles take up and use amino acids for growth. Resistance exercise, as you know, provides the stimulus for muscle hypertrophy by promoting protein synthesis, which may be elevated for up to 48 hours following just a single bout of strenuous exercise. Eating in close association with resistance exercise is important because protein breakdown also increases after exercise, and food intake helps the body make more muscle than it degrades. Thus, the timing of nutrient delivery relative to the bout of exercise is also important. The general thinking is that feeding should occur 20 to 30 minutes after exercise, or as soon as possible thereafter.

Should You Really Be Trying to Gain Weight?

The ultimate goal for many athletes engaged in heavy strength training is to increase muscle mass. For some athletes—such as wrestlers and baseball players—an increase in muscle with minimal increase in fat mass is desirable. For others—such as powerlifters or football linemen—the absolute mass is important. Vegetarian athletes are no different in this respect. Often included in the trying to gain weight group are athletes who "leaned up" after the transition to a vegetarian diet, most likely because they did not eat enough calories initially, and now want to put this weight back on. See box 13.2 to dispel the myth that vegetarian diets lower testosterone levels and are not compatible with gaining muscle mass.

Similar to athletes with weight-loss goals, many athletes have unrealistic expectations about weight gain. They or their coach have the idea that they can put on 20 to 30 pounds (9-13 kg) of solid muscle during the preseason. They also feel that bigger is almost always better, which follows the movement in certain sports like football and baseball for athletes to become bigger and more muscular. This movement has led to an increase in the number of athletes wanting to gain weight, sometimes at the expense of good health. An example of this is a college football player I worked with for weight loss during my first year as a collegiate sports dietitian. This athlete had deep-red stretch marks over many areas of his body, including his chest and shoulders. Upon inquiry, he told me that he had been on the weight-gain list the year before. He had overdone it by eating a lot of pizza, burgers, fries, and sausage and now was on the weight-loss list. Unfortunately, this athlete and others like him are at increased risk for future struggles with long-term weight maintenance.

Although vegetarian athletes are not likely to overdo the sausage and burgers, athletes trying to gain weight should seriously consider whether their weight-gain goals are realistic based on their genetics, current training regimen, prior training regimen, age, sex, and sport. Expecting to look like Arnold Schwarzenegger in his prime when you come from a family of men who look like Fred Astaire is probably not a realistic goal. However, hoping to gain 20 pounds (9 kg) during your first year of college—the first year you engage in heavy resistance training—certainly may be. One study of 18- to 25-year-old bodybuilders and football players showed that an increase of 20 percent in body mass was possible during one year of heavy resistance training.[36] And although most of the weight gain was in lean mass, individual responses were variable. Such large initial gains, however, quickly taper off and may be as little as 1 to 3 percent after several years of training. This is a common training phenomenon, whereby athletes tend to reach their genetic potential early during a targeted training program and experience only small gains thereafter.

Adapting the Plan to Promote Weight Gain

As with weight reduction, the eating plan for weight gain should be similar to the meal plan you would follow if you were trying to maintain weight, but contain extra calories to support lean-tissue gain. Exactly how much extra has not been established, but the general recommendation is to increase energy intake by about 500 calories per day above daily needs, and to meet your protein and carbohydrate needs.[7] Protein, of course, supplies the amino acids needed for growth, and carbohydrate spares the amino acids so that they can be used to build muscle rather than be converted to blood sugar.

Increasing calories above those of an already high intake, however, is easier said than done. You need to be diligent in your efforts, refrain from skipping

Box 13.2

Low Testosterone Myth

The popular media has spread the rumor that a vegetarian diet might not be appropriate for strength and power athletes because plant-based diets reduce testosterone levels. Although these reports might scare some strength athletes, I can assure you that they mean little to your performance and muscle-gaining abilities, and, in fact, may not be true at all.

- **Testosterone may be lowered when switching to a drastically different diet.** A handful of small-scale studies have found that the concentration of total testosterone in blood tends be lowered when people switch to either a vegetarian diet[37,38] or a low-fat omnivorous diet.[39] Unbound testosterone concentrations—the small fraction that is free to enter target cells—are not typically affected, however, unless the diet is extremely low in fat. Why this drop in total concentration occurs is not well understood but may be related to the reduced fat and cholesterol content of the diet[39] or to the sudden and substantial change in dietary habits.[38,40] Testosterone levels were also found to drop in black South African men who switched from their usual vegetarian diet to a Western diet.[41]

- **Vegan and vegetarian men do not have lower testosterone levels.** Larger-scale comparisons between long-term vegetarians and meat eaters have found that neither total-testosterone nor free-testosterone concentrations are different among vegans, vegetarians, or meat eaters.[40,42] In fact, if anything, total testosterone has been noted by several investigators to be slightly elevated in long-term vegetarians compared to omnivores,[43] and in vegans compared to both vegetarians and omnivores.[42] Thus, it appears that if testosterone levels are lowered during the transition to a vegetarian or vegan diet, this drop is probably short lived.

- **What does it mean if testosterone levels drop?** In the aforementioned studies, total testosterone was lowered in the blood when people switched to a different type of diet, but this reduction was just a small dip and did not fall below the normal range of 300 to 1,200 nanograms per deciliter (ng/dl) for total testosterone. Free testosterone did not drop and remained within the normal range of 9 to 30 ng/dl. Because there is no relationship between muscle gain or strength and variable total testosterone in blood within the normal range, this small dip is meaningless for athletic performance but may be advantageous for cancer prevention. Certainly, if testosterone drops below the normal range, muscle and bone loss may ensue. On the other hand, elevating testosterone beyond the normal physiological range through anabolic steroid use promotes gains in muscle mass. Neither, however, is the issue here.

- **What if I am concerned?** If you are concerned about your testosterone level, ask your personal or team physician to measure total and free testosterone from a blood sample at your next physical. (You may have to pay out of pocket for this.) If it is on the lower range of normal, assess your intake of dietary fat and total energy and increase smart fat choices as needed. The most likely reason for lower testosterone, however, is lack of calorie intake. See chapter 2 for more information and tips on increasing energy intake. Most likely, however, the test will put you at ease.

meals, and pay attention to meal timing. I was always amazed when I asked the college athletes I counseled for weight gain about their food intake immediately before our appointment, which was typically in the late morning or early afternoon following practice. "Nothing for breakfast," they would say. "Nothing after practice," they would follow. "Really?" I always responded. "You are trying to gain weight but you have not eaten anything yet today." These athletes were ignoring some of the basics of gaining weight, which include spreading food intake throughout the day and taking advantage of postexercise meal timing. Ingesting carbohydrate and protein following training promotes muscle protein synthesis because of the improved anabolic hormone environment,[44] so you don't want to miss this window when your goal is to maximize weight gain.

You can take in an extra 500 or so calories each day by eating larger-than-normal portions of healthy foods as part of a well-balanced diet or by adding an extra snack or two (of approximately 250 calories each) to your current intake. Keep bulky low-calorie foods such as whole-grain cereal, salads, and soup to a minimum because they are too filling in relation to the calories they provide. In contrast, healthy shakes, smoothies, fruit juice, and other liquid supplements along with dried fruit and nuts provide an easy way to squeeze the calories in (see box 2.3 on page 27). Healthy sources of fat, including olive oil, avocado, flaxseed oil, low-trans-fat margarine, and nuts and seeds (including nut and seed butters), can be added if you have already met your carbohydrate and protein needs (see box 13.3).

Beyond that, how much weight you gain depends on the many factors discussed earlier, including your genetics, body type, and training regimen and the number of years you have been training. These are factors I typically review with athletes during their initial visit. Athletes who are just starting a new training regimen, such as freshmen football players, are more likely to note significant gains in muscle mass as a result of their resistance training than are more senior players. Along these same lines, athletes who come from families with more muscular (or mesomorphic) body types are more likely to show results than those who come from families with lean (ectomorphic) body types. To this day, I still recall working with an African American football player who had been trying to gain weight for several years. At our first session, we discussed his family background and I learned that not only were his dad, brother, and uncle trying to gain weight, but so was his mother. Although I was able to help him gain about 5 pounds (2.25 kg) before the spring game, which protected him a bit more from the contact on the field, it was apparent he was fighting his genes.

A lot of liquid supplements for weight-gain promise immediate benefits. These liquid formulas are a bit easier to consume than solids and may work simply by increasing an athlete's energy intake. Liquid supplements for weight gain, however, are also packed with various combinations of amino acids that not only taste "supplementy," but also may be produced using nonvegan or nonvegetarian sources. The best bet for a health-conscious vegetarian athlete is to make smoothies and shakes at home (see recipe in chapter 14) so you can control the ingredients. With that said, several plant-based protein powders on the market contain various combinations of plant proteins, including soy, pea,

Box 13.3

Tips for Adopting a Plan to Promote Weight Gain

- Eat a well-balanced vegetarian diet that provides approximately 500 calories per day more than you need in combination with an intense strength or resistance training program.
- Ensure adequate protein intake in the upper range recommended for athletes. Intake beyond this, however, will not promote muscle growth.
- Increase energy intake by selecting larger portion sizes of healthy foods or by adding one or two 250-calorie snacks to your current eating regimen.
- Spread food intake throughout the day and don't skip meals. Eating three meals a day plus two to four snacks is typically needed. Some sources suggest that five to nine eating occasions are required to promote gains in lean mass.[45]
- Consume a high-carbohydrate, protein-containing snack or liquid meal 20 to 30 minutes after exercise to provide the building blocks and anabolic hormone environment.[44]
- Sneak in additional calories by consuming liquids, including smoothies, shakes, and fruit juice. Grape and cranberry juice typically have more calories per cup than other juices.
- Add healthy fats to your diet by snacking on peanuts, nuts, and seeds. Dipping bread in olive oil; spreading peanut butter, other nut butters, or no-trans-fat margarine on crackers, toast or bagels; and adding avocado slices to salads and sandwiches or as a topping on crackers are all great options.
- Keep bulky low-calorie foods such as whole-grain cereal, salads, and soup to a minimum. They are too filling in relation to the calories they provide.
- Do not go overboard. Consuming more than 1,000 calories per day in excess of your normal required intake will lead to fat deposition.
- Strength train, strength train, strength train; and also ensure adequate rest and sleep.[45]
- Remember that muscle can only be gained through intense strength or resistance training several times a week, coupled with the consumption of additional calories.
- Don't overdo it.[46] Excess calorie consumption that results in rapid weight gain may produce mainly adipose tissue, or fat. Athletes should be warned against sudden or excessive gains in body fat—even if it is the culture in some sports.[8]

and brown rice. Additionally, it may be useful to supplement creatine depending on your training phase, goals, and situation. See chapter 10 for additional information on creatine. If you want to try a creatine or protein supplement, evaluate it with great scrutiny as discussed in chapter 10.

This chapter has focused on how you can alter your vegetarian meal or nutrition plan if necessary to promote weight loss or weight gain and also provided tips for changing your habits to maintain a healthy body weight. You are now ready for the remaining step—learning how to whip up quick meals and snacks that fit into your customized meal plan.

14 | Whipping Up Quick Plant-Based Meals and Snacks

She was an junior on the women's soccer team and came to see me in hopes of improving her eating habits. "I don't feel good about myself," she said as she walked in the door to my office, "I need to eat better." Indeed, when we started through her typical day, it was easy to see that her eating habits were irregular and inconsistent. She typically skipped breakfast and admitted it was because she liked to leave the house quickly. She then found herself having to grab a vending-machine snack right before practice because she was ravenous. Lunch was equally haphazard. "I eat a good meal with my roommate at night," she told me. As our discussion proceeded, I realized that she had a good understanding of nutrition and knew what she needed to do, but that she needed specific how-tos—simple how-tos at that, because she claimed she could not cook. We came up with a list of ideas for high-carbohydrate, nutrient-dense meals that were easy to prepare on a budget. We also scheduled a grocery store tour that would focus on how to select nutritious snacks and foods for use in quickly prepared meals. Our most immediate goal, however, was to come up with ideas for quick, healthy breakfasts that she could eat while running out the door. These simple but important changes would start her off on the right track nutritionally.

– Enette

Many athletes get off track when faced with preparing their own meals. In fact, for many athletes it is easy to eat right when their only responsibility is to make good choices from the training table, mess hall, cafeteria, or sorority dining room—unless of course the quality of the food is not up to par. Entering the kitchen and having to prepare healthy meals on a schedule, a budget, or both, however, can be challenging. Wouldn't it be great if we could just hire a personal chef with extensive experience in plant-based cuisine? Because this is unlikely for most of us, this chapter provides tips and ideas to help you set a kitchen PR (preparation record) creating healthy plant-based meals. If you are a novice or feel you just can't cook, this chapter aims to take some of the uncertainty out of meal preparation and start you on your way to performing your best in the kitchen. The last chapter contains a handful of our favorite go-to recipes that are simple but delicious.

Different Tastes for Different Folks

Throughout this book, we have tried to emphasize that there is not a one-size-fits-all approach. As an active vegetarian, you have different taste preferences, eating philosophies, cultures, and lifestyles, and you practice different sports. As such, you may find many of the following tips helpful and directed right at you but find others completely futile. This is to be expected, given that some of you are in school, some are single, some are married, and some have 10 kids (or on some days it seems like there are 10). Some of you frequent your city supermarket, and others shop exclusively at the local co-op or health food store. Some of you garden or shop at the farmers market, while others rely on mostly packaged food. Some of you train in the early-morning hours, and others sneak in workouts before dinner or whenever the 10 kids allow. Some of you are trying to shed a few pounds, and others need ideas to keep eating healthfully. No matter your situation, pick and choose the tips most helpful to you—remembering that things can and do change—and you will be well on your way to whipping up healthy plant-based meals.

Getting Started

As with most exercise and sport training, it is a good idea to start with a plan rather than to dive right in unprepared. Although you won't be concerned with purchasing properly fitting sport equipment, you will need to evaluate the organization of your kitchen, pantry, and cupboards; learn the layout of your favorite food store; and get in the habit of making a weekly game plan.

Organize the Pantry Louis Parrish, a general medicine practitioner who promotes cooking as therapy, once said "If you can organize your kitchen, you can organize your life." This is particularly true for the athlete who eats a plant-based diet. It may take an entire weekend, but it is definitely worth the effort. If your pantry is organized and well stocked, you can easily find the ingredients needed to prepare a quick meal. Start by taking everything out of the cupboards and putting things back so that they are easy to see and reach and fit logically into the flow of how you cook and eat in the kitchen. Oh, and while you're at it, toss out those spices and ingredients you have held onto for years.

Think Ergonomics Athletes are well aware of ergonomics in their own sport but not necessarily in their kitchen. Cyclists are trained to cut corners closely during criterium races, and team athletes intuitively know the shortest path to take to the ball or the opponent. Apply this same type of thinking to your kitchen. Before putting things back into your cupboard, think about where in the kitchen you cook, where you clean up, and where you eat—the three principal work centers in the kitchen. Ideally, your cooking or food-preparation center should be close to the stove, have adequate counter space for chopping and mixing, and be close to the sink and refrigerator. The most-used items—knives, pots and pans, mixing bowls, spices, and cooking utensils—should be stored in the cooking and prep area so that you do not have to do intervals across your kitchen during food preparation. Ideally, the storage pantry should be close to the work area. Because this is not always possible, stock it with the foods and ingredients you use least often during day-to-day food preparation. These might include items such as flour, cornmeal, dried beans, dried fruit, and snack foods. Items used most frequently can be put in a kitchen cupboard as space permits, on the easiest to reach shelves in the pantry, or in another creative and close-by location.

If you are not sure how to come up with a plan, try thinking about the way your coach comes up with playing strategies. It may help to diagram things and trace the path you would walk during dinner preparation. Also, consider the cleanup and serving areas. Dish soap, cleaning supplies, and the dish drainer should be close to the sink; silverware, plates, and glasses should be close to the table. If you have to walk across the kitchen to get a spatula or spices while prepping foods, they're not stored in the most ergonomic spot. If your kitchen is not ideally laid out and you cannot devise "the perfect plan," your goal then should be to come up with the most logical plan. For example, if your sink, refrigerator, and pantry are not close to the prep area, then your plan could be to wash all the vegetables and place them in the prep area by the stove, then gather everything from the pantry and refrigerator and put them in the prep area. Right now my family lives in an old Victorian-style house and despite some remodeling, I don't have a kitchen pantry. My storage pantry is down some stairs, but I also have two sets of attractive wooden kitchen shelves (think Williams-Sonoma or Ikea) in a large hall right off the kitchen. Although I sometimes welcome the idea of an extra stair workout or hallway sprint, I have to be organized if I want to prepare dinner in a timely manner. Luckily, my sink, stove, and chopping block form a nice triangle close to the refrigerator.

Invest in Storage Containers There is a lot to be said for storing ingredients in attractive, airtight containers that fit neatly into cupboards and pantries. To conserve space, they should be square or rectangular, not round. They should also be labeled and preferably clear if you are okay with glass or high-quality plastic. More than 10 years ago, I purchased clear stackable containers that fit in my panty in a modular fashion. I filled them with dry goods, including our most-used grains, textured vegetable protein (TVP), and dried beans. I have never regretted the time investment. In my upstairs hallway pantry, I store dried lentils, beans, and grains along with roasted walnuts, almonds, pumpkin seeds, and flaxseed in square storage containers attractively arranged with a tea collection in an antique Dr Pepper crate and a few infrequently used (but still important) appliances. In my downstairs pantry, I store canned goods (tomatoes, tomato sauce, olives, coconut milk, and an assortment of every kind of bean found in a can) along with fresh onions, unopened grains such as rice, oatmeal and some breakfast cereals, snack items, and corn chips. Pasta, which we use more than rice, is stored upstairs in cupboards in the prep area along with the spices, oils, vinegars, and other basic ingredients. My flour collection, raw sugar, cornmeal, and master mix (a homemade all-purpose baking mix) are stored in a roundabout in the cupboards below my prep area because these ingredients fit there and because I use these items with surprising regularity.

Don't Bury the Herbs and Spices   Another hint I learned when we lived in a new home in Louisiana (that had lots of kitchen drawers), was the benefit of the spice drawer. Keeping spices and herbs in similarly sized containers in a drawer near the stove is a tremendous time saver because you can easily locate the spices you need without having to take everything out of the spice cupboard. My favorite containers are the small glass jars that are round on top with slightly squared bottoms that keep them from rolling. Organizing them in the drawer, however, should be done by personal preference. I typically go with the Simon and Garfunkel approach and put parsley next to sage, rosemary, and thyme and follow with basil and the other spices in a functional order that is probably only logical to me. Others simply alphabetize. If you don't have a spice drawer, which I don't in my Victorian home, you need to find a dedicated cupboard or purchase an attractive spice rack that won't take away your food-preparation space. All in all, you want to arrange the spices you use regularly in a way that you can find them quickly and easily.

Take a Self-Guided Grocery Store Tour   Somewhere in the process of organizing, it might be wise to visit your favorite supermarket or health food store or drop in at Costco to both stock up on ingredients and familiarize yourself with products for vegetarians. This is a great idea even for veteran vegetarians because new foods come onto the market regularly. Before making this trip, take stock of what you have in your pantry and what types of items you are looking for. For example, you might be curious about which food products are fortified with vitamin B_{12} or have added flax, or what healthy snacks, pre-mixes, or bean varieties are available. You might also want to see what foods are available in the bulk foods section of your supermarket or co-op. You may be interested in everything, which is fine; just go prepared to be there a while (and don't take the kids). Table 14.1 lists suggestions for basic items to keep stocked in your pantry or freezer. Box 14.1 provides ideas for your self-guided grocery store tour.

TABLE 14.1 Suggestions for Stocking a Healthful Pantry

Grains	Vegetables	Fruit	Protein	Nuts and oils
Pasta Couscous Brown rice White rice Wild rice Polenta Bulgur or barley Whole-grain and healthy crackers Quinoa Ancient grains Whole-wheat flour Enriched, unbleached white flour Cornmeal All-purpose baking mix (homemade or commercially prepared)	Onions Garlic Sweet potatoes Potatoes Canned tomato products (whole and chopped tomatoes, puree, sauce, paste) Dried mushrooms Sun-dried tomatoes Frozen vegetables (including kale, leafy greens, brussels sprouts, pumpkin puree, roasted tomatoes) Frozen sweet peppers, chopped Frozen roasted chilies and hot peppers Frozen pesto cubes	Dried fruit (cranberries, raisins, cherries, apricots, prunes, dates, figs) Selected canned fruit (in its own juice) Frozen strawberries, berries, peaches Canned local jams, fruit preserves, chutneys	Textured vegetable protein (TVP) Dry beans and peas (lentils, split peas, chickpeas, black, pinto, white, kidney, black-eyed, fava, adzuki) Frozen plant-based protein analogues Frozen edamame	Almonds Cashews Peanuts Pecans Pine nuts Pumpkin seeds Sunflower seeds Nut butters Tahini Olive oil Canola or grapeseed oil Flaxseed oil Flax seeds Hemp oil Sesame seed oil Other flavorful oils

Note: Because many of these items have a limited shelf life, it is a good idea to date foods when purchased and stock only those that you use regularly. If you are a gardener, your frozen vegetable collection can come from surplus harvest at the end of the growing season.

Box 14.1

Taking a Self-Guided Grocery Store Tour

Spending a little time in your grocery store or health food store will help make you aware of the vegetarian products available and their nutritional value. Although the layout of each store differs, the following will help as you take your tour.

Fresh Produce

- Fresh produce is always a good choice. Look for seasonal and locally grown produce.
- Look for a variety of fruits and vegetables and make the effort to try those you have not tasted before.
- Most stores now sell organic produce, which is slightly more expensive. You can also check with the produce manager to learn where produce is purchased and whether the store buys goods from local farmers. Another option is shopping for produce at your local farmers market.
- Look for time savers such as presliced mushrooms and packages of mixed greens and baby spinach. Major grocery stores regularly sell these at reasonable prices—for example, buy one, get one free.

(continued)

Taking a Self-Guided Grocery Store Tour *(continued)*

Bread and Cereal Shelves

- Look for cereal with at least 2 grams of fiber, 8 grams or less of sugar (~ 2 tsp), and 2 grams or less of fat per serving. Compare portion sizes and carbohydrate content on the nutrition facts label; servings range from a 0.25 cup to 1.25 cups. Many cereals are available with added flax or hemp.
- Look for bread that is made from whole grain or partially whole grain. If selecting white bread, choose enriched or unmilled versions, including real sourdough and ciabatta.
- Check ingredient labels for animal products or fully hydrogenated oils.

Canned-Food Aisle

- Canned beans, peas, and tomato products are a must for the plant-based pantry. Choose brands with firm beans or peas of good quality. Use reduced-sodium products if desired, and remember to rinse all beans before use. Also look for vegetarian varieties of baked beans.
- Choose 100 percent pure fruit juices instead of fruit cocktails or punches. If you select a juice that needs sugar, such as cranberry juice or lemonade, look for brands without high-fructose corn syrup.
- Look for canned fruit in its own juice and unsweetened applesauce. These make good staples in the winter months.

Cracker and Cookie Aisle

- Check out the selection of cookies and crackers. You can locate brands that are healthy, but most are loaded with high-fructose corn syrup, sugar, or highly processed oils.
- Good bets for crackers include table water crackers and whole-grain crackers made without fully or partially hydrogenated oils. Check out the emerging variety of wheat-free crackers, including sweet potato and rice crackers and those made with ancient grains (as one of the first few ingredients).
- Best bets for cookies include fruit bars like Fig Newtons; oatmeal cookies; cookies sweetened mostly with fruit purees; and cookies that contain whole grains, nuts, or dried fruit. However, it may be more nutritious (and economical) to whip up a healthy batch at home.

Bulk-Foods Section

- The bulk foods section is a great place to find muesli, granola, and other interesting and healthy cereals; hard-to-find grains; dried fruit; TVP; nutritional yeast; fair-trade teas; and organic candy.
- It is worth a stop every time you are in the store.

Dairy Case

- Organic full-fat milk, cottage cheese, and yogurt provide rich flavor and may contain more desirable bioactive conjugated linoleic acids (CLAs), particularly if the cows were grass fed,[1] that may offer some health benefit. On the other hand, milk, buttermilk, cottage cheese, and yogurt that are nonfat or have 1 percent milk fat offer low-saturated-fat options for athletes who need to watch intake of saturated fat.

- Many brands of plant milks are available in the dairy case or in a nearby case or aisle. Be sure to check the protein content because many nut milks are not as high in protein as you might think.

- Look for strongly flavored cheeses, where a little cheese goes a long way, or cheeses that are made partly with nonfat milk. Cashew-based cheeses are available now more than ever and may be found in health food stores or the specialty section of grocery stores. Be mindful that both the fat content and price may be higher than those of dairy products.

Frozen Foods

- Check out the selection of frozen fruits and vegetables. Because these foods are frozen soon after picking, their nutritional value is often higher than that of fresh. Frozen vegetables are also convenient to keep on hand and lower in sodium than canned. In addition, some stores do not carry certain varieties of fresh products, for example turnip or collard greens, but do offer frozen versions.

- Look for plant-based protein analogues and vegetarian frozen entrees. Many health food store brands have gone mainstream and can be found in local grocery stores.

- The varieties of plant-based protein analogues continue to grow. Check out new and interesting products that fit your taste preferences. Not all tofu dogs and veggie burgers taste alike.

Other

- Learn the layout of your store and which foods are stocked where; this facilitates quick shopping.

- Meander the aisles and read nutrition labels on new or interesting-looking foods. Some seemingly nonvegetarian items, such as premixes, might be vegetarian and might even have vegetarian cooking suggestions on the back.

- In your wanderings, also check out salad dressings, vinegars, flavorful oils, and vegetarian broth offerings. Finding a flavorful salad dressing made with healthy oils and no high-fructose corn syrup and flavorful not-so-salty broth will drastically improve how your meals and foods taste. If you don't find a dressing you like, you can always make your own from flavorful vinegars and oils (see the Add a Salad to the Menu section).

Keep the Cookbooks in Check   The final things you need to organize are your recipes and cookbooks. Although many of you probably have quite a cookbook collection and are maybe even considering purchasing a few more, having cookbooks does not mean you will be efficient cooks with many healthy meal ideas. If only it were that simple! Instead, just the opposite often occurs, because people either become overwhelmed with their collection or spend valuable time looking through cookbooks but are somehow unable to make the connection between the cookbook and the dinner table. What my husband and I started doing years ago (because he wanted a list of tried-and-true recipes he could pass on to patients and colleagues) was to keep files of practical recipes we wanted to try that I organized by categories, such as main dish beans, main dish pasta, main dish other, vegetables, salads, sandwiches, breakfast items, and holiday. When we wanted to try a new recipe, one of us would pull it from the file or look one up in a cookbook and prepare it. If we loved it and it was easy to prepare, I would type it into a word-processing program, noting modifications, meal serving suggestions, and the original source. If we thought it was *just OK* or did not really enjoy it, we tossed it into the recycling bin. If we loved it but found it too tedious, it went back into the file drawer in a folder labeled "special occasion." Alternately, if you seek out recipes online, you can do something similar using an electronic filing system that works for you.

Over the years, we have developed our collection of easy-to-prepare preferred recipes. Although we keep adding to the file, I print it out periodically and stick the pages in plastic protectors that we keep in a stainless steel file holder right in the kitchen. And the word-processed files are easy to email to my mother-in-law, interested friends, patients, and colleagues (in a way silently recruiting them into the vegetarian world). Although I occasionally consult my favorite cookbooks, it is typically only to look up a standard recipe like cornbread or bran muffins, or to seek out a new recipe idea. I have also narrowed my collection tremendously and only keep the cookbooks that have recipes we *love.* After a while you begin to notice that there are some cookbooks you

---

Vegan View: New Plant-Based Options Abound

It seems like every day a new plant-based product to replace meat and dairy hits the market, from cashew yogurts to fancy French cheeses. It's incredible what you can now get; this makes eating a plant-based diet today quite different, and much easier, than it was in the 1970s! It's no longer just soy and gluten; coconut, cashews, almonds, pea, hemp, oats, and more are being turned into plant milks, cheeses, ice creams, and meats. A veggie burger that bleeds (thanks to the added heme) may not be your cup of tea, but these new options can replace the dairy and meat you may currently eat. Of course, as a discerning athlete, you must check the label: They don't all have the equivalent nutritional composition of the products they are replacing. Check the protein, fat, iron, and calcium content. And remember that there is a wide variety in tastes and textures, so try a few companies and versions to find one you like.

always reach for and others that collect dust. This does not mean they are not good cookbooks, just that they don't match your taste preference and style.

Sticking to the Basics

Although you don't want to wait until you are fully organized to start whipping up healthy meals, it certainly helps to start out somewhat on the right foot. Once you are organized or are in the process of organizing, you can begin thinking about daily meal preparation.

Work Out the Plan   The number one reason athletes eat haphazardly is that they fail to plan. In chapter 12, we discussed custom meal plans—which help you learn to eat right—but you also need a weekly or bimonthly menu plan to assist with dinner, portable lunches, and grab-and-go breakfasts. Unlike the eating plan, however, the meal plan is something you, along with the rest of the members of your household, should create regularly. Although you can go about this in many ways, it may be less daunting if you dedicate time once a week for menu planning and follow a basic structure. The basic structure might look something like the sample shown in table 14.2, where you would tentatively plan to serve certain types of dishes once a week and even on specific nights if it helps. Another alternative is a soup and salad night, veggie burger night, Mexican or Indian night, pasta night, stir-fry or quick-skillet night, and slow-cooker night, for example. It depends on your preferences. If you are semivegetarian, you might build off of the plant foods you are already eating and limit meat-containing dishes to once or twice a week.

Once you have a workable form, select main dish recipes that fit the theme and add in—just like you did with your eating plan—bread, side vegetables or salads, fruits, and healthy desserts as appropriate. Often with vegetarian cuisine, the vegetables are part of the main dish, so you may simply need to add bread or a fruit or leafy green salad and you are done. For example, a bowl of vegetarian chili goes great with whole-wheat soda crackers or homemade cornbread and sliced fresh fruit drizzled with fresh lime juice, whereas most bean and vegetable soups and pasta dishes need just a leafy green salad and some bread. A tofu and vegetable stir-fry with fresh ginger is complete. Just serve it over rice or Asian noodles with a glass of water and white wine if desired. Add a fresh or baked pear for dessert or freshly popped (add-your-own-oils) popcorn as a late-night snack if you are still hungry.

Think About Planned-Overs   Give yourself a break at least once a week by eating "planned-overs." You can do this simply by eating vegetarian chili on both Monday and Wednesday or creatively by serving Monday's chili over a baked or microwaved potato on Wednesday or even freezing Monday's chili and eating it on Wednesday a few weeks later. I do this a lot with vegetable soups, such as pumpkin or butternut squash. I broil a few small pumpkins or squash from the garden and sauté with onions, sage, and olive oil in vegetable

TABLE 14.2   Sample Menu Rotation

Sunday	Monday	Tuesday	Wednesday	Thursday	Friday	Saturday
Hearty bean dish	Tofu or tempeh	Pasta	Planned-overs	Vegetable dish	Protein analogues	Rice or grain

YEAR-ROUND AND WINTER SUGGESTIONS

Hearty bean dishes

Lentil tacos*
Vegetarian chili*
Red beans and rice
Sloppy joes*
Minestrone*
Hoppin' john
White-bean soup
Lentil dahl over Indian rice
Spicy chickpeas over rice
Jamaican black beans with broiled plantain
Hearty bean skillet dish or casserole (see table 14.3)

Tofu or tempeh dishes

Tofu vegetable stir-fry with cashews
Tofu with peanut sauce and Asian noodles*
Tofu, onion, and vegetable fajitas
Tofu and vegetable pot pie
Baked tempeh with mashed potatoes and mushroom gravy
Asian noodles with marinated tempeh and snow peas

Pasta dishes

Spaghetti with marinara sauce or lentil–tomato sauce
Pasta primavera
Penne with roasted vegetables
Spinach lasagna
Black bean and cilantro lasagna*
Rigatoni with caramelized winter squash, shallots and fresh herbs

Vegetable dishes

"Cream" of carrot, broccoli, or cauliflower soup (see table 14.4 for recipe ideas)
Roasted pumpkin or butternut soup
Potato dill soup
Parsnip and carrot soup with leeks
Beet greens and vegetarian sausage soup
Winter squash stuffed with pine nuts and feta cheese (served over brown rice)
Stuffed peppers (served with rice)
Spaghetti squash with red or white pasta sauce and toasted pine nuts
Baked potato or sweet potato with toppings

Protein-analogue dishes

Veggie burger on whole-grain bun with sweet potato fries
Veggie "chicken" nuggets with broccoli slaw and pumpernickel rolls
Mushroom and "burger" crumbles stroganoff
Vegetarian sausage with potato pancakes and homemade applesauce
Tofu pigs in a blanket

Rice or grain dishes

Couscous with winter vegetable stew
Mushroom and barley soup
Spinach risotto (made in pressure cooker)
Smoked-chipotle rice with pinto beans
Wild rice soup
Mixed vegetable and rice pilaf with toasted nuts* (also great with other grains)

SUMMER SUGGESTIONS

Hearty bean dishes

Three-bean salad
Black bean and corn salad
White bean and goat cheese tostadas with tomato-mango salsa
Tofu or tempeh dishes
Greek tofu salad
Asian cabbage and noodle salad with tofu
Sesame tofu over cold rice noodles
Tofu and vegetable kabobs
Tofu, grapes, and red-leaf-lettuce salad (served with toasted flat bread)

Pasta dishes

Penne and roasted pepper and tomato salad
Italian pasta salad (with chickpeas)
Pasta with homemade pesto* and fresh tomatoes

Vegetable dishes

Main dish chef's salad (with greens, beans, cottage cheese, and vegetables)
Tomato gazpacho with avocado
Grilled portobello mushroom burger
Baked (or microwaved) potato or sweet potato with fresh vegetables and soy sour cream

Protein-analogue dishes

Grilled vegetarian burger on whole-grain bun with grilled summer vegetables
Coney Island vegetarian dog and slaw

Rice or grain dishes

Couscous salad with cucumber, peppers, and tomatoes
Tabouli
Wheat-berry and orange salad with vinaigrette
Polenta triangles with fresh saffron tomatoes

*See chapter 15 for recipes.

broth and, after pureeing, I freeze quite a bit in pint or quart bags. I then stir in the milk, soy milk, or silken tofu along with it for the current night's dinner and do the same with the defrosted mixture for a quick meal a few weeks later. Another way to use planned-overs is to cook up a huge pot of dried beans and use them in several meals throughout the week, giving you black bean week, pinto bean week, and cannellini bean week. Cooked beans can also be frozen and tossed in recipes a few weeks later.

Keep the Plans Quick and Simple   During the week and on busy race or game weekends, don't be afraid to keep the plan simple. Although I cook from our recipe list many nights, I also make many throw-together meals such as vegetarian burgers and broiled sweet potato fries or simple skillet meals or casseroles (see table 14.3). I also make quick meals by adding frozen vegetables and either tofu or canned and rinsed beans to commercially available premixes. For several of my current favorites, I toss tofu into Thai peanut or other Thai-style mixes and steam Chinese cabbage. Or I whip up one of the "impossible pies" or pizza bakes listed on the Bisquick box (using the new Bisquick Heart Smart made with canola oil or homemade master mix—see box 14.2). My kids

TABLE 14.3   Quick Skillet Meals

Grains	Sauce	Beans, TVP, or burger crumbles	Vegetables	
1 cup uncooked	1 can soup plus 1-1/2 cans water or milk	1 can beans, or 3/4 cup dry TVP, or 1-1/2 cups burger crumbles, or 1 package tofu	1-1/2 to 2 cups frozen or raw	1. Choose one food from each of the four groups in the table. If desired, sauté vegetables first. Stir in remaining ingredients. 2. Season to taste with salt, pepper, soy sauce, fresh or dehydrated minced onion, and fresh garlic. 3. Bring water to boil.
Whole-wheat macaroni shells, fiore, rotini, or other small pasta Brown rice Bulgur	Canned chopped tomatoes with herbs Cream of celery soup Cream of mushroom soup Tomato soup Onion soup Vegetable soup or broth	Kidney beans Pinto beans Black beans White beans Chickpeas Black-eyed peas TVP "Burger" crumbles Extra-firm tofu	Onions Celery Green peppers Mushrooms Carrots Peas Corn Green beans Broccoli Spinach Mixed vegetables	4. Reduce heat to lowest setting; cover and simmer 30-40 min until pasta or rice is tender. Stir occasionally to prevent sticking. 5. Stir in up to 1/2 cup cheese at the very end (optional). Example 1: Macaroni mixed with canned tomatoes and herbs, kidney beans, and a combination of onion, celery, and bell or hot peppers Example 2: Shells mixed with mushroom soup, TVP, and mixed vegetables (no cheese) *Note:* These ingredients also work well in a casserole. Mix all ingredients and bake in a covered casserole dish at 350 °F (177 °C) for 35-45 minutes.

Note: Refer to appendix F for guidance on converting English units to metric.

Adapted from *Wyoming Cent$ible Nutrition News,* a publication of the Wyoming Food Stamp Nutrition Education Program, University of Wyoming.

loved my version of salsa "chicken" fiesta even when they were little, which I prepare with one can of pinto beans and one can of light-red kidney beans instead of chicken. Other ideas include making fajitas with a commercial fajita mix and tofu, onion, bell pepper, and summer squash; tossing black-eyed peas into a dirty-rice mix or pinto beans into a smoked-chipotle rice mix; or using TVP, portabella mushrooms, or "burger" crumbles instead of hamburger in noodle or rice dishes. A favorite of my oldest daughter is to toss extra-firm tofu into the Asian peanut salad mix available at Costco. A final idea is to create a quick dragon bowl (see front cover) for a quick dinner or to take for lunch. Begin with a base of fresh greens lightly tossed with Asian dressing (see page 257, Add a Salad to the Menu). Cover with a pile of noodles, quinoa, or brown rice tossed with a little sesame oil, ginger, tamari or Sriracha sauce. Pile on assorted fresh, roasted, or steamed veggies, fruit, tofu, legumes, and nuts. Vegetarians can also consider tossing in a hard or soft cooked egg.

Although a clear disadvantage to some of these mixes is their content of sodium, processed fats, or unrecognizable ingredients, you can look for brands that have no monosodium glutamate or added hydrogenated oils and use just half to three-quarters of the salt-containing flavor packet. For the Bisquick meals, you can also make your own baking premix (see box 14.2), using a

TABLE 14.4 Quick and Hearty "Cream" Soups

Onion	Vegetable	Garlic and spices	"Milk and cream"	
1 onion or large leek 1 bunch green onions or shallots Celery (All roughly chopped)	1 large head broccoli or cauliflower 1 roasted butternut squash or small pumpkin 3-4 cups potatoes, carrots or other vegetable	2 or 3 cloves of garlic 1 tsp salt or vegetable bullion (more to taste) 1/2 tsp curry powder or dry mustard (broccoli) 1-3 tbsp fresh sage (winter squash) or dill (potatoes)	1-2 cups cows' milk, soy milk, rice milk, coconut milk, or onion-based "dairy-free cream"* or 1 package silken tofu. *to make dairy-free cream, roast whole onions in oven for 1 hour at 400 °F (204 °C). Remove skins and blend with a few splashes of oil and lemon juice until smooth.	1. Choose food from each of the four groups in the table. 2. Sauté onion or leek in 1-2 tsp olive oil until soft. 3. Stir in roughly chopped vegetables or pulp from roasted winter squash or pumpkins. Add 2-3 cups water (more for raw vegetables and less for roasted squash) and garlic or spices 4. Simmer uncovered over medium-low heat for 10-20 min until vegetables are soft. 5. Puree in batches in a blender or food processor until smooth (or use an immersion blender). Blend in tofu or "milk" choice and more water as needed. 6. Return to pan. Heat on low until warm 7. Stir in 1 cup grated cheese (optional) for soups such as cauliflower, broccoli, and potato. Top with sliced green onions, roasted pumpkin seeds, or a dollop of yogurt.

Note: Refer to appendix F for guidance on converting English units to metric.

combination of whole and white flours and healthy oils. This works perfectly for making quick meals and breads for dinner as well as breakfast.

Add a Salad to the Menu   Add a mixed green salad to dinner or lunch at least a few times a week. Salads are easy to make—particularly if you use the prepared green mixes—and pack in the nutrients, including calcium, vitamin C, vitamin E, vitamin K, vitamin A, the carotenoids, iron, zinc, magnesium, and healthy fats. Tossing in fresh and dried fruit adds more carbohydrate. If you are tired of the traditional lettuce and tomato salad, try some of the following salads made with greens, fruits, vegetables, nuts, healthy oils, and optional cheese. Also note that the oil in the dressing helps enhance absorption of the fat-soluble vitamins and phytochemicals[2] (as does avocado[2,3] and cooked eggs), whereas vinegar may aid in absorption of iron, zinc, and calcium.

- Mixed greens with tangerines, dried cranberries, and slivered almonds. Serve with honey and Dijon mustard vinaigrette.
- Spinach and arugula with chopped apple, dried cranberries, and toasted walnuts. Serve with red wine and olive oil vinaigrette.
- Spinach and red leaf lettuce with strawberries, red onions, and toasted walnuts. Serve with champagne and olive oil vinaigrette.
- Arugula with grilled apple, bread, blue cheese, and grapes. Serve with basic or raspberry vinaigrette.
- Watercress with fennel, oranges, and walnuts. Serve with sweet orange dressing (made with orange juice and olive or hemp oil).
- Arugula with Bartlett pears and grated fresh Parmesan or Gorgonzola cheese. Serve with lemon juice and hazelnut oil or walnut oil vinaigrette.
- Watercress with red pears and walnuts. Serve with honey and Dijon mustard dressing.
- Mixed greens with caramelized onions, baked goat cheese, toasted walnuts, and fresh or dried figs. Serve with rosemary honey vinaigrette.
- Boston or Bibb lettuce and dandelion greens with chopped apricots, toasted pecans, and smoked Gouda. Serve with raspberry vinaigrette.
- Mixed greens with blueberries, toasted pecans, and Gorgonzola or blue cheese. Serve with white wine and olive oil vinaigrette.
- Baby kale or fresh spinach with avocado, grated carrot, and sunflower seeds. Serve with tomato and herb dressing.
- Kale (finely chopped) with toasted pumpkin seeds, Parmesan cheese (optional), and finely chopped red onion, fresh apples or peaches. Serve with red wine or white balsamic vinaigrette. Rice vinegar, minced ginger, fresh garlic, tamari sauce, toasted sesame oil, orange juice, peanut butter, mango chutney, olive oil, and dash of sugar. Makes an excellent base for a dragon bowl.

Box 14.2

Master Mix and Recipes

Master mix (MIX)

4 cups enriched flour
3-3/4 cups whole-wheat flour
1/4 cup double-acting baking powder
3 tbsp sugar
1 tbsp iodized salt
1-1/3 cups nonfat dry milk powder[a]
1 cup canola oil

Sift enriched flour with baking powder, sugar, and salt. Stir in dry milk. Cut in oil with pastry blender or fingers until it looks like coarse cornmeal. Stir in whole-wheat flour; stir well. Makes about 10 cups.

Note: Keeps about three months in refrigerator.

To measure MIX: Stir lightly and pile into cup (do not shake or level off).

Cornbread

1 cup MIX
1 cup cornmeal
2 tbsp sugar
1/2 tsp baking soda
1 egg beaten[a]
1 cup buttermilk, sour milk, or soy milk

Blend dry ingredients thoroughly. Combine beaten egg and buttermilk; stir into dry ingredients. Pour into greased 8-inch (20 cm) square pan.

Bake at 425 °F (218 °C) for 25 to 30 minutes.

Biscuits

2 cups MIX
1/3 to 1/2 cup water

Stir MIX and water together in bowl. Knead gently about 12 times on floured surface. Roll or pat to 1/2-inch (12 mm) thickness. Cut into circles using a floured biscuit cutter or glass. Bake at 450 °F (232 °C) for 12 to 15 minutes.

Makes 10 to 12 biscuits

Banana bread

2 eggs[b]
1/4 cup sugar
1/2 tsp baking soda
1-1/4 cups mashed banana
2-1/2 cups MIX

Beat eggs and sugar together in a bowl until well blended. Mix in soda and mashed banana. Stir in MIX just until all dry ingredients are coated. Pour into a greased loaf pan that is 9 × 5 × 3 inches (23 × 13 × 8 cm). Bake at 350 °F (171 °C) for 45 to 55 minutes or until brown.

Variation: For pumpkin bread, use 1/2 cup sugar plus 1/2 tsp cinnamon, 1/4 tsp nutmeg, 1/4 tsp ginger, 1/4 cup water, and 1 cup canned or cooked mashed pumpkin or squash. For zucchini bread use 1-1/2 cups shredded zucchini and 2/3 cup sugar.

Muffins

3 cups + 2 tbsp MIX
4 tbsp raw sugar or brown sugar
1 egg, beaten[b]
1 cup water
1 cup fruit (mashed banana, blueberries, pumpkin puree, applesauce, or rhubarb)
1 tsp cinnamon, vanilla, or pumpkin pie spice (optional)

Combine MIX and sugar. Blend egg and water; add to MIX. Stir gently just until dry ingredients are moistened. Mixture should be lumpy. Bake in well-greased muffin pans at 425 °F (218 °C) for about 20 minutes. Makes 12 muffins.

Note: Refer to appendix F for guidance on converting English units to metric. Additional recipes for using homemade master mix or Bisquick Heart Smart (made with canola oil) can be found at www.bettycrocker.com/products/bisquick.

[a]May use nondairy dry milk substitutes such as Vances DariFree or or NutQuick powder.

[b]May use vegan egg replacer.

Adapted from *Wyoming Cent$ible Nutrition News,* a publication of the Wyoming Food Stamp Nutrition Education Program, University of Wyoming.

Keep in mind, however, that because the dressing can make or break the salad, you should use fresh homemade vinaigrettes or your favorite commercial dressing prepared with healthy oils and without high-fructose corn syrup. The basic dressing has one part vinegar plus juice, if desired, and one to two parts oil plus added favorites such as black pepper, herbs, finely chopped scallions, green onions or chives, Dijon mustard, maple syrup, honey, or other flavorings. Using different vinegars such as rice, balsamic, red wine, raspberry, or tangerine will also impart different flavors when paired with different oils such as olive, walnut, or hazelnut. It is worth it to splurge on high-quality vinegar and oil.

Prepare Grab-and-Go Breakfasts   Because many athletes struggle with the need for grab-and-go breakfasts, coming up with a list of options and posting them on the refrigerator or in the notes on your smart phone is a big help. See box 14.3 for a list of ideas to get you started. Believe it or not, this is much easier than planning lunch or dinner. Before you go to the store each week, simply take stock of what you have and make your list accordingly. For example, if you are happy having English muffins all week, you just need to add fresh fruit and English muffins to your list and make sure you are not out of jam or low-trans-fat margarine. If you like the idea of homemade hearty muffins, set aside time on the weekend and make up a batch or two and freeze them (see box 14.2 and chapter 15 for recipes). You can then pop one or two in the microwave before leaving the house or when you get to work. Remember to add juice or fresh fruit or even a glass of soy milk or a hard-boiled egg. Also remember that when you have more time—like your off day or Sunday morning after your long run—you might enjoy experimenting with cooked hearty grains, tofu, or egg and vegetable skillet dishes. Ideas include fruit crepes, waffles with apricot and ginger compote, scrambled tofu with vegetables, tofu breakfast burrito, and hot porridge with fruit puree and roasted nuts.

Plan Portable Lunches   Lunches are also a challenge for many vegetarian athletes, myself included. I remember living in Birmingham, Alabama, where many restaurants served delicious and reasonably priced vegetarian fare just a short walk from my lab. Currently, however, I have no such luxury. If I am not prepared, I end up eating sport bars and dried fruit and coming home starved. Although I can get away with this on rest days, it is worse than awful on days I run at noon or stop at the dance studio after work for Irish dance practice. The solution, of course, is to stock your pantry with lunch options and spend five or so minutes after dinner preparing the next day's lunch (see box 14.4 for ideas). My youngest daughter, Marlena, is a pro at planning lunches and honestly should have guest edited the lunch-planning section. If it helps, set up a rotating lunch schedule and use what you learned in chapter 12 to plan your lunches. Marlena aims for a main meal item, a fruit or two, pretzels, nuts or chips, and sometimes a healthy dessert. Remember that leftovers are also a great lunch option. In my house, however, Marlena often comes to the table with her lunch container so no one else can snag the leftovers.

Box 14.3

Ideas for Grab-and-Go Breakfasts

Keep fresh or dried fruit and juice in small reusable containers on hand, ready to grab along with one of the following:

- Homemade muffins, made with grapeseed or canola oil and whole or unmilled grains
- Trail mix or granola in portion-sized baggies
- Whole-grain English muffin with low-trans-fat margarine or nut butter and jam (making a sandwich using both halves reduces the mess)
- Fresh or toasted bagels with nut butter or Neufchatel cheese
- Fruit bread such as pumpkin, zucchini, or banana, made with canola oil
- Toaster sticks or waffles (hold the syrup); some versions now add flax
- Fruit smoothie with added flax or flaxseed oil (see table 14.5)
- Dairy or soy yogurt, fruit, and granola parfait (made the night before in a to-go container)
- Breakfast cookies (Make your favorite oatmeal cookies with half the sugar, orange juice as the liquid, and added dried fruit and ground flaxseed. Who said you can't have cookies for breakfast? See recipe in chapter 15.)
- Healthier granola or breakfast bars made with whole grains and healthy oils and without high-fructose corn syrup (usually available at health food stores)
- Cereal and soy milk in a large portable cup (Believe it or not, I used to run down a huge hill in Brookline, Massachusetts, with cereal and sliced banana in a cup to catch the mass-transit train. I then devoured it seated or standing. Don't try this while driving, however.)
- Overnight oatmeal in a to-go container (Toss in nuts, dried fruit, and a splash of sweetener right before you eat.)

Think Healthy Snacks   Thinking about healthy snacks is similar to planning a grab-and-go breakfast and a portable lunch. Make a list of healthy snacks and keep several varieties in stock at home, at your office, and in your workout bag. Because your energy needs vary considerably from day to day, it helps to have healthy snacks available when you are hungry. If you are a fan of less-healthy snacks, it is best to buy them in individual-sized portions.

Compose a Store List   The final piece of weekly meal planning is to make a grocery store list, but you probably saw this coming. To do this properly, check your organized pantry for what is in stock and make a list of what you will need to make quick breakfasts and lunches and prepare dinner meals. If you always shop at the same grocery store, you may find that it is easiest to make up your list based on the store layout. For example, when I make my list, I try to list the foods in the order I find them as I walk through the store: bakery section, breakfast cereal, canned vegetables, dairy, produce, and the vegetarian section. Believe me, it takes me almost twice as long to shop at the store across town, where I am not familiar with the layout.

Box 14.4

Ideas for Quick Portable Lunches

Pack one of the following lunches with fresh fruit, whole-grain crackers, whole-wheat pretzels or chips baked or made with healthy oils, and healthy cookies. Add water, soy milk, fruit juice, or Gatorade to drink.

Tomato, avocado, and spicy sprouts on a sesame-seed bagel

Black beans, lettuce, avocado or Neufchatel cheese, and salsa in a spinach or whole-wheat roll-up

Home-grown tomato, fresh large-leaf basil, and mozzarella drizzled with balsamic vinegar on sour dough (my summertime favorite)

Hummus and sliced vegetables in a pita or on grilled focaccia bread

Chickpeas, vegetables, cottage cheese (optional), and Italian dressing in a whole-wheat pita

Black-eyed-peas spread (1 can beans, 1/2 cup parsley, 2 tbsp olive oil, 2 tbsp lemon juice, 1/2 tsp tarragon, and garlic and pepper to taste) on flat bread or leftover cornbread

Chili bean spread (1 cup pinto beans, 1 tsp chili powder, 1 tsp onion powder, 1 tsp chopped green chili peppers, and 1/4 tsp red-pepper flakes) on flat bread or in a whole-wheat roll-up

Red-pepper bean spread (1 cup white beans, 3 tsp finely chopped roasted sweet peppers, 1 tsp finely chopped scallions) on focaccia or flat bread

Kidney beans, chopped sweet peppers, and celery with Italian dressing in a pita

Fresh spinach, cashews, cranberry sauce, and chickpeas in a whole-wheat roll-up

Grilled or roasted peppers, eggplant, and squash with olive oil and feta on sourdough or Italian bread

Tofu "egg" salad (firm tofu mixed with celery, sweet peppers, mustard, mayonnaise, and dill) in a whole-wheat pita with lettuce and tomato

Marinated tofu, lettuce, and vegetables in a whole-grain pita

Herbed cottage cheese or tofu filling (1/2 cup cottage cheese or mashed tofu, 1 tsp lemon juice, 1 tbsp minced green onion, 1 tsp dill or 2 tbsp chopped chives) in a whole-wheat pita with shredded vegetables

Tempeh-salad sandwich (tempeh mixed with mayonnaise, yogurt, celery, and mustard) on whole-grain bread or in a whole-wheat pita with lettuce and tomato

Grilled or roasted eggplant spread (1 large roasted eggplant blended with 1/4 cup chopped parsley, 1 tbsp green onion, 2 tsp lemon juice, 1 tbsp olive oil, and salt and pepper to taste) on sourdough or Italian bread

Dark leafy greens in a pita with chickpeas, kidney beans, or white beans and honey-mustard dressing

Peanut butter, sliced banana, raisins, and walnuts on whole-wheat bread

Nut butter and jam on whole-wheat bread

Peanut butter and pickles on mixed-grain bread (delicious after long endurance races or when pregnant)

Refer to appendix F for guidance on converting English units to metric.

For other ideas, take note of the menu next time you eat at your favorite restaurant, deli, coffee shop, or natural food store.

TABLE 14.5 Whipping Up Healthy Smoothies

Fruit (~1 cup fresh or frozen)	Fruit juice (~1/2 cup)	Tofu or dairy	Extras (small amounts for flavor)	
Bananas	Apple	Milk (1 cup)	Honey	1. Select ingredients.
Pineapples	Orange	Buttermilk (1 cup)	Maple syrup	2. If using flaxseeds, blend on high until ground. Add ingredients and blend until smooth.
Mangos	Pineapple	Yogurt (1 cup)	Vanilla	
Berries	Grape	Silken tofu (1 cup)	Flaxseed or peanut butter (1 tbsp)	3. If using flax or hemp oils, blend all ingredients except oil until smooth. Turn blender to low and slowly drizzle in oil.
Kiwi fruits	Cranberry	Soy milk (1 cup)	Flaxseed oil (1-3 tsp)	
Nectarines		Powdered milk (2 tbsp)	Grape nuts or wheat germ (1-2 tbsp)	4. For all other combinations, place all ingredients in blender and mix until smooth.
Cherries		Isolated soy protein (1-3 tbsp)	Fresh mint	5. Experiment with different combinations of fruit, vegetables, fluids and extras.
Papayas		Calcium-rich greens such as kale	Fresh lime or fresh lemon zest	
Peaches				
Apricots				Example 1: Bananas with orange juice, yogurt, and flaxseed
Melon				Example 2: Peaches with cranberry juice, tofu, and fresh mint
Fruit cocktail				
Kale				Example 3: Pineapple, orange juice, kale, almond milk, and crushed ice
Spinach				*Note:* Ice cubes or crushed ice may be added to make a slushier frozen smoothie.

Note: Refer to appendix F for guidance on converting English units to metric.

Adapted from WIN the Rockies (Wellness IN the Rockies, http://www.uwyo.edu/wintherockies).

Keeping It Exciting

Creating healthy meals is a lifelong process and one you need to fit into your regular routine—just like your training. Once you have the basics down, however, you will find that it does not take much work, and the work is, for the most part, enjoyable. Although I must admit, my favorite meals are those I prepare with my husband on relaxed nights, perhaps while enjoying a glass of wine, after a good workout earlier in the day. When the kids were little, I also heartily enjoyed making quick meals they could help with. If only I could get them to do that as teenagers. The following information provides a few more suggestions for effective meal planning for vegetarian athletes.

Periodize Your Meal Plan Eating the same thing every week can get pretty boring. This and the fact that different foods are available during different seasons—particularly locally grown foods—are reasons to periodize your menus, much like you periodize your training. In our family, we tend to eat a lot of hearty soups in the winter, which we serve with salad and whole grain or European-style bread. In the summer, we make a lot of hearty salads and meals that can be prepared without heating the house (see table 14.2). We also take advantage of seasonal produce, whether it comes from our garden, the farmers market, or the store. As an athlete, however, you may also find your menu choices vary a bit depending on your training season. If you are training at a high volume, you might find that you prefer eating main dishes with pasta, rice, or other grains most of the time and then enjoy soup and salad when your training volume is lower. This is also something to consider when planning your weekly menus. Think about what you prefer to eat after a weight workout compared to an aerobic workout. Hopefully, if you live with a roommate, spouse, or partner, your training schedules and menu preferences will coincide. If not, aim to make the same main dish and vary the side selection and portions according to your training. See the Athlete's Plates food guide for visual examples (appendix B).

Try a New Cooking Technique or a Class   There is much more to cooking than an oven, a skillet, and a microwave. If you are not using them already, try experimenting with a slow cooker, pressure cooker, grill, or wok or enroll in a cooking class. Slow cookers are great if you have time in the morning; you can throw in a vegetarian stew, dahl, soup, curry, or pasta sauce and come home to find dinner ready to go. On the other hand, pressure cookers can cook a meal, including risotto, quinoa, or bean soup in less than 20 minutes. Unlike your grandma's pressure cooker, new technology makes current models safer to use. Grills—both outdoor or the indoor type—are perfect for grilling tasty fresh veggies, marinated tofu, and even fruit—yum! My oldest daughter, Lindsey, was amazed to learn how fancy-looking and tasty an indoor grill makes peanut butter and banana or hummus and veggie sandwiches. (OK, I have to admit the grill had been collecting dust for several years until she rediscovered it.) Woks and rice cookers are also convenient if you make stir-fry often and cook a lot of rice.

To enroll in a class, check out those offered by hospitals, cooking stores, or college or university cooperative extension or outreach programs. And, don't be afraid to take a class if it is not specifically vegetarian. Many times the instructor will provide vegetarian suggestions if he or she knows up front that you are vegetarian. And usually you can modify the recipes so that they are vegan or vegetarian. Cooking classes not only give you ideas, but often also improve your chopping and cooking skills. By the way, when was the last time you sharpened your vegetable-chopping knives?

Don't Be Afraid to Modify Delicious-Sounding Omnivorous Recipes
Several of our favorite recipes in our recipe packet are ones I modified from meat-based recipes or dishes I saw on restaurant menus. Although you will get better at this the more you cook and eat vegetarian meals, here are a few tricks of the trade. Marinated tofu works well in place of chopped chicken or turkey. Marinate the tofu in the sauce or spices used in the recipe and if desired, use previously frozen tofu. Freezing the tofu removes some of the water and makes the texture a bit chewier. TVP, tempeh, seitan, or "burger" crumbles (a ground-beef analogue) typically work well in place of ground beef in many dishes. The burger crumbles have more flavor but also add salt. Thus, TVP works better in dishes with stronger flavors and burger crumbles work better when the flavor of the dish depends on the quality of the protein analogue. Fresh

or dried mushrooms, particularly porcini, portobello, and crimini, also work well as beef substitutes. In many recipes, different beans work well either alone or in combination with TVP. Just experiment, and it should become second nature. Finally, many spicy versions of vegetarian sausages can be sliced and added in place of meat sausage. However, these dishes will taste fine without sausage as long as you add a flavorful lower-salt vegetarian broth. In my family, I always add the veggie sausages at the end because two of my kids hate them. The rest of us like them more than we should.

Grow Herbs and Leafy Greens   Although many vegetarian athletes are interested in gardening—and may even be master gardeners—others do not have the space or the time. My suggestion for all athletes, however, is to experiment with learning to grow the minimal amount during the growing season in your area. This includes herbs such as basil, cilantro, mint, and darker leafy greens such as California mix, arugula, spinach, kale, and dandelion greens. Once you establish kale, for example, it grows like a weed and can supply an abundance of this calcium-rich green for salads, smoothies, and soup (later in season). You can also blanch it for two minutes in boiling water and freeze it for use later in the winter. In just a small space, you can have access to fresh herbs and greens. Also you can grow herbs year-round in pots in your house. If this is not feasible or of no interest to you, joining a CSA (community supported agriculture) or regularly frequenting your farmers market will connect you with the seasonality of food and expose you to more plant-based foods. A movement is growing to connect elite athletes to their food and how it is grown. The Olympic Training Center, for example, encourages resident athletes to spend time in the garden on the Colorado campus.

Become a Foodie   Becoming a vegetarian athlete foodie takes time and dedication. As your training and lifestyle allow, make the effort to expose yourself to new foods by strolling through farmers markets (looking for foods you have not tried), watching the Food Network (warning, this can be addictive), spending quality time with your cookbook collection, and frequenting trendy vegetarian restaurants. I may be biased, but there are many more options for vegetarians than omnivores; they just need to be discovered. Concerning the cookbooks (see box 14.5), one idea is to try a new recipe every few weeks. Find a reasonable-sounding recipe as quickly as possible, commit to make the recipe, and put needed ingredients on your shopping list. You could also purchase a new-to-you vegetable at the farmers market and search for a recipe using this vegetable. Again, you can approach this in a variety of ways, but the point is to find a way to expose yourself to new foods and vegetarian dishes.

Congratulations Are in Order

Congratulations on making it to the end of the book and making the effort to learn about more healthy choices and going for the plant-based advantage.

Good planning and attention to food and diet details are hard work but worth it! While you should be well on your way to better health and performance, the final chapter is packed with some of our recipe staples to assist you along your path. Good luck, optimal performance, and good health!

Box 14.5

Selected Cookbooks and References

Enette's Favorite Cookbooks

A variety of great vegan and vegetarian cookbooks are available. These are my favorites and most used. OK, I rarely buy a new cookbook, but these are my standbys.

Bishop, Jack. *Vegetables Every Day: The Definitive Guide to Buying and Cooking Today's Produce, With More than 350 Recipes.* New York: HarperCollins, 2001.

Bronfman, David, and Rachelle Bronfman. *CalciYum! Delicious Calcium-Rich Dairy-Free Vegetarian Recipes.* Toronto, Ontario: Bromedia, 1998.

Graimes, Nicola. *The Greatest Ever Vegetarian Cookbook.* New York: Hermes House, 1999.

Irvine, Heather Mayer. *The Runner's World Vegetarian Cookbook: 150 Delicious and Nutritious Meatless Recipes.* New York: Rodale Press, 2018.

McIntosh, Susan M. (editor). *Low-Fat Ways to Cook Vegetarian.* Birmingham, AL: Oxmore House, 1996.

Ray, Rachel. *Rachael Ray's 30-Minute Veggie Meals.* New York: Lake Isle Press, 2001.

Rivera, Michelle. *The Simple Little Vegan Slow Cooker.* Summertown, TN: Book Publishing Co., 2005.

Sass, Lorna J. *Great Vegetarian Cooking Under Pressure: Two-Hour Taste in Ten Minutes.* New York: William Morrow, 2013.

Shaw, Diana. *The Essential Vegetarian Cook Book: Your Guide to the Best Foods on Earth. What to Eat. Where to Get It. How to Prepare It.* New York: Clarkson Potter, 1997.

Williams, Chuck. (editor). *Williams-Sonoma Kitchen Library: Vegetarian.* San Francisco: Time-Life Custom Publishing, 1996.

Matt's Book Recommendations

Cookbooks

Bryant, Terry. *Afro-Vegan: Farm-Fresh African, Caribbean, and Southern Flavors Remixed.* Emeryville, CA: Ten Speed Press, 2014.

Hingle, Richa. *Vegan Richa's Everyday Kitchen: Epic Anytime Recipes With a World of Flavor.* Woodstock, VA: Vegan Heritage Press, 2017.

Mason, Taymer. *Caribbean Vegan: Meat-Free, Egg-Free, Dairy-Free Authentic Island Cuisine for Every Occasion.* New York, NY: The Experiment, 2016.

(continued)

Selected Cookbooks and References *(continued)*

Moran, Victoria, and J.L. Fields. *The Main Street Vegan Academy Cookbook: Over 100 Plant-Sourced Recipes Plus Practical Tips for the Healthiest, Most Compassionate You.* Dallas, TX: BenBella, 2017.

Moskowitz, Isa, and Matt Ruscigno. *Appetite for Reduction: 125 Fast and Filling Low-Fat Vegan Recipes.* Boston, MA: Da Capo Press, 2010.

Nussinow, Jill. *Vegan Under Pressure: Perfect Vegan Meals Made Quick and Easy in Your Pressure Cooker.* Boston, MA: Houghton Mifflin Harcourt, 2016.

Palmer, Sharon. *Plant-Powered for Life: Eat Your Way to Lasting Health with 52 Simple Steps and 125 Delicious Recipes.* New York, NY: The Experiment, 2014.

Romero, Terry Hope. *Salad Samurai: 100 Cutting-Edge, Ultra-Hearty, Easy-to-Make Salads You Don't Have to Be Vegan to Love.* Boston, MA: Da Capo Lifelong Book, 2014.

Schinner, Miyoko. *Artisan Vegan Cheese.* Summertown, TN: Book Publishing Co, 2012.

Sobon, Jackie. *Vegan Yack Attack on the Go! Plant-Based Recipes for Your Fast-Paced Vegan Lifestyle - Quick and Easy, Portable, Make-Ahead, and More!* Beverly, MA: Fair Winds Press, 2018.

Nutrition

Davis, Brenda, and Vesanto Melina. *Becoming Vegan: Comprehensive Edition.* Summerton, TN: Book Publishing Co., 2014.

Davis, Garth, and Howard Jacobson. *Proteinaholic. How Our Obsession with Meat is Killing Us and What We Can Do About It.* New York, NY: HarperCollins, 2015.

Greger, Michael. *How Not to Die: Discover the Foods Scientifically Proven to Prevent and Reverse Disease.* New York, NY: Flatiron Books, 2015.

Mangels, Reed, and Ginny Messina. *The Dietitian's Guide to Vegetarian Diets: Issues and Applications.* Burlington, NJ: Jones & Bartlett Learning, 2010.

Norris, Jack, and Ginny Messina. *Vegan for Life: Everything You Need to Know to Be Fit and Healthy on a Plant-Based Diet.* Boston, MA: Da Capo Press, 2011.

Other

Frazier, Matt, and Matthew Ruscigno. *No Meat Athlete: Run on Plants and Discover Your Fittest, Fastest, Happiest Self.* Beverly, MA: Fair Winds Press, 2013.

Roll, Rich. *Finding Ultra, Revised and Updated Edition: Rejecting Middle Age, Becoming One of the World's Fittest Men, and Discovering Myself.* New York, NY: Random House, 2012.

Resources and Organizations

Vegetarian Resource Group, Baltimore, Maryland, www.vrg.org

Vegetarian Nutrition Dietetic Practice Group, www.vndpg.org

15 | Recipes

This chapter features simple, flexible recipes for quick and healthy plant-based dishes for athletes.

MAIN COURSES

Lentil Tacos

This is a standby family favorite. Most meat eaters are surprised by how good this recipe is. Don't omit the raisins or currants because they are key ingredients. Serve with fresh fruit squeezed with lime or a lime sorbet for dessert. —Enette

Instructions

1. In a large frying pan, sauté onions, celery, and garlic over medium heat in the olive oil for 5 to 6 minutes.
2. Stir in the lentils, chili powder, cumin, and oregano. Cook for 1 minute.
3. Add the broth and raisins, currants, or cranberries. Cover and cook for 20 minutes or until the lentils are tender. Remove the lid and cook, stirring often, until the lentils are thickened, about 10 minutes. Stir in the salsa.
4. Spoon the lentil mixture into warmed, softened tortillas. Top with shredded lettuce, tomatoes, onions, additional salsa, and cheese (optional).

Makes filling for 6 servings (enough to fill three corn tortillas or one large whole-grain tortilla).

Nutrition Content of Filling (and Three Small Corn Tortillas)

158 calories (328 kcal) • 29 g carbohydrate (61.2 g) (2 grains) • 9 g protein (12.4 g) (1 protein) • 2 g fat (3.8 g) (~½ cup + serving vegetables [more with toppings]) • 5.6 g fiber (13.3g) • 2.9 mg iron (76 g) • 48 mg calcium (76 g) 1.3 mg zinc (1.71 mg)

Ingredients List

1 cup onions, minced
1/2 cup celery, minced
1 clove garlic, minced
1 tsp olive oil
1 cup lentils, dry
1 tbsp chili powder
2 tsp ground cumin
1 tsp dried oregano
1 cup vegetable broth
1 tbsp raisins, black currant, or dried cranberries, finely chopped
1 cup mild to hot salsa
Corn tortillas (warmed in microwave, oven, or unoiled pan)
Shredded lettuce*
Chopped tomatoes*
Shredded cheese (optional)*

*Toppings not included in the nutrient content list.

Sloppy Joes

I have never been sure who Joe is, but this sloppy joe recipe is quick and easy and is as good in the middle of winter as it is on a hot summer day. Serve on hearty-grain buns with coleslaw or kale salad and a fruit-based dessert. –Enette

Instructions

1. Pour boiling water over the TVP and set aside.
2. In a large skillet, sauté the onions and green pepper in the oil until tender. Add the garlic and cook 1 to 2 minutes more. Add the TVP, spices, and tomato sauce and stir until well mixed.
3. Stir in the beans. Simmer for 15 to 20 minutes.
4. Serve over hamburger buns.

Makes 6 sloppy joes.

Nutrition Content per Sloppy Joe, Filling and Bun

308 calories • 49 g carbohydrate (3 grains) • 15 g protein (2 protein)
5 g fat (~3/4 cup serving vegetables) • 10 g fiber • 4.7 mg iron
163 mg calcium • 1.7 mg zinc

Ingredients List

1 cup dry texturized vegetable (TVP) or soy protein (TSP)
7/8 cup boiling water
1-2 tsp canola or Mediterranean-blend oil (grapeseed, canola and olive oil blend)
1 cup onions, finely chopped
1 green or red pepper, finely chopped
2 cloves garlic, finely minced
1 can (2 cups) tomato sauce
1/2 cup water
1-1/2 tbsp chili powder
1 tsp soy sauce
2 tbsp sugar
1 can pinto or light-red kidney beans (rinsed and drained)
Salt and pepper to taste
6 whole-grain hamburger buns

Vegetarian Chili

Honestly, all you need is one good vegetarian recipe that you can modify with the seasons. I make this chili in the summer with green onions, fresh tomatoes, cannellini beans, and a little more water, less cocoa, and fresh corn when available. After the fall harvest, I make it with pumpkin puree, roasted chilies and black beans. In the winter, I use whatever veggies are available, including green pepper, jalapeno, and pinto beans. Add a few more cayenne peppers or jalapenos to turn up the heat. Add a teaspoon of sugar to cut the acidity if cocoa powder is not available. Top with green onions, shredded cheddar cheese, or a dollop of sour cream (optional). Serve with cornbread, soda crackers, and sliced fresh fruit with a squeeze of lime. –Enette

Instructions

1. In a large pot, briefly sauté white or green onion, green or red pepper, and jalapenos or cayenne peppers until soft (5-6 min). If using green onions, reserve usable green tops. Add half of the garlic and let sizzle for a few seconds.
2. Stir in tomato sauce, tomatoes, vegetables, beans, and spices. Cover and simmer for 25 to 45 minutes. Add remaining garlic to simmering chili during the last few minutes of cooking for full garlic flavor (or omit this step if you prefer less garlic flavor). Garnish with a dab of yogurt or low-fat sour cream, green onions, or cheddar cheese. To make a meal, serve with fruit or green salad and bread or saltine crackers.

Makes 6 large bowls.

Nutrition Content per Serving

404 calories • 63 g carbohydrate (4 carbohydrate/ starchy vegetable)
24 g protein (3 protein) • 5.9 g fat (1-2 servings vegetables [more with toppings]) • 21 g fiber • 6.7 mg iron • 143 mg calcium • 2.0 mg zinc

Ingredients List

2 tsp olive oil or Mediterranean blend (grapeseed, canola, and olive blend)
3 bunches of green onions or 1 medium onion, chopped
1 green or red pepper, chopped
1-2 roasted mild chilies, chopped (more to taste)
1-3 jalapenos or cayenne peppers, fresh or roasted and frozen, finely chopped (optional)
2-3 cloves garlic, minced or finely chopped (optional)
15 oz can tomato sauce
15 oz can chopped tomatoes or 2 cups fresh finely chopped tomatoes
2-3 cups of water (more if thinner chili is desired)
2 24 oz cans of beans (black beans, kidney beans, pinto beans, or cannellini beans
1 cup of TVP
2-3 cups vegetable in combination, such as corn, sliced carrots, zucchini, pureed pumpkin, sliced olives, or prickly pear cactus
2-3 tsp cumin
1 tsp oregano
2-3 tbsp chili powder
1-2 tbsp cocoa powder

Hearty Minestrone Soup

This recipe was modified from Liz Applegate's grandmother's recipe (www.runnersworld.com/nutrition-weight-loss/a20782344/soups-grandma-berneros-minestrone-soup). It is seriously so good and versatile and can accommodate whatever you have in your garden, refrigerator, or freezer. Thanks, Liz, but we don't miss the meat. This modified version is one of my daughter Lindsey's absolute favorites. It also is a great source of well-absorbed calcium. Serve with hearty bread and a salad if desired (we, however, just eat more soup and skip the salad). –Enette

Instructions

1. Sauté onions, garlic, and celery in large soup pot with olive oil.
2. Add water, salt, bay leaves, tomato sauce, beans, mixed vegetables, and TVP. Simmer on low for 15 to 20 minutes until all vegetables are tender.
3. Add pasta and kale. Simmer another 10 to 15 minutes. Stir in the pesto. Note that pasta can also be cooked separately and added at end with the pesto if a firmer texture is desired.
4. Serve warm, topped with freshly grated Parmesan or Asiago if desired.

Makes six large bowls or eight smaller bowls.

Nutrition Content per large bowl

421 calories • 65 g carbohydrate (4 grains/ starchy vegetables) • 21 g protein (3 protein) • 10 g fat (1 cup + serving vegetables [more with toppings]) 19 g fiber • 5.5 mg iron • 244 mg calcium • 2.4 mg zinc

Ingredients List

1 tbsp olive oil
1 large onion, chopped,
5 stalks celery, chopped in thin slices
3 cloves of garlic, minced
2 bay leaves
10 cups of water
1-2 tsp iodized salt
15 oz can (2 cups) tomato sauce (or 2 cups fresh)
3 15 oz cans beans (combination of kidney, garbanzo, cannellini, butter, or lima beans)
3 cups total of chopped seasonal or frozen vegetables (examples: carrots, green beans, potatoes, corn, zucchini, and okra) cut in 1/2-inch pieces or smaller
1/2 cup TVP (optional)
2 cups fresh or frozen kale cut in 1/2-inch strips
2 cups of small shaped pasta, cooked
3 tbsp pesto
Parmesan or Asiago cheese, freshly grated (optional, not included in nutrition content list)

Nutty Tofu Crisp Over Asian Noodles

This is one of my family's favorite recipes. Serve with a heaping portion of steamed greens (e.g., chard, bok choy, Chinese cabbage) and sparkling water or a glass of white wine. This recipe is an excellent source of calcium with or without the calcium-rich greens. –Enette

Instructions

1. Mix the first eight ingredients with a fork to create marinade.
2. Cut pressed tofu halves a second time, diagonally. Place tofu quarters in marinade for at least 15 minutes on each side.
3. Cook noodles according to package directions.
4. Dip the marinated tofu into the chopped peanuts to fully coat one side. Heat 1 tsp of peanut oil in a nonstick skillet. Cook tofu, with the peanut side down, until golden brown (~ 1-1/2 min) and repeat on the other side.
5. Heat remaining marinade over the stove or in the microwave and pour over the hot noodles. Divide noodles into four equal servings, place nutty tofu cakes on top, and serve.

Makes 4 servings.

Nutrition Content per serving

338 calories • 36 g carbohydrate (2 grains) • 30 g protein (4 protein) • 12.5 g fat • 3.9 g fiber • 3.7 mg iron • 238 mg calcium • 0.8 mg zinc

Ingredients List

1/4 cup rice or balsamic vinegar
1 tbsp soy sauce
2 tbsp natural peanut butter
2 cloves garlic, minced
1 bunch of green onions, finely chopped
1 tsp Asian chili paste
1 tbsp water
1 tsp sugar
16 oz extra-firm tofu, cut in half horizontally, pressed to remove extra water
1 tbsp finely chopped peanuts
1 tsp peanut or canola oil
12 oz thin spaghetti cut in half (regular or whole wheat)

Mike's Veggie and Tofu Stir Fry

This is a recipe my husband has perfected over the years. I have honestly never attempted to make it, which gives me an excuse to take the night off from cooking. He uses a combination of carrots, broccoli, peppers, bok choy, snap peas, and young green beans. Served over brown or white rice, it is a meal in itself. It goes nicely with a glass of white wine or sparkling water and a scoop of sorbet for dessert. –Enette

Instructions

1. In large glass measuring cup, mix water with cornstarch slowly to avoid lumps. Stir in the broth granules, ginger, lemon grass, soy sauce, garlic, chili paste, and chili peppers. Pour into a flat dish and set aside.
2. Sauté the vegetables in large pan or wok in 1 tablespoon oil until soft, starting with peppers and carrots and adding in stages every few minutes to prevent overcooking the broccoli, greens, and peas. When soft, remove from pan and set aside.
3. Add 2 tablespoons canola or Mediterranean oil to pan or wok. When oil sizzles, add tofu and continue cooking over medium heat until slightly browned. If using a pan, avoid stirring for several minutes until the side down has time to brown.
4. Turn heat off. Add liquid mixture to tofu and let set about 10 minutes. This will thicken sauce and allow some of the browned tofu scraps to loosen from the pan.
5. Stir in vegetables and heat over low just until warmed. Stir in sesame oil.
6. Serve over brown or white rice topped with cashews.

Makes 6 servings.

Nutrition Content for Stir Fry (and 1 Cup White Rice)

387 calories (581 calories) • 20.8 g carbohydrate (62 g) (4 grains)
19.8 g protein (21.4) (3 protein) • 25.9 g fat (26.4 g) (1-1/2 cup serving vegetables) • 5.3 g fiber (6.7 g) • 4.5 mg iron (7.3 mg) • 304 mg calcium (334 mg) • 1.6 mg zinc (2.2 mg)

Ingredients List

1 tbsp corn starch
2-1/2 cups water
1 tsp vegetable broth granules
1 tbsp ginger paste (or fresh, finely chopped ginger)
1 tbsp lemon grass paste (or fresh, tender, finely chopped lemon grass)
2 tbsp soy sauce
3 cloves garlic
1 tsp hot chili paste
2-3 Thai chilies or 1 cayenne pepper (optional) to taste, crushed
1 tbsp plus 2 tbsp canola or Mediterranean oil
1 red, orange, or yellow bell pepper, thinly sliced
1 green bell pepper, thinly sliced
6-7 small carrots or 3-4 large carrots, thinly sliced
2 small or 1 large head broccoli, separated into small florets (smaller heads are easier to separate)
1 cup other vegetable such as snap peas, sliced zucchini, small green beans
2 cups greens such as bok choy, swiss chard, cabbage, cut in thin strips
2 packages extra-firm tofu, cut into cubes
2 tsp sesame oil
1 cup roasted cashews

Can't Be Beat Borscht

This borscht has chocolate in it! Beets are a unique source of the phytonutrients betanin and vulgaxanthin, which may help with recovery. And chocolate is an excellent source of antioxidants and micronutrients, so together this is a powerful recovery food. This recipe originates from my friend and culinary genius, Joshua Ploeg. –Matt

Instructions

1. Bring all ingredients, except the cacao powder and lemon juice, to a boil in a large soup pot.
2. Lower the heat to a simmer and cook for 20 minutes.
3. Add the cocoa powder and cook for another 20 minutes, stirring often.
4. Add the lemon juice and remove from heat.

Makes 8 servings.

Nutrition Content per Serving

86 calories • 20 g carbohydrate (1 starchy vegetable) • 3 g protein • 1 g fat (3/4 cup vegetables) • 5 g fiber • 2 mg iron • 40 mg calcium • 1 mg zinc

Ingredients List

8 cups vegetable broth (or 8 cups water with 1 or 2 bouillon cubes)
1 to 1-1/2 teaspoons salt
2 cups potatoes, diced
5 cups beets, diced
1/2 cup red onion, chopped
1/2 cup carrots, diced
2 garlic cloves, minced
1 tsp dill
1/2 tsp paprika
1/2 tsp caraway or cumin seed, crushed
1/3 cup raw cacao powder or 1/2 dark chocolate bar
3 tbsp lemon juice

Black Bean and Cilantro Lasagna

OK, this recipe is technically not quick, but it is one of our favorites to make for company. It has been a routine for years to make this with my daughter Marlena. I prep the food, and she assembles the lasagna. When my daughter Lindsey omitted dairy from her diet, we started making her a small separate lasagna without the cheeses. She tells us it is just as good without the cheese. Serve with a green salad and crusty bread. –Enette

Instructions

1. Whirl tomatoes in blender or food processor with cilantro and garlic until smooth. This may be done in batches.
2. Cook noodles according to package directions (for firmer noodles, I try to cook noodles about 2 min less than directions). Drain and immediately immerse noodles in cold water. Blot dry.
3. In a bowl, combine beans, cumin, and chili powder. With a potato masher or the back of a large spoon, coarsely mash beans mixing in 1/4- to 1/2-cup of the tomato sauce as necessary.
4. In another bowl, mix the ricotta (optional), tofu, and half of the pepper jack cheese.
5. Arrange five noodles, slightly overlapping, to cover the bottom of a lightly oiled 9- × 13-inch baking dish. Top with half each of the beans, ricotta mixture, and tomato sauce. Repeat layers to use remaining noodles, beans, ricotta and tofu, and sauce. Sprinkle top with cheese. If made ahead, cover and chill up until the next day.
6. Bake uncovered at 375 °F (190 °C) until top is browned and casserole is bubbling, about 40 minutes (45-50 min if chilled). Let stand 10 minutes before serving.

Makes 8 hearty servings.

Ingredients List

2 28 oz cans chopped tomatoes (or 7 cups fresh, roasted tomatoes, chopped after roasting)
2 cloves garlic, minced or finely chopped
1 cup firmly packed fresh cilantro
10 dry wide lasagna noodles
3 15 oz cans black beans, drained and rinsed, or 6 cups freshly cooked dried beans (best and less salty if made with fresh black beans)
2 tsp ground cumin
1 tsp chili powder
1 15 oz carton part-skim ricotta cheese or 8 ounce package vegan cream cheese
1 16 oz package firm tofu
4 oz pepper jack cheese or cashew pepper cheese (optional)

Nutrition Content per Serving

431 calories • 49 g carbohydrate (3 grains/ starchy vegetables) • 30 g protein (3 protein) • 12.5 g fat (1-1/2 dairy) (1 cup vegetables) • 14.5 g fiber • 7 mg iron • 486 mg calcium • 2 mg zinc

Mean Bean Burgers

What do you mean burgers made from beans? We mean *mean bean burgers*! Beans truly are magical in that there are so many ways to consume them. These homemade burgers are much cheaper than buying them ready-made and can be just as—or more—delicious. –Matt

Instructions

1. Add all ingredients in a large bowl, mix well, and mash with a potato masher or fork until chunky.
2. Scrape out to a cutting board and form the loaf into 2 or 3 patties.
3. Heat a nonstick pan on medium-high heat and add oil.
4. When the oil is hot, cook the patties, flipping occasionally until brown on both sides, roughly 10 minutes.
5. Serve on whole-wheat buns with lettuce, tomatoes, onions, pickles, and jalapenos as you would other burgers.

Tip: Freeze them for later! After forming, store patties separated by parchment paper. To prepare, simply sauté the same as other frozen patties, being careful they don't stick.

Variations

• Turn them into meatballs by adding oregano or generic Italian spice and form into balls before cooking in pan.

Makes 3 burgers.

Ingredients List

1 tsp olive or preferred oil
1 can kidney, black, or other beans, drained and rinsed
1/2 cup cooked brown rice
1/2 cup rolled oats
2 tbsp salsa, ketchup, or BBQ sauce
1 tsp garlic powder
1/4 tsp salt
1 tsp cumin powder
1 tsp paprika or chili powder
Bind with 1 tbsp ground flaxseeds (optional)

Nutrition Content per Serving

255 calories • 43 g carbohydrate (3 grains/ starchy vegetables) • 12 g protein (1 protein) • 5 g fat • 10 g fiber • 4 mg iron • 81 mg calcium • 1 mg zinc

Tofu Tacos

One of the most common critiques of veganism is that you can't get enough calcium without drinking cows' milk, but this recipe proves that you can get plenty in one meal. Kale and leafy greens are high in calcium, as most people know, but so are the corn tortillas and the tofu, because of how they are made. The masa for corn tortillas is treated with limewater (calcium hydroxide) that adds bioavailable calcium and increases the absorption of B vitamins and amino acids. Tofu production requires a coagulant, and the most commonly used is calcium sulfate, also a bioavailable source of calcium. Check the packages of your favorite brands for these ingredients. –Matt

Instructions

1. Heat a large skillet on medium heat and add the oil.
2. Allow oil to warm for 1 minute, and then add the onion and garlic. Sauté for 2 minutes, stirring as needed.
3. Add the bell pepper, cabbage, and leafy green stems. Sauté for 2 minutes.
4. Move the ingredients to the outer edges of the pan so that the center is clear.
5. Add the tofu in quarterly increments, crumbling with your hand or a wooden spoon. Make sure the tofu doesn't stick; turn as needed. Add the turmeric, black pepper, and hot sauce. When the tofu is thoroughly heated, mix and sauté for 5 minutes.
6. Add the greens, zucchini, and mushrooms and continue to cook for 3 minutes or until the vegetables are soft, stirring as needed.
7. Combine the cornstarch and water in a small dish. Add to the pan and mix well until the water disappears. Add the black Himalayan salt and nutritional yeast, mix, and turn heat off. The scramble should be slightly gelatinized.
8. Serve hot with salsa and avocado slices in warm corn tortillas.

Makes 4 servings.

Variation

- Add a few leaves of arugula, aka rocket lettuce, to each taco for even more leafy greens!

Nutrition Content per Serving

209 calories • 25 g carbohydrate (1-1/2 grains) • 13 g protein (1 protein)
9 g fat (~2 cups vegetables) • 13 g fiber • 3 mg iron • 192 mg calcium
3 mg zinc

Ingredients List

1 tbsp olive oil
1/2 onion, diced
4 cloves garlic, minced
1 bell pepper, diced
4 cups curly kale or collard greens, chopped (separate stems if using)
1 14 oz package of firm tofu
1 tsp turmeric
1 tsp black pepper
Hot sauce, to taste
1 zucchini, diced
1/2 cup red cabbage, sliced
1 cup mushrooms, sliced
1 tbsp cornstarch
1/4 cup water
1 tsp black Himalayan salt (or regular salt, to taste)
1/4 cup nutritional yeast (optional)
1/2 cup salsa
1 avocado, sliced
8 corn tortillas

Fish-Free Tuna Salad

Chickpea tuna is a delightful bean dip variation. The seaweed gives it that taste of the sea you may be craving, while the celery and carrots give it a nice crunch. Use it as a sandwich spread or to top salads to turn them into a filling meal. –Matt

Instructions

1. In a medium salad bowl, mash chickpeas, mayo, and salt with a potato masher or fork.
2. Fold the chopped vegetables into the chickpea mash.
3. Add liquid from pickle jar as needed to reach desired consistency.

Makes 3 servings.

Nutrition Content per Serving

256 calories • 38 g carbohydrate (3 starchy vegetables) • 11 g protein (1 protein) • 7 g fat (~1/2 cup vegetables) • 11 g fiber • 2 mg iron • 99 mg calcium • 1 mg zinc

Ingredients List

1 15 oz can chickpea, drained
2 tbsp vegan mayo
1 tsp salt
1 sheet seaweed (e.g., nori)
2 celery stalks, chopped
2 carrots, chopped
1/4 small red onion, finely chopped
1 pickle spear, chopped
Pickle jar liquid, as needed

Eugene's Kale Salad

Eugene was a student in one of my local food courses. He was a great student and, as it turned out, also vegan. He shared this kale salad recipe because he thought I might like it. I have modified it a bit to make it my own, but whenever I make it—which is almost weekly in the summer and fall—I think fondly of Eugene. You can cut the olive oil in half if you prefer less fat. –Enette

Instructions

1. Remove tough stems from washed kale and chop into bite-sized pieces. Sprinkle with salt and let set 20 to 30 minutes. Place in salad bowl and massage between fingers for several minutes. Kale will soften and change to a slightly different color of green.
2. Meanwhile, pulse olive oil, lemon juice, and vinegar in food processor until smooth and emulsified. Or place in a glass bowl and mix vigorously with a fork.
3. Toss kale with dressing, diced onions, diced fruit, cheese, and pumpkin seeds or almonds. Top with croutons and serve immediately. Use commercially available croutons or make your own. Cut day-old bread into crouton-sized pieces, drizzle with olive oil, and bake at 375 °F (190 °C) for 10 to 15 minutes.

Makes 6 servings.

Nutrition Content per Serving

188 calories • 11 g carbohydrate (1/2 protein) • 4.6 g protein (1-1/2 cup serving vegetables) • 14.8 g fat • 6.9 g fiber • 1.4 mg iron • 147 mg calcium 0.7 mg zinc

Ingredients List

1 bunch fresh kale (~ 1 lb, tough stems removed)
1/2 to 1 tsp iodized salt
1/3 cup olive oil
Juice of 1 lemon (~ 3 tbsp) or fruit-infused white balsamic vinegar
1 tbsp Dijon mustard
1/2 red onion, finely diced
1/2 cup apple or grapes or 1/4 cup dried cranberries, apricots, or black currants, very finely chopped
2 tbsp Parmesan cheese (optional)
1/4 cup pumpkin seeds or toasted sliced almonds
Croutons (optional)

SIDES AND OTHER ITEMS

Garden Rice Pilaf with Toasted Nuts

This is an easy and versatile carbohydrate-rich recipe that can be made to fit your cravings or with what you find in your garden, refrigerator, or freezer. If you don't have wild rice, experiment with other rice or ancient grains. The Minnesotans in my family, however, are partial to the wild rice. Some of our favorites include classic pilaf with bell peppers, peas, carrots, and lima beans; mushroom pilaf with green peppers, assorted mushrooms, and toasted almonds; and Mexican rice with poblano peppers, tomatoes, spinach, and black beans. Serve with a fresh green salad and fruit bubbly (fruit juice mixed with sparkling water). –Enette

Instructions

1. Sauté onions, peppers, and garlic in a large skillet with oil.
2. Add water, salt, vegetable base, and wild rice and simmer, covered over medium heat for 30 minutes.
3. Add the remaining ingredients except nuts and simmer, covered for an additional 40 minutes or until all grains are soft. Add water if necessary. Remove lid and cook uncovered if necessary to remove additional water.
4. Top with toasted almonds, walnuts, or pine nuts.

Makes 6 servings.

Nutrition Content per Serving

478 calories • 78 g carbohydrate (5 grains) • 15.7 g protein (2 protein) • 10.9 g fat 1 cup serving vegetables • 11.5 g fiber • 2.9 mg iron • 114 mg calcium 3.6 mg zinc

Ingredients List

1 tbsp olive oil
1 onion, finely chopped
2 bell or large poblano peppers, finely chopped (green, yellow, orange, or red or a combination)
3-4 cloves garlic, minced or finely chopped
1 jalapeno or 1/2 cayenne pepper, finely chopped (optional)
1 cup wild rice
8 cups water
2 tsp vegetable base
1 tsp iodized salt
1-1/2 cups brown rice, quinoa, or other grain (adjust water as necessary)
3-4 cups fresh vegetables, such as chopped carrots, green peas, spinach, swiss chard, assorted mushrooms, celery, and tomatoes
2 cups cooked beans or peas such as chickpeas, edamame, lima beans, and black beans
2 tbsp tomato paste (optional for certain rice combinations)
1 cup toasted sliced almonds, walnuts, or pine nuts (optional)
1 tsp toasted sesame oil added after cooking

Matt's Recipe Notes

If I've learned anything over all of my years working in food and nutrition, it's that we all have our own cooking style. Some people pick a few recipes, buy each specific ingredient, and then follow the directions exactly. This is an effective way to approach new ways of cooking as you learn what you like (both in preparation and taste) and do not like. Cookbook authors develop specific flavor profiles and pass on the way they think is best. But following directions exactly isn't for everyone. You probably already know who you are: Do you follow a training plan to the letter, or do you glance at it and aim to be close while doing it your own way? I'm in the latter camp and my recipes reflect this. There are a lot of variations and my goal is to guide you toward making new foods in your own style and taste. –Matt

Pesto Sauce

I make this in large batches when basil is plentiful in the garden and serve over pasta. I freeze the rest in ice cube trays, pop them out when frozen, and store in plastic bags in the freezer for use in soups and other dishes during the winter and spring. –Enette

Instructions

1. Place basil leaves (along with parsley and spinach) and garlic in a blender or food processor and mince well.
2. Add the nuts and continue to blend until nuts and basil are ground.
3. Drizzle in the olive oil, as you keep the machine running, until mixture becomes a fine paste.
4. Transfer to a bowl and stir in Parmesan or nutritional yeast. Season with salt and pepper.
5. Toss over hot pasta (allow 2-3 tbsp pesto per serving) or use as an accent in soup and salads. Freeze leftovers in ice cube tray, and transfer into plastic bags when frozen for use in recipes throughout the season.

Makes ~1-1/2 cups or 24 tbsp.

Nutrition Content per Serving

44 calories per tbsp • 1 g carbohydrate • 1 g protein • 4.3 g fat • <0.5 g fiber • 0.3 mg iron • 19 mg calcium (10 for vegan version) • 0.1 mg zinc

Ingredients List

3 cups packed fresh basil leaves (or a combination of basil, fresh parsley, and spinach)

3-4 cloves garlic

1/3 cup pine nuts, chopped walnuts, or almonds, lightly toasted

1/3 cup olive oil

1/3 cup grated Parmesan or Asiago cheese (traditional version) or 1/4 cup nutritional yeast plus 1-1/2 tbsp lemon juice (vegan version)

1/4 tsp salt

1/8 tsp cayenne pepper (optional)

"You Won't Believe These Are Potatoes" Cheeze Sauce

A creamy sauce made from potatoes and carrots? Yes! This delicious sauce goes great with whole-grain pasta, drizzled over steamed vegetables, or as a dip for fresh veggies. Not peeling the potatoes has a few advantages: higher antioxidant and nutrient content, and it saves you time. The same is true for the carrots. –Matt

Instructions

1. In a saucepan, add the potatoes, carrots, onion, and enough water to cover and bring to a boil.
2. Cover the pan and simmer for about 15 minutes, or until the potatoes are soft. Save cooking water.
3. Meanwhile, blend remaining ingredients. Add the vegetables and cooking water, as needed, to the blender and process until perfectly smooth.

Variations

- After the sauce is done, add 1 jar of chunky salsa and use it to top Mexican-style meals or in burritos.
- Make mac and cheese by covering cooked pasta in a casserole dish and adding bread crumbs.
- This can be made easily in an instant pot. Add all ingredients, cook for 5 minutes, then blend!

Makes 4 servings.

Nutrition Content per Serving

318 calories • 51 g carbohydrate (3 starchy vegetables) • 16 g protein (2 protein) • 9 g fat (1/2 cup vegetables) • 11 g fiber • 2 mg iron • 50 mg calcium • 5 mg zinc

Ingredients List

4 medium, white potatoes, quartered

2 carrots, peeled and chopped

1 small white onion, peeled and chopped

1/2 cup raw cashews, soaked 2 hours or overnight, if not using a high-speed blender

2 tsp sea salt

2-3 cloves garlic, minced

1 tsp mustard, such as Dijon

1 lemon, juiced, about 4 tbsp

1 tsp black pepper

1 tsp paprika

Cayenne or hot sauce to taste (optional)

Add 1/4 cup nutritional yeast to the blender ingredients in step 3

Perfect Peanut Sauce

Instructions

1. Combine ingredients in a blender and blend until smooth. Add vegetable broth or water until desired consistency is reached.
2. Pour liberally over sautéed vegetables, tofu, and noodles.

Variations

- If time is tight (or let's be real: you don't want to wash the blender) you can make this sauce in the pan you cook the vegetables in. I make a little section on the side of the pan and combine the ingredients while constantly stirring so it doesn't stick. If you use fresh garlic and ginger, start with those, otherwise start with the peanut butter and broth mix and stir in the remaining ingredients. –Enette

Makes 4 servings.

Nutrition Content per Serving

216 calories • 12 g carbohydrate • 8 g protein (1 protein) • 17 g fat • 2 g fiber
1 mg iron • 23 mg calcium • 1 mg zinc

Ingredients List

1/2 cup peanut butter
1/2 cup vegetable broth or water
1-2 tbsp soy sauce
2 tsp rice vinegar (or other mild vinegar)
1 tbsp sweetener (agave, maple syrup, unrefined sugar)
2-4 cloves garlic or 1 tsp powdered garlic
1 tbsp-sized piece of fresh ginger or 1 tsp powdered ginger
Sriracha or other hot sauce to taste (optional)

White Bean Spread

I love hummus, but it's time for its monopoly on bean spreads to come to an end. Once you make a few of these and dial in the recipe, you'll be adding it to everything. Burritos? Check. Pasta sauce? Why not? Straight out of the container with a spoon while the fridge is still open? Yes, but you should probably step away from the fridge and close the door because you are going to eat more than one spoonful. –Matt

Instructions

1. In a medium bowl, combine the beans, lemon juice, herbs, salt, pepper, and nutritional yeast if using. Roughly mash the mixture with the back of a fork.
2. Fold in chopped red onion to the mixture.

Variations

- Black bean spread with cumin and oregano
- Peruvian bean (canary or peruano) spread with marjoram or 1/2 teaspoon liquid smoke

Makes 8 servings.

Nutrition Content per Serving

137 calories • 25 g carbohydrate (1-1/2 starchy vegetables) • 10 g protein
0 g fat • 6 g fiber • 4 mg iron • 91 mg calcium • 2 mg zinc

Ingredients List

2 15 oz cans white beans, rinsed and drained
1 bunch of fresh herbs (or 1 tsp dried) such as basil, thyme, or dill
Pinch of salt
Pinch of black pepper
1 small red onion, thinly diced
Juice of half a lemon
2 tbsp nutritional yeast (optional)

Base Mile Quinoa

The ingredient list is short, but don't underestimate this dish as a super nutritious, easy, and fast way to up your plant-based game. Green peas are eaten like vegetables, but are technically a legume and high in fiber, protein, and phytochemicals. Red cabbage is unique in that it contains two beneficial phytochemical groups: polyphenols and glucosinolates. I like this dish because these ingredients have a long shelf life. It's often what I make when I don't have much else in the kitchen.

Once prepared and stored in the fridge, this quinoa can be added to salads, used as the grain in a bowl with beans, added to canned soup to turn it into a complete meal, or, honestly, eaten straight with nutritional yeast and hot sauce. –Matt

Ingredients List

2 cups quinoa, rinsed
3 cups water or broth
1 cup frozen peas
1 cup red cabbage, diced
Salt, to taste

Instructions

1. Rinse quinoa.
2. Add all ingredients to medium-sized pot.
3. Bring to a boil.
4. Turn heat to low, let simmer for 15 minutes or according to quinoa package instructions.

Makes 8 servings.

Variation

- This is great for the instant pot, if you have one. Combine all ingredients, cook for 5 minutes on high.

Nutrition Content per Serving

100 calories • 18 g carbohydrate (1 grain) • 4 g protein • 1 g fat (1/4 cup vegetables) • 3 g fiber • 1 mg iron • 24 mg calcium • 1 mg zinc

Balsamic Strawberry Dressing

A tasty dressing goes a long way, and the marriage of sweet fruit and vinegar may have you eating more salads than you are prepared for. Don't fight it, give in to your new life as someone who makes salad dressing at home! I make this when I have fresh berries that need to be used soon. Frozen berries can be used, but it changes the texture slightly. This dressing will keep in the refrigerator for several days. –Matt

Ingredients List

1 cup raspberries or strawberries, fresh
2 tbsp raspberry or other fruit vinegar
1 tbsp regular or golden balsamic vinegar
2 tbsp water
2 tsp liquid sweetener
2 tsp Dijon mustard
Freshly ground pepper, to taste

Instructions

1. Combine all ingredients in a food processor and blend well.

Makes 5 servings.

Nutrition Content per Serving

22 calories • 5 g carbohydrate • 0.5 g protein • 0 g fat (1/4 cup fruit) 1 g fiber • 0 mg iron • 8 mg calcium • 0 mg zinc

Ginger Tahini Sauce

This versatile sauce can be used for salads or warm bowls. Tahini creates a rich base in both flavor and texture and can be easily adjusted for caloric needs. Without a blender, you can grate or finely dice the ginger and garlic. –Matt

Instructions

1. Roughly chop the ginger and garlic.
2. Place all ingredients into a blender or small food processor.
3. Blend until smooth, adding water as needed.

Makes 2 servings.

Nutrition Content per Serving

148 calories • 11 g carbohydrate • 11 g protein (1 protein) • 9 g fat • 6 g fiber 2 mg iron • 73 mg calcium • 4 mg zinc

Ingredients List

2 tbsp tahini
2 garlic cloves, chopped
1 tbsp ginger, chopped
Lemon juice, from 1/2 to 1 lemon
2 tbsp nutritional yeast
1 tbsp soy sauce
Water, as needed

BAKED GOODS

Fruit Crisp

This recipe works well with a variety of fresh or frozen fruit, including apples, peaches, blueberries, rhubarb, and cranberries. I often keep the crisp part in a container in the refrigerator so it is ready for an impromptu dessert or to top muffins (see previous recipe). Serve hot or cold with a dollop of vanilla ice cream or sweet tofu cream. –Enette

Instructions

1. Preheat oven to 350 °F (177 °C). Lightly grease a 9-inch square baking pan, and set aside.
2. In a small bowl, stir together sugar, flour, oatmeal, and cinnamon. With a pastry blender or fork, cut in oil until mixture is crumbly.
3. Chop fruit (if appropriate) and place in baking dish. For less-sweet fruits such as rhubarb or fresh cranberries, stir in sugar to coat or sweeten. (Note: Most ripe fruits do not require this step.) Sprinkle with lemon peel and lemon juice.
4. Sprinkle crumb mixture evenly over the top.
5. Bake, uncovered 40 to 60 minutes until fruit is soft and bubbly. Let cool about 15 minutes before serving.

Makes 12 servings.

Nutrition Content per Serving

275 calories • 45 g carbohydrate (2 grains) • 3.4 g protein • 11 g fat (~1/3-1/2 cup fruit) • 4.3 g fiber • 1.2 mg iron • 38 mg calcium • 0.3 mg zinc

Ingredients List

1 cup firmly packed brown sugar (or 3/4 cup other sweetener such as agave, honey, or maple syrup)
1 cup whole-wheat or other whole-grain flour
2 cups rolled oats
2 tsp ground cinnamon (can add sprinkle of nutmeg or ginger depending on the fruit)
1/2 cup canola oil or Mediterranean-blend oil (it also works with unsalted butter, but I rarely use butter)
4-5 cups fresh or frozen fruit
1 tsp lemon juice
1 tsp grated lemon peel (optional)
1-6 tbsp raw sugar to taste (optional)

Cocoa-Quinoa Endurance Bars

Mastering a homemade bar to take on long training days or for after a workout is an opportunity to get the flavors you like or to mix it up when you are bored. And it can save you money! This recipe is a guideline; the nuts, fruits, and most other ingredients can all be swapped or altered. –Matt

Instructions

1. Preheat oven to 350 °F (177 °C).
2. Spread quinoa on a cookie sheet and toast for 7 to 8 minutes.
3. In a large bowl, combine quinoa, nuts, coconut, and dried fruit.
4. In a saucepan, combine remaining ingredients except the chocolate chips. Bring to a simmer over medium heat for 2 minutes.
5. Pour over quinoa mixture and combine until dry ingredients are evenly coated.
6. Mix in chocolate chips.
7. Spoon into a greased 9- ×13-inch baking dish. Press mixture into pan. Bake for 15 minutes.
8. Let cool and then cut and serve or store in an airtight container.

Makes 12 bars.

Nutrition Content per Serving

300 calories • 32 g carbohydrate (1 grain) • 7 g protein (1 protein) • 17 g fat (1 fruit) • 5 g fiber • 2 mg iron • 57 mg calcium • 1 mg zinc

Ingredients List

1-1/2 cups uncooked quinoa
1/2 cup ground almonds or other nuts
1/2 cup grated or shredded dried coconut
1/2 cup dried cranberries
1/2 cup dried apples or other dried fruit, chopped
1/4 tsp salt or to taste
1/2 cup almond or peanut butter
2 tbsp coconut oil
1/4 cup liquid sweetener such as agave
1/2 cup fruit-sweetened chocolate chips or dark chocolate pieces

BREAKFAST OR ANYTIME

Vegan Omelet

The increased interest in plant-based diets is challenging the definition of foods, and one example is the omelet. Made without eggs, this version uses the magic of chickpea flour to hug the veggies and make a vegan omelet. It is similar to bánh xèo, a Vietnamese pancake that uses rice flour. –Matt

Instructions

1. Heat oil in a sauté pan on medium heat.
2. When warm, add the onions, mushrooms, chili, and garlic.
3. Meanwhile, in a mixing bowl combine the chickpea flour and spices and stir in plant milk until the texture resembles batter.
4. Once the vegetables are soft, about 5 minutes, pour the batter right over them.
5. Cook on a medium heat 6 to 8 minutes, until the edges are brown.
6. Using a spatula, flip the omelet.
7. Cook until the outside is lightly brown and cooked thoroughly, 3 to 4 minutes.

Makes 2 omelets.

Nutrition Content per Serving

215 calories • 27 g carbohydrate (2 starchy vegetables) • 10 g protein (1 protein) • 8 g fat (1/2 cup vegetables) • 7 g fiber • 4 mg iron • 181 mg calcium • 1 mg zinc

Ingredients List

2 tsp olive oil
6 spring onions, sliced
1/2 cup mushrooms, sliced
1 small pepper, finely chopped (e.g., jalapeno)
2 cloves garlic, minced
3/4 cup of chickpea flour
1 tsp turmeric
1 tsp yellow curry powder
1/4 tsp salt
1/2 cup unsweetened plant milk

Overnight Oats

Made the night before, this dish is ready for you as you rush out the door in the morning. It can be made in any container with a lid and works well in a mason jar. Experiment with different grains and fruit combinations. –Enette

Instructions

1. Combine oats, chia seeds, and sweetener in mason jar or other container with a lid. Stir in plant-based milk, yogurt, citrus juice, and citrus zest.
2. Top with fresh fruit, cover, and refrigerate overnight.
3. Toss in nuts and serve. (Note: Some fruit will preserve better if added right before serving; nuts can be added overnight but they may become less crisp).

Makes 1 serving.

Nutrition Content per Serving

566 calories • 87 g carbohydrate (4 grain) • 20 g protein (3 protein) • 19.5 g fat
1 cup fruit • 6.9 g fiber • 3.1 mg iron • 147 mg calcium • 1.2 mg zinc

Ingredients List

1/3 cup old-fashioned oats
1 tsp chia seeds
1 tbsp brown sugar or honey
1/3 cup plain, Greek yogurt
1/3 cup soy milk (or other plant-based milks)
Juice from 1 lemon, lime, or small orange (1-1/2 to 2 tbsp)
Lemon, lime, or orange zest
1 cup fruit such as sliced banana, kiwi, fresh berries, or mandarin oranges
1/4 cup nuts (e.g., sliced almonds, pecan pieces, walnuts)

Breakfast in a Cookie

This is a fun recipe that was published in my hometown newspaper many years ago. Like everything, I have modified the recipe a bit over the years. Cookies can be frozen in groups of two or three and accompanied with fresh fruit or soy milk. –Enette

Instructions

1. Combine bran and orange juice in a small bowl. Set aside.
2. In another bowl, cream the butter, fruit puree, and sugar. Add the egg and beat until light. Blend in honey or maple syrup, vanilla, and the bran–orange mixture.
3. Combine flour, baking powder, baking soda, salt, dry milk, orange rind, oatmeal, nuts, and raisins. Stir this dry mixture into creamed mixture.
4. Drop by level tablespoons onto greased cookie sheets (~ 2 in. apart). Bake at 350 °F (177 °C) for 10 to 12 minutes or until golden brown.

Makes 3 dozen cookies.

Nutrition Content per Serving

106 calories • 16 g carbohydrate (1/2 grain) • 2.3 g protein • 3.9 g fat (1 fruit serving) • 1.2 g fiber • 0.5 mg iron • 31 mg calcium • 0.3 mg zinc

Ingredients List

1/3 cup whole-bran cereal
1/4 cup orange juice
1/4 stick softened butter or margarine or 1/4 cup coconut oil
1/4 cup canola oil
1 cup fruit puree including apple sauce or pumpkin puree
1/4 cup raw sugar
1 egg (or the equivalent vegan egg replacer)
1/4 cup maple syrup or honey
1-1/2 tsp vanilla extract
1 cup unbleached flour
1 tsp baking powder
1/2 tsp baking soda
1/2 tsp iodized salt
1/3 cup nonfat dry milk
2 tsp grated orange or lemon rind
1 cup regular oatmeal
1 cup finely chopped walnuts (or other nuts)
1 cup raisins, cranberries, or other dried fruit, finely chopped

Hearty Whole-Grain Muffins With Streusel Topping

I have always loved hot homemade muffins for breakfast, and my kids are addicted to them. I love to change the muffins by the season. This is one of my favorite recipes, and it is as versatile as it is delicious. —Enette

Instructions

1. Preheat oven to 375 °F (190 °C). Line muffin cups with paper liners.
2. Mix together flour, sugar, baking powder, cinnamon, salt, and nutmeg a bowl.
3. In a separate larger bowl, combine fruit and eggs and mix in the liquid (juice, milk, or soy milk) and oil.
4. Add the flour mixture to the liquid mixture. Stir just until moistened.
5. Fill muffin tins about three-quarters full, dividing batter evenly among muffin tins.
6. Sprinkle with approximately 2 teaspoons of the streusel topping plus 1 teaspoon finely chopped nuts. Bake for 20 to 25 minutes or until lightly browned. Freeze leftover muffins.

Makes 24 muffins.

Nutrition Content for One Muffin

175 calories • 26 g carbohydrate (2 grains) • 3 g protein • 7.1 g fat • 1.4 g fiber
1 mg iron • 71 mg calcium • 0.4 mg zinc

Ingredients List

2 cups unbleached flour
1-1/2 cups whole-wheat flour
1 cup dark-brown sugar (packed) or raw sugar
1 tbsp baking powder
1-1/2 tsp cinnamon
1 tsp nutmeg
1 tsp iodized salt
1-1/2 cups finely chopped or pureed fruit such as pumpkin puree, mashed banana, chopped or pureed apples, grated zucchini, finely chopped rhubarb, or blueberries
1 tsp grated citrus peel (omit for pumpkin muffins)
2 large eggs, beaten
1 cup milk, soy milk, or fruit juice (or a combination)
2/3 cup canola or Mediterranean oil
Streusel topping (see crisp recipe on page 278)
1/2 cup finely chopped nuts (optional)

APPENDIX A

Energy Costs of Physical Activity

TABLE A.1 Approximate Caloric Expenditure (above rest) per Minute for Rest and Various Exercise and Sport Activities

Weight in kg	45	52	59	66	73	80	86	93	100
Weight in lb	100	115	130	145	160	175	190	205	220
Baseball, player	2.1	2.5	2.8	3.0	3.4	3.8	4.0	4.4	5.7
Baseball, pitcher	2.9	3.4	3.8	4.2	4.7	5.2	5.5	6.0	6.4
Basketball, vigorous or competition	5.5	6.4	7.2	8.0	8.9	9.8	10.6	11.5	12.3
Bicycling, 15 mph	6.3	7.3	8.2	9.0	10.0	11.0	11.9	12.9	13.8
Bicycling, 20 mph	9.7	11.2	12.6	14.0	15.5	17.0	18.4	19.9	21.3
Calisthenics, light	2.4	2.9	3.2	3.5	3.9	4.4	4.7	5.1	5.5
Calisthenics, timed, vigorous	8.7	10.0	11.3	12.6	14.0	15.4	16.7	18.0	19.3
Dancing, active (square/disco)	3.5	4.1	4.6	5.1	5.7	6.2	6.7	7.3	7.8
Dancing, aerobic (vigorously)	5.0	5.9	6.6	7.3	8.1	8.9	9.6	10.4	11.1
Football, touch, vigorous	4.5	5.3	5.9	6.5	7.3	8.0	8.7	9.4	10.0
Hiking, 3 mph with pack	3.5	4.1	4.6	5.1	5.7	6.2	6.7	7.3	7.8
Hockey, field	4.0	5.9	6.6	7.3	8.1	8.9	9.6	10.4	11.1
Hockey, ice	5.6	6.5	7.4	8.2	9.1	10.0	10.8	11.8	12.6
Martial arts (judo/karate)	7.5	8.7	9.7	10.8	12.0	13.2	14.3	15.5	16.6
Mountain climbing	5.5	6.4	7.2	8.0	8.9	9.8	10.6	11.5	12.3
Racquetball	5.5	6.4	7.1	7.9	8.8	9.7	10.5	11.4	12.2
RUNNING, STEADY STATE									
6 mph (10:00 min/mile)	6.2	7.3	8.2	9.1	10.1	11.1	11.9	13.0	14.0
7 mph (8:35 min/mile)	7.5	8.7	9.7	10.8	12.0	13.2	14.3	15.5	16.6
8 mph (7:30 min/mile)	8.7	10.1	11.3	12.6	14.0	15.4	16.6	18.0	19.3
9 mph (6:40 min/mile)	9.8	11.3	12.7	14.2	15.7	17.3	18.7	20.2	21.7
10 mph (6:00 min/mile)	11.1	12.8	14.4	16.1	17.8	19.6	21.2	22.8	24.5
11 mph (5:28 min/mile)	12.3	14.2	16.0	17.9	19.8	21.7	23.5	25.5	27.3
12 mph (5:00 min/mile)	13.5	15.6	17.6	19.6	21.7	23.9	25.9	28.0	30.0
Skating, ice, 9 mph	3.2	3.7	4.2	4.6	5.2	5.7	6.2	6.7	7.2
Skating, inline, 13 mph	8.5	9.8	11.1	12.4	13.7	15.1	16.2	17.5	18.8
Skiing, cross country, 5 mph	6.7	7.7	8.7	9.6	10.7	11.6	12.8	13.8	14.8
Skiing, downhill	5.5	6.4	7.2	8.0	8.9	9.8	10.6	11.5	12.3
Soccer	4.9	5.8	6.5	7.2	8.0	8.8	9.5	10.3	11.0

(continued)

TABLE A.1 *(continued)*

Weight in kg	45	52	59	66	73	80	86	93	100
Weight in lb	100	115	130	145	160	175	190	205	220
SWIMMING, YARDS/MIN									
Backstroke, 30	2.5	3.0	3.3	3.6	4.0	4.5	4.8	5.2	5.4
Backstroke, 35	3.5	4.1	4.6	5.1	5.7	6.2	6.7	7.3	7.6
Backstroke, 40	4.5	5.3	5.9	6.5	7.3	8.0	8.7	9.4	9.8
Breaststroke, 30	3.7	4.3	4.9	5.4	6.0	6.6	7.2	7.8	10.3
Breaststroke, 40	5.3	6.2	7.0	7.8	8.6	9.5	10.3	11.1	11.9
Front crawl, 25	3.0	3.5	3.9	4.3	4.8	5.3	5.7	6.2	6.4
Front crawl, 35	3.8	4.5	5.1	5.5	6.2	6.8	7.3	7.9	8.2
Front crawl, 45	4.7	5.5	6.2	6.9	7.7	8.4	9.1	9.9	10.3
Front crawl, 50	6.0	7.0	7.9	8.8	9.7	10.7	11.6	12.5	13.0
Tennis, competition	5.4	6.3	7.1	7.9	8.8	9.7	10.5	11.4	12.2
Volleyball, vigorous or competition	5.5	6.4	7.1	7.9	8.8	9.7	10.5	11.4	12.2
WALKING, BRISK OR RACE									
4 mph (15:00 min/mile)	3.2	3.7	4.2	4.6	5.2	5.7	6.2	6.7	7.2
5 mph (12:00 min/mile)	4.4	5.2	5.8	6.4	7.1	7.8	8.5	9.2	9.8
5.8 mph (10:20 min/mile)	6.7	7.7	8.7	9.6	10.7	11.8	12.8	13.8	14.8
Weight training	4.2	4.9	5.5	6.1	6.7	7.4	8.0	8.7	9.3
Wrestling	8.5	8.7	9.7	10.8	12.0	13.2	14.3	15.5	16.6
Lying quietly	1.0*	1.1*	1.3*	1.5*	1.6*	1.7*	1.9*	2.0*	2.2*
Standing with light work	1.7	2.0	2.2	2.4	2.8	3.1	3.3	3.6	3.8

Keep the following in mind when using this table:

1. The figures are approximate values above rest or resting energy expenditure (REE) and thus can be calculated and added to your daily REE value as discussed in chapter 2. To obtain these values, REE* was subtracted from the total cost of the activity to get net activity cost, or calorie expenditure above rest. The values in the table are only for the time you are performing the activity. For example, during an hour of a basketball game you may play strenuously for only 35 or 40 minutes, as you may take time-outs and rest during foul shots. In general, record only the amount of time that you are actually exercising during the activity. You can also include time spent standing but do not need to estimate time spent sitting.

2. The energy cost, expressed in calories per minute, will vary for different activities in a given individual depending on several factors. For example, the caloric cost of bicycling will vary depending on the type

of bicycle, going uphill and downhill, and wind resistance. Energy cost for swimming at a certain pace will depend on swimming efficiency, so the less efficient swimmer will expend more calories. Thus, the values expressed here are approximations and may be increased or decreased depending on various factors that influence energy cost for a specific physical activity.

3. Not all body weights could be listed, but you may approximate by using the closest weight listed or using a value between the two closest values.

4. There may be small differences between men and women, but not enough to make a significant difference in the total caloric value for most exercises.

5. Not all physical activities and sports could be listed. For a more extensive list see the original source.

Adapted from M. Williams, E. Rawson, and D. Branch, *Nutrition for Health, Fitness & Sport,* 11th ed. (New York: McGraw-Hill, 2017), by permission of The McGraw-Hill Companies.

APPENDIX B

Food Guidance Systems

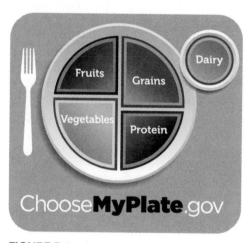

FIGURE B.1 American MyPlate

USDA Center for Nutrition Policy and Promotion

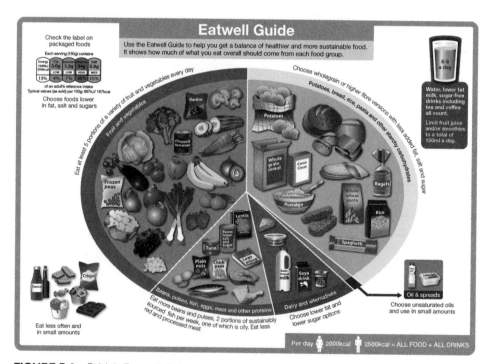

FIGURE B.2 British Eatwell Guide

Department of Health in association with the Welsh Government, the Scottish Government, and the Food Standards Agency in Northern Ireland. © Crown copyright 2016

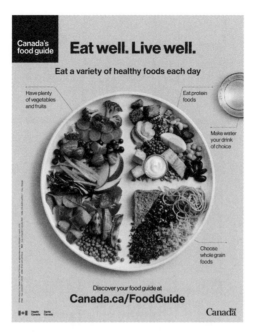

FIGURE B.3   Canadian Food Guide

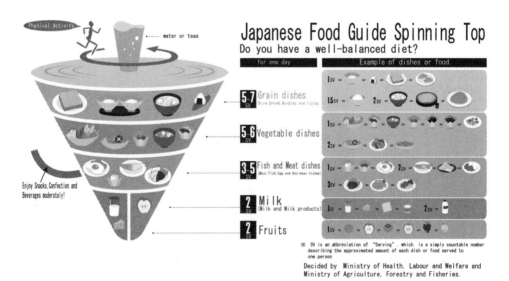

FIGURE B.4   Japanese Food Guide

Source: Ministry of Agriculture, Forestry and Fisheries Web site, http://www.maff.go.jp/e/data/publish/.

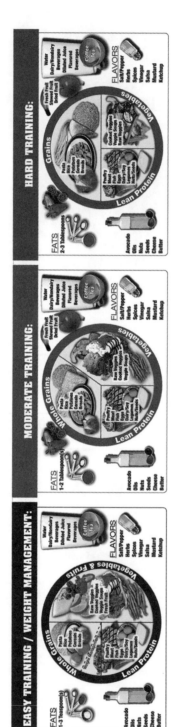

FIGURE B.5 Athlete's Plate

Used with permission of Nanna Meyer, University of Colorado at Colorado Springs (UCCS) Sport Nutrition Graduate Program (https://www.uccs.edu/swell/theathletesplate).

APPENDIX C

Foods Containing FODMAPs

Foods suitable on a low-FODMAP diet

Fruit	Vegetables	Grain foods	Milk products	other
Fruit Banana, blueberry, boysenberry, cantaloupe, cranberry, durian, grape, grapefruit, honeydew melon, kiwifruit, lemon, lime, mandarin orange passionfruit, pawpaw, raspberry, star anise, strawberry, tangelo Note: If fruit is dried, eat in small quantities	**Vegetables** Alfalfa, bamboo shoots, bean shoots, bok choy, carrot, celery, choko, choy sum, endive, ginger, green beans, lettuce, olives, parsnip, potato, pumpkin, red capsicum (bell pepper), silverbeet spinach, squash, swede, sweet potato, taro, tomato, turnip, yam, zucchini **Herbs** Basil, chili, coriander, ginger, lemongrass, marjoram, mint, oregano, parsley, rosemary, thyme	**Cereals** Gluten-free bread or cereal products **Bread** 100% spelt bread **Rice** **Oats** **Polenta** **Other** Arrowroot, millet, psyllium, quinoa, sorghum, tapioca	**Milk** Lactose-free milk*, oat milk*, rice milk*, soy milk* *check for additives **Cheeses** Hard cheeses, and brie and camembert **Yoghurt** Lactose-free varieties **Ice-cream substitutes** Gelati, sorbet **Butter substitutes** Olive oil	**Tofu** **Sweeteners** Sugar* (sucrose), glucose, artificial sweeteners not ending in "-ol" **Honey substitutes** Golden syrup*, maple syrup*, Molasses, treacle *small quantities

Eliminate foods containing FODMAPs

Excess fructose	Lactose	Fructans	Galactans	Polyols
Fruit Apple, mango, nashi, tinned fruit in natural juice, watermelon **Sweeteners** Fructose, high fructose corn syrup **Large total fructose dose** Concentrated fruit sources, large serves of fruit, dried fruit, fruit juice **Honey** Corn syrup, fruisana	**Milk** Milk from cows, goats or sheep, custard, ice cream, yoghurt **Cheeses** Soft unripened cheeses (e.g., cottage, cream, mascarpone, ricotta)	**Vegetables** Artichoke, asparagus, beetroot, broccoli, Brussels sprouts, cabbage, eggplant, fennel, garlic, leek, okra, onion (all), shallots, spring onion **Cereals** Wheat and rye, in large amounts (e.g., bread, crackers, cookies, couscous, pasta) **Fruit** Custard apple, persimmon, watermelon **Miscellaneous** Chicory, dandelion, inulin, pistachio	**Legumes** Baked beans, chickpeas, kidney beans, lentils, soy beans	**Fruit** Apple, apricot, avocado, blackberry, cherry, longan, lychee, nashi, nectarine, peach, pear, plum, prune, watermelon **Vegetable** Cauliflower, green capsicum (bell pepper), mushroom, sweet corn **Sweeteners** Sorbitol (420) Mannitol (421) Isomalt (953) Maltitol (965) Xylitol (967)

APPENDIX D

Glycemic Index of Common Foods

High glycemic–index foods (GI > 85)		Moderate glycemic–index foods (GI = 60-85)		Low glycemic–index foods (GI < 60)
Angel food cake	Rice Krispies	Sponge cake	White rice (long grain)	Barley kernel bread
Croissant	Shredded wheat	Pastry	Basmati rice	Barley
Muffins	Cornmeal	Popcorn	Parboiled rice	Rice bran
Melba toast	Millet	Oat bran bread	Wild rice	Wheat kernels
Cake doughnut	Ice cream	Rye kernel bread	Sweet potatoes and yams	Milk (whole or skim)
Soft drinks	Brown rice	Pita bread, white	Wheat, cooked	Yogurt (all types)
Waffles	Rice cakes	Bulgur bread	Ice cream, low fat	Apples
Cheese pizza	Soda crackers	Mixed-grain bread	Banana	Apricots (dried)
Bagel, white	Oatmeal	All-Bran cereal	Fruit cocktail	Cherries
Barley flour bread	Total cereal	Bran Chex cereal	Grapefruit juice	Grapefruit
White bread	Couscous	Oat bran cereal	Grapes	Peaches (fresh)
Rye flour bread	Watermelon	Special K cereal	Kiwi fruit	Pears (fresh)
Whole-wheat bread	Potatoes	Cracked barley	Mango and papaya	Plums
Cheerios	Hard candy	Buckwheat	Orange (whole or juice)	Beans (all types)
Corn bran cereal	Sucrose	Bulgur	Durum spaghetti	Lentils
Corn Chex cereal	Carrots	Sweet corn	Linguine	Dried peas
Cornflakes	Glucose			Spaghetti
Cream of wheat	Maltose			Peanuts
Crispix cereal	Corn chips			Tomato soup
Grape-Nuts	Honey and syrups			Fructose
Raisins	Sport drinks			
Mueslix	Molasses			

White bread (50 g) was used as the reference food and has a GI of 100.

Adapted from K. Foster-Powell and J.B. Miller, "International Table of Glycemic Index," *The American Journal of Clinical Nutrition* 62, no. 4 (1995): 871S-890S.

APPENDIX E

Dietary Reference Intakes
for Vitamins and Minerals

TABLE E.1   Dietary Reference Intakes: Recommended Vitamin Intakes for Individuals

Age	MEN			WOMEN			Pregnancy (19-50)	Lactation (19-50)
	19-50	51-70	Over 70	19-50	51-70	Over 70		
Vitamin A (mcg/day)[a]	900	900	900	700	700	700	770	1,300
Vitamin C (mg/day)	90	90	90	75	75	75	85	120
Vitamin D (mcg/day)[b,c]	5*	10*	15*	5*	10*	15*	5*	5*
Vitamin E (mg/day)[d]	15	15	15	15	15	15	15	19
Vitamin K (mcg/day)	120*	120*	120*	90*	90*	90*	90*	90*
Thiamin (mg/day)	1.2	1.2	1.2	1.1	1.1	1.1	1.4	1.4
Riboflavin (mg/day)	1.3	1.3	1.3	1.1	1.1	1.1	1.4	1.6
Niacin (mg/day)[e]	16	16	16	14	14	14	18	17
Vitamin B_6 (mg/day)	1.3	1.7	1.7	1.3	1.5	1.5	1.9	2.0
Folate (mcg/day)[f]	400	400	400	400[i]	400	400	600[j]	500
Vitamin B_{12} (mcg/day)	2.4	2.4[h]	2.4[h]	2.4	2.4[h]	2.4[h]	2.6	2.8
Pantothenic acid (mg/day)	5*	5*	5*	5*	5*	5*	6*	7*
Biotin (mcg/day)	30*	30*	30*	30*	30*	30*	30*	35*
Choline (mg/day)[g]	550*	550*	550*	425*	425*	425*	450*	550*

Note: This table (taken from the dietary reference intake reports; see www.nap.edu) presents recommended dietary allowances (RDAs) in **bold type** and adequate intakes (AIs) in ordinary type followed by an asterisk (*). RDAs and AIs may both be used as goals for individual intake. RDAs are set to meet the needs of almost all (97-98%) individuals in a group. For the ages presented here, the AI is believed to cover needs of all individuals in the group, but lack of data or uncertainty in the data prevent being able to specify with confidence the percentage of individuals covered by this intake.

[a]As retinol activity equivalents (RAEs). 1 RAE = 1 mcg retinol, 12 mcg beta-carotene, 24 mcg alpha-carotene, or 24 mcg beta-crypto-xanthin. The RAE for dietary provitamin A carotenoids is twofold greater than retinol equivalents (RE), whereas the RAE for preformed vitamin A is the same as RE.

[b]As cholecalciferol. 1 mcg cholecalciferol = 40 IU vitamin D.

[c]In the absence of adequate exposure to sunlight.

[d]As a.-tocopherol. a.-tocopherol includes RRR-a.-tocopherol, the only form of a.-tocopherol that occurs naturally in foods, and the 2R-stereoisomeric forms of a.-tocopherol (RRR-, RSR-, RRS-, and RSS-a.-tocopherol) that occur in fortified foods and supplements. It does not include the 2S-stereoisomeric forms of a.-tocopherol (SRR-, SSR-, SRS-, and SSS-a.-tocopherol), also found in fortified foods and supplements.

[e]As niacin equivalents (NE). 1 mg of niacin = 60 mg of tryptophan.

[f]As dietary folate equivalents (DFE). 1 DFE = 1 mcg food folate = 0.6 mcg of folic acid from fortified food or as a supplement consumed with food = 0.5 mcg of a supplement taken on an empty stomach.

[g]Although AIs have been set for choline, little data exists to assess whether a dietary supply of choline is needed at all stages of the life cycle, and it may be that the choline requirement can be met by endogenous synthesis at some of these stages.

[h]Because 10 to 30 percent of older people may absorb food-bound B_{12} poorly, it is advisable for people older than 50 years to meet their RDA mainly by consuming foods fortified with B_{12} or a supplement containing B_{12}.

[i]In view of evidence linking folate intake with neural tube defects in the fetus, it is recommended that all women capable of becoming pregnant consume 400 mcg from supplements or fortified foods in addition to intake of food folate from a varied diet.

[j]It is assumed that women will continue consuming 400 mcg from supplements or fortified food until their pregnancy is confirmed and they enter prenatal care, which ordinarily occurs after the end of the periconceptional period—the critical time for formation of the neural tube.

Sources: Dietary Reference Intakes for Calcium, Phosphorous, Magnesium, Vitamin D, and Fluoride (1997); Dietary Reference Intakes for Thiamin, Riboflavin, Niacin, Vitamin B6, Folate, Vitamin B12, Pantothenic Acid, Biotin, and Choline (1998); Dietary Reference Intakes for Vitamin C, Vitamin E, Selenium, and Carotenoids (2000); Dietary Reference Intakes for Vitamin A, Vitamin K, Arsenic, Boron, Chromium, Copper, Iodine, Iron, Manganese, Molybdenum, Nickel, Silicon, Vanadium, and Zinc (2001); and Dietary Reference Intakes for Water, Potassium, Sodium, Chloride, and Sulfate (2004). These reports may be accessed via www.nap.edu.

Adapted with permission from Dietary Reference Intakes for Vitamin A, Vitamin K, Arsenic, Boron, Chromium, Copper, Iodine, Iron, Manganese, Molybdenum, Nickel, Silicon, Vanadium and Zinc, © 2000 by the National Academy of Sciences, courtesy of the National Academies Press, Washington, DC.

TABLE E.2   Dietary Reference Intakes: Recommended Element Intakes for Individuals

Age	MEN			WOMEN				
	19-50	51-70	Over 70	19-50	51-70	Over 70	Pregnancy (19-50)	Lactation (19-50)
Calcium (mg/day)	1,000*	1,200*	1,200*	1,000*	1,200*	1,200*	1,000*	1,000*
Chromium (mcg/day)	35*	30*	30*	25*	20*	20*	30*	45*
Copper (mcg/day)	**900**	**900**	**900**	**900**	**900**	**900**	**1,000**	**1,300**
Fluoride (mg/day)	4*	4*	4*	3*	3*	3*	3*	3*
Iodine (mcg/day)	**150**	**150**	**150**	**150**	**150**	**150**	**220**	**290**
Iron (mg/day)	**8**	**8**	**8**	**18**	**8**	**8**	**27**	**9**
Magnesium (mg/day)	**400** (ages 19-30) **420** (ages 31-50)	**420**	**420**	**310** (19-30) **320** (31-50)	**320**	**320**	**350** (19-30) **360** (31-50)	**310** (19-30) **320** (31-50)
Manganese (mg/day)	2.3*	2.3*	2.3*	1.8*	1.8*	1.8*	2.0*	2.6*
Molybdenum (mcg/day)	**45**	**45**	**45**	**45**	**45**	**45**	**50**	**50**
Phosphorus (mg/day)	**700**	**700**	**700**	**700**	**700**	**700**	**700**	**700**
Selenium (mcg/day)	**55**	**55**	**55**	**55**	**55**	**55**	**60**	**70**
Zinc (mg/day)	**11**	**11**	**11**	**8**	**8**	**8**	**11**	**12**
Potassium (g/day)	4.7*	4.7*	4.7*	4.7*	4.7*	4.7*	4.7*	5.1*
Sodium (g/day)	1.5*	1.3*	1.2*	1.5*	1.3*	1.2*	1.5*	1.5*
Chloride (g/day)	2.3*	2.0*	1.8*	2.3*	2.0*	1.8*	2.3*	2.3*

Note: This table presents recommended dietary allowances (RDAs) in **bold type** and adequate intakes (AIs) in ordinary type followed by an asterisk (*). RDAs and AIs may both be used as goals for individual intake. RDAs are set to meet the needs of almost all (97-98%) individuals in a group. For the ages presented here, the AI is believed to cover needs of all individuals in the group, but lack of data or uncertainty in the data prevents being able to specify with confidence the percentage of individuals covered by this intake.

Sources: *Dietary Reference Intakes for Calcium, Phosphorous, Magnesium, Vitamin D, and Fluoride (1997); Dietary Reference Intakes for Thiamin, Ribo-flavin, Niacin, Vitamin B6, Folate, Vitamin B12, Pantothenic Acid, Biotin, and Choline (1998); Dietary Reference Intakes for Vitamin C, Vitamin E, Selenium, and Carotenoids (2000); Dietary Reference Intakes for Vitamin A, Vitamin K, Arsenic, Boron, Chromium, Copper, Iodine, Iron, Manganese, Molybdenum, Nickel, Silicon, Vanadium, and Zinc (2001); and Dietary Reference Intakes for Water, Potassium, Sodium, Chloride, and Sulfate (2004).* These reports may be accessed via www.nap.edu.

Adapted with permission from *Dietary Reference Intakes for Vitamin A, Vitamin K, Arsenic, Boron, Chromium, Copper, Iodine, Iron, Manganese, Molyb-denum, Nickel, Silicon, Vanadium and Zinc,* © 2000 by the National Academy of Sciences, courtesy of the National Academies Press, Washington, D.C.

APPENDIX F

Metric Conversions for Common Measures

TABLE F.1 Metric Conversions for Common Measures

Measurement		Conversion formula	Metric equivalent
Teaspoon	Liquid	× 5 =	5 ml
	Solid	× 4.7 =	4.7 g
Tablespoon	Liquid	× 15 =	15 ml
	Solid	× 14.2* =	14.2 g
Cup	Liquid	× 236 =	236 ml
	Solid	× 230* =	230 g
Ounce	Liquid	× 29 =	29 ml
	Solid	× 28* =	28 g
Inch		× 2.5 =	2.5 cm

*These are general conversion factors. To accurately convert cups to grams, a different factor is necessary depending on the type of food. For example, 1 cup of flour is 120 grams, and 1 cup of peanut butter is 258 grams. To accurately convert measurements for specific foods, use an online conversion tool such as the one at the GourmetSleuth site, www.gourmetsleuth.com/conversions/grams/grams-to-cups-conversions/calculator-help.

REFERENCES

Chapter 1

1. Vegetarian Resource Group. How many adults in the U.S. are vegetarian and vegan? The Vegetarian Resource Group asks in a 2016 national poll conducted by Harris Poll. www.vrg.org/nutshell/Polls/2016_adults_veg.htm. Published 2016. Accessed April 15, 2017.

2. Vegetarian Resource Group. How many teens and other youth are vegetarian and vegan? The Vegetarian Resource Group asks in a 2014 national poll conducted by Harris Poll. www.vrg.org/blog/2014/05/30/how-many-teens-and-other-youth-are-vegetarian-and-vegan-the-vegetarian-resource-group-asks-in-a-2014-national-poll. Published May 30, 2014.

3. Vegetarian Resource Group. How often do Americans eat vegetarian meals? And how many adults in the U.S. are vegan. https://www.vrg.org/journal/vj2011issue4/vj2011issue-4poll.php. Published 2012. Accessed July 23, 2018.

4. Leahy E, Lyons S, Tol SJ. An estimate of the number of vegetarians in the world. www.esri.ie/pubs/WP340.pdf. *Working Paper No. 340.* 2010(March):1-44.

5. Pelly FE, Burkhart SJ. Dietary regimens of athletes competing at the Delhi 2010 Commonwealth Games. *Int J Sport Nutr Exerc Metab.* 2014;24(1):28-36.

6. American College of Allergy, Asthma, and Immunology. Meat allergy. https://acaai.org/allergies/types/food-allergies/types-food-allergy/meat-allergy, 2014. Accessed November 4, 2018.

7. Tick bites linked to red meat allergy. WebMD website. www.webmd.com/allergies/news/20140813/tick-bites-red-meat-allergy. Published August 13, 2014.

8. Humane Research Council. Study of current and former vegetarians and vegans. https://faunalytics.org/wp-content/uploads/2015/06/Faunalytics_Current-Former-Vegetarians_Full-Report.pdf. Published December 2014. Accessed June 6, 2018.

9. Meyer N, Reguant-Closa A. Eat as if you could save the planet and win! Sustainability integration into nutrition for exercise and sport. *Nutrients.* 2017;9(4).

10. Gonzalez-Garcia S, Esteve-Llorens X, Moreira MT, Feijoo G. Carbon footprint and nutritional quality of different human dietary choices. *Sci Total Environ.* 2018;644:77-94.

11. Barr SI, Chapman GE. Perceptions and practices of self-defined current vegetarian, former vegetarian, and nonvegetarian women. *J Am Diet Assoc.* 2002;102(3):354-360.

12. Brown C, Mathew J, Wolf I, Kerckhoff A. What does "plant-based" actually mean? *Vegetarian Journal.* 2018;37(4):24-27.

13. Hanne N, Dlin R, Rotstein A. Physical fitness, anthropometric and metabolic parameters in vegetarian athletes. *J Sports Med Phys Fitness.* 1986;26(2):180-185.

14. Grandjean AC. The vegetarian athlete. *Phys Sportsmed.* 1987;15(5):191-194.

15. Harris HA. Nutrition and physical performance. The diet of Greek athletes. *Proc Nutr Soc.* 1966;25(2):87-90.

16. Longo UG, Spiezia F, Maffulli N, Denaro V. The best athletes in ancient Rome were vegetarian! *J Sports Sci Med.* 2008;7(4):565.

17. Simopoulos AP. Opening address. Nutrition and fitness from the first Olympiad in 776 BC to 393 AD and the concept of positive health. *Am J Clin Nutr.* 1989;49(5 Suppl):921-926.

18. Boyl M. *Community Nutrition in Action: An Entrepreneurial Approach.* Boston, MA: Cengage Learning; 2017.

19. Newby PK, Tucker KL, Wolk A. Risk of overweight and obesity among semivegetarian, lactovegetarian, and vegan women. *Am J Clin Nutr.* 2005;81(6):1267-1274.

20. Dinu M, Abbate R, Gensini GF, Casini A, Sofi F. Vegetarian, vegan diets and multiple health outcomes: a systematic review with meta-analysis of observational studies. *Crit Rev Food Sci Nutr.* 2017;57(17)3640-3649:0.

21. Yokoyama Y, Nishimura K, Barnard ND, et al. Vegetarian diets and blood pressure: a meta-analysis. *JAMA Intern Med.* 2014;174(4):577-587.

22. Melina V, Craig W, Levin S. Position of the Academy of Nutrition and Dietetics: Vegetarian Diets. *J Acad Nutr Diet.* 2016;116(12):1970-1980.

23. Orlich MJ, Fraser GE. Vegetarian diets in the Adventist Health Study 2: a review of initial published findings. *Am J Clin Nutr.* 2014;100 Suppl 1:353S-358S.

24. Fraser GE. Associations between diet and cancer, ischemic heart disease, and all-cause mortality in non-Hispanic white California Seventh-day Adventists. *Am J Clin Nutr.* 1999;70(3 Suppl):532S-538S.

25. Willett WC. Convergence of philosophy and science: the third international congress on vegetarian nutrition. *Am J Clin Nutr.* 1999;70(3 Suppl):434S-438S.

26. Lippi G, Mattiuzzi C, Sanchis-Gomar F. Red meat consumption and ischemic heart disease. A systematic literature review. *Meat Sci.* 2015;108:32-36.

27. Micha R, Wallace SK, Mozaffarian D. Red and processed meat consumption and risk of incident coronary heart disease, stroke, and diabetes mellitus: a systematic review and meta-analysis. *Circulation.* 2010;121(21):2271-2283.

28. Snowdon DA, Phillips RL. Does a vegetarian diet reduce the occurrence of diabetes? *Am J Public Health.* 1985;75(5):507-512.

29. Kouvari M, Notara V, Kalogeropoulos N, Panagiotakos DB. Diabetes mellitus associated with processed and unprocessed red meat: an overview. *Int J Food Sci Nutr.* 2016;67(7):735-743.

30. Lippi G, Mattiuzzi C, Cervellin G. Meat consumption and cancer risk: a critical review of published meta-analyses. *Crit Rev Oncol Hematol.* 2016;97:1-14.

31. Helmus DS, Thompson CL, Zelenskiy S, Tucker TC, Li L. Red meat-derived heterocyclic amines increase risk of colon cancer: a population-based case-control study. *Nutr Cancer.* 2013;65(8):1141-1150.

32. Kruger C, Zhou Y. Red meat and colon cancer: a review of mechanistic evidence for heme in the context of risk assessment methodology. *Food Chem Toxicol.* 2018;118:131-153.

33. Takachi R, Tsubono Y, Baba K, et al. Red meat intake may increase the risk of colon cancer in Japanese, a population with relatively low red meat consumption. *Asia Pac J Clin Nutr.* 2011;20(4):603-612.

34. Aune D, Giovannucci E, Boffetta P, et al. Fruit and vegetable intake and the risk of cardiovascular disease, total cancer and all-cause mortality-a systematic review and dose-response meta-analysis of prospective studies. *Int J Epidemiol.* 2017;46(3):1029-1056.

35. Bhupathiraju SN, Wedick NM, Pan A, et al. Quantity and variety in fruit and vegetable intake and risk of coronary heart disease. *Am J Clin Nutr.* 2013;98(6):1514-1523.

36. Rimm EB, Ascherio A, Giovannucci E, Spiegelman D, Stampfer MJ, Willett WC. Vegetable, fruit, and cereal fiber intake and risk of coronary heart disease among men. *JAMA.* 1996;275(6):447-451.

37. Souza RG, Gomes AC, Naves MM, Mota JF. Nuts and legume seeds for cardiovascular risk reduction: scientific evidence and mechanisms of action. *Nutr Rev.* 2015;73(6):335-347.

38. Cho SS, Qi L, Fahey GC Jr., Klurfeld DM. Consumption of cereal fiber, mixtures of whole grains and bran, and whole grains and risk reduction in type 2 diabetes, obesity, and cardiovascular disease. *Am J Clin Nutr.* 2013;98(2):594-619.

39. Makarem N, Nicholson JM, Bandera EV, McKeown NM, Parekh N. Consumption of whole grains and cereal fiber in relation to cancer risk: a systematic review of longitudinal studies. *Nutr Rev.* 2016;74(6):353-373.

40. Jacobs DR Jr., Marquart L, Slavin J, Kushi LH. Whole-grain intake and cancer: an expanded review and meta-analysis. *Nutr Cancer.* 1998;30(2):85-96.

41. Kushi LH, Meyer KA, Jacobs DR Jr. Cereals, legumes, and chronic disease risk reduction: evidence from epidemiologic studies. *Am J Clin Nutr.* 1999;70(3 Suppl):451S-458S.

42. de Vogel J, Jonker-Termont DS, van Lieshout EM, Katan MB, van der Meer R. Green vegetables, red meat and colon cancer: chlorophyll prevents the cytotoxic and hyperproliferative effects of haem in rat colon. *Carcinogenesis.* 2005;26(2):387-393.

43. Fleury S, Riviere G, Alles B, et al. Exposure to contaminants and nutritional intakes in a French vegetarian population. *Food Chem Toxicol.* 2017;109(Pt 1):218-229.

44. Appleby PN, Key TJ, Thorogood M, Burr ML, Mann J. Mortality in British vegetarians. *Public Health Nutr.* 2002;5(1):29-36.

45. Giem P, Beeson WL, Fraser GE. The incidence of dementia and intake of animal products: preliminary findings from the Adventist Health Study. *Neuroepidemiology.* 1993;12(1):28-36.

46. Key TJ, Fraser GE, Thorogood M, et al. Mortality in vegetarians and nonvegetarians: detailed findings from a collaborative analysis of 5 prospective studies. *Am J Clin Nutr.* 1999;70(3 Suppl):516S-524S.

47. Nieman DC. Vegetarian dietary practices and endurance performance. *Am J Clin Nutr.* 1988;48(3 Suppl):754-761.

48. Fisher I. The influence of flesh eating on endurance. *Yale Medical Journal.* 1907;XIII:204-221.

49. Berry E. The effects of a high and low protein diet on physical efficiency. *American Physical Education Review.* 1909;14:288-297.

50. Craddock JC, Probst YC, Peoples GE. Vegetarian and omnivorous nutrition - comparing physical performance. *Int J Sport Nutr Exerc Metab.* 2016;26(3):212-220.

51. Nieman DC, Underwood BC, Sherman KM, et al. Dietary status of Seventh-Day Adventist vegetarian and non-vegetarian elderly women. *J Am Diet Assoc.* 1989;89(12):1763-1769.

52. Rizzo NS, Jaceldo-Siegl K, Sabate J, Fraser GE. Nutrient profiles of vegetarian and nonvegetarian dietary patterns. *J Acad Nutr Diet.* 2013;113(12):1610-1619.

53. Jonvik KL, Nyakayiru J, Pinckaers PJ, Senden JM, van Loon LJ, Verdijk LB. Nitrate-rich vegetables increase plasma nitrate and nitrite concentrations and lower blood pressure in healthy adults. *J nutr.* 2016;146(5):986-993.

54. Lynch HM, Wharton CM, Johnston CS. Cardiorespiratory fitness and peak torque differences between vegetarian and omnivore endurance athletes: a cross-sectional study. *Nutrients.* 2016;8(11).

55. Raben A, Kiens B, Richter EA, et al. Serum sex hormones and endurance performance after a lacto-ovo vegetarian and a mixed diet. *Med Sci Sports Exerc.* 1992;24(11):1290-1297.

56. Richter EA, Kiens B, Raben A, Tvede N, Pedersen BK. Immune parameters in male athletes after a lacto-ovo vegetarian diet and a mixed Western diet. *Med Sci Sports Exerc.* 1991;23(5):517-521.

57. Krajcovicova-Kudlackova M, Ursinyova M, Blazicek P, et al. Free radical disease prevention and nutrition. *Bratisl Lek Listy.* 2003;104(2):64-68.

58. Rauma AL, Mykkanen H. Antioxidant status in vegetarians versus omnivores. *Nutrition.* 2000;16(2):111-119.

59. Powers S, Nelson WB, Larson-Meyer E. Antioxidant and vitamin D supplements for athletes: sense or nonsense? *J sports sci.* 2011;29 Suppl 1:S47-55.

60. Powers SK, DeRuisseau KC, Quindry J, Hamilton KL. Dietary antioxidants and exercise. *J sports sci.* 2004;22(1):81-94.

61. Trapp D, Knez W, Sinclair W. Could a vegetarian diet reduce exercise-induced oxidative stress? A review of the literature. *J sports sci.* 2010;28(12):1261-1268.

62. Krajcovicova-Kudlackova M, Dusinska M. Oxidative DNA damage in relation to nutrition. *Neoplasma.* 2004;51(1):30-33.

63. Krajcovicova-Kudlackova M, Spustova V, Paukova V. Lipid peroxidation and nutrition. *Physiol Res.* 2004;53(2):219-224.

64. Urso ML, Clarkson PM. Oxidative stress, exercise, and antioxidant supplementation. *Toxicology.* 2003;189(1-2):41-54.

65. Connolly DA, McHugh MP, Padilla-Zakour OI, Carlson L, Sayers SP. Efficacy of a tart cherry juice blend in preventing the symptoms of muscle damage. *Br J Sports Med.* 2006;40(8):679-683; discussion 683.

66. Bell PG, McHugh MP, Stevenson E, Howatson G. The role of cherries in exercise and health. *Scand J Med Sci Sports.* 2014;24(3):477-490.

67. Coelho Rabello Lima L, Oliveira Assumpcao C, Prestes J, Sergio Denadai B. Consumption of cherries as a strategy to attenuate exercise-induced muscle damage and inflammation in humans. *Nutr Hosp.* 2015;32(5):1885-1893.

68. Ammar A, Turki M, Hammouda O, et al. Effects of pomegranate juice supplementation on oxidative stress biomarkers following weightlifting exercise. *Nutrients.* 2017;9(8).

69. Trombold JR, Reinfeld AS, Casler JR, Coyle EF. The effect of pomegranate juice supplementation on strength and soreness after eccentric exercise. *J Strength Cond Res.* 2011;25(7):1782-1788.

70. Hutchison AT, Flieller EB, Dillon KJ, Leverett BD. Black currant nectar reduces muscle damage and inflammation following a bout of high-intensity eccentric contractions. *J Diet Suppl.* 2016;13(1):1-15.

71. Morillas-Ruiz JM, Villegas Garcia JA, Lopez FJ, Vidal-Guevara ML, Zafrilla P. Effects of polyphenolic antioxidants on exercise-induced oxidative stress. *Clin Nutr.* 2006;25(3):444-453.

72. Ricker MA, Haas WC. Anti-inflammatory diet in clinical practice: a review. *Nutr Clin Pract.* 2017;32(3):318-325.

73. Zhu F, Du B, Xu B. Anti-inflammatory effects of phytochemicals from fruits, vegetables, and food legumes: a review. *Crit Rev Food Sci Nutr.* 2018;58(8):1260-1270.

74. Newcomer BR, Sirikul B, Hunter GR, Larson-Meyer E, Bamman M. Exercise over-stress and maximal muscle oxidative metabolism: a 31P magnetic resonance spectroscopy case report. *Br J Sports Med.* 2005;39(5):302-306.

75. Orlich MJ, Singh PN, Sabate J, et al. Vegetarian dietary patterns and the risk of colorectal cancers. *JAMA Intern Med.* 2015;175(5):767-776.

76. Johnson JR, Sannes MR, Croy C, et al. Antimicrobial drug-resistant Escherichia coli from humans and poultry products, Minnesota and Wisconsin, 2002-2004. *Emerg Infect Dis.* 2007;13(6):838-846.

77. Brown, JM, Hazen, SL. Microbial modulation of cardiovascular disease. *Nat Rev Microbiol.* 2018;16(3):171-181.

78. Lang JM, Pan C, Cantor RM, et al. Impact of Individual Traits, Saturated Fat, and Protein Source on the Gut Microbiome. *MBio.* 2018;9(6).

79. What does Tom Brady eat? How the star stays on the field in his 40s. https://www.cbsnews.com/news/tom-brady-football-player-diet-nutrition. Published September 19, 2017.

Chapter 2

1. Goran M, Poehlman E, Johnson R. Energy requirements across the life span: new findings based on measurement of total energy expenditure with doubly labeled water. *Nutrition Research.* 1994;15(1):115-150.

2. Goran M. Variation in total energy expenditure in humans. *Obesity Research.* 1995;3(1):59-66.

3. Ebine N, Feng JY, Homma M, Saitoh S, Jones PJ. Total energy expenditure of elite synchronized swimmers measured by the doubly labeled water method. *Eur J Appl Physiol.* 2000;83(1):1-6.

4. Hill RJ, Davies PS. Energy intake and energy expenditure in elite lightweight female rowers. *Med Sci Sports Exerc.* 2002;34(11):1823-1829.

5. Anderson L, Orme P, Naughton RJ, et al. Energy intake and expenditure of professional soccer players of the English Premier League: evidence of carbohydrate periodization. *Int J Sport Nutr Exerc Metab.* 2017;27(3):228-238.

6. Sagayama H, Kondo E, Shiose K, et al. Energy requirement assessment and water turnover in Japanese college wrestlers using the doubly labeled water method. *J Nutr Sci Vitaminol (Tokyo).* 2017;63(2):141-147.

7. Hill RJ, Davies PS. Energy expenditure during 2 wk of an ultra-endurance run around Australia. *Med Sci Sports Exerc.* 2001;33(1):148-151.

8. Toth MJ, Poehlman ET. Sympathetic nervous system activity and resting metabolic rate in vegetarians. *Metabolism.* 1994;43(5):621-625.

9. Montalcini T, De Bonis D, Ferro Y, et al. High vegetable fats intake is associated with high

10. LaForgia J, Withers RT, Gore CJ. Effects of exercise intensity and duration on the excess post-exercise oxygen consumption. *J Sports Sci.* 2006;24(12):1247-1264.

11. Manore M, Thompson J. *Sport Nutrition for Health and Performance*. Champaign, IL: Human Kinetics; 2000.

12. Mountjoy M, Sundgot-Borgen J, Burke L, et al. The IOC consensus statement: beyond the female athlete triad—relative energy deficiency in sport (RED-S). *Br J Sports Med.* 2014;48(7):491-497.

13. Cunningham J. A reanalysis of the factors influencing basal metabolic rate in normal adults. *Am J Clin Nutr.* 1980;33:2372-2374.

14. Thompson J, Manore MM. Predicted and measured resting metabolic rate of male and female endurance athletes. *J Am Diet Assoc.* 1996;96(1):30-34.

15. Brouns F, Saris WH. Diet manipulation and related metabolic changes in competitive cyclists. Paper presented at American College of Sports Medicine Annual Meeting 1990.

16. Nattiv A, Loucks AB, Manore MM, et al. American College of Sports Medicine position stand. The female athlete triad. *Med Sci Sports Exerc.* 2007;39(10):1867-1882.

17. Manore MM, Kam LC, Loucks AB. The female athlete triad: components, nutrition issues, and health consequences. *J Sports Sci.* 2007;25 Suppl 1:S61-71.

18. Ackerman KE, Slusarz K, Guereca G, et al. Higher ghrelin and lower leptin secretion are associated with lower LH secretion in young amenorrheic athletes compared with eumenorrheic athletes and controls. *Am J Physiol Endocrinol Metab.* 2012;302(7):E800-806.

19. Deuster PA, Kyle SB, Moser PB, Vigersky RA, Singh A, Schoomaker EB. Nutritional intakes and status of highly trained amenorrheic and eumenorrheic women runners. *Fertil Steril.* 1986;46(4):636-643.

20. Kaiserauer S, Snyder AC, Sleeper M, Zierath J. Nutritional, physiological, and menstrual status of distance runners. *Med Sci Sports Exerc.* 1989;21(2):120-125.

21. Nelson ME, Fisher EC, Catsos PD, Meredith CN, Turksoy RN, Evans WJ. Diet and bone status in amenorrheic runners. *Am J Clin Nutr.* 1986;43(6):910-916.

22. Barr SI. Vegetarianism and menstrual cycle disturbances: is there an association? *Am J Clin Nutr.* 1999;70(3 Suppl):549S-554S.

23. Brooks SM, Sanborn CF, Albrecht BH, Wagner WW Jr. Diet in athletic amenorrhoea. *Lancet.* 1984;1(8376):559-560.

24. Slavin J, Lutter J, Cushman S. Amenorrhoea in vegetarian athletes. *Lancet.* 1984;1(8392):1474-1475.

25. Timko CA, Hormes JM, Chubski J. Will the real vegetarian please stand up? An investigation of dietary restraint and eating disorder symptoms in vegetarians versus non-vegetarians. *Appetite.* 2012;58(3):982-990.

26. Klopp SA, Heiss CJ, Smith HS. Self-reported vegetarianism may be a marker for college women at risk for disordered eating. *J Am Diet Assoc.* 2003;103(6):745-747.

27. O'Connor MA, Touyz SW, Dunn SM, Beumont PJ. Vegetarianism in anorexia nervosa? A review of 116 consecutive cases. *Med J Aust.* 1987;147(11-12):540-542.

28. Robinson-O'Brien R, Perry CL, Wall MM, Story M, Neumark-Sztainer D. Adolescent and young adult vegetarianism: better dietary intake and weight outcomes but increased risk of disordered eating behaviors. *J Am Diet Assoc.* 2009;109(4):648-655.

29. Bardone-Cone AM, Fitzsimmons-Craft EE, Harney MB, et al. The inter-relationships between vegetarianism and eating disorders among females. *J Acad Nutr Diet.* 2012;112(8):1247-1252.

30. Barnard ND, Levin S. Vegetarian diets and disordered eating. *J Am Diet Assoc.* 2009;109(9):1523; author reply 1523-1524.

31. Fisak B Jr., Peterson RD, Tantleff-Dunn S, Molnar JM. Challenging previous conceptions of vegetarianism and eating disorders. *Eat Weight Disord.* 2006;11(4):195-200.

32. Ackerman KE, Cano Sokoloff N, DE Nardo Maffazioloi G, Clarke HM, Lee H, Misra M. Fractures in relation to menstrual status and bone parameters in young athletes. *Med Sci Sports Exerc.* 2015;47(8):1577-1586.

Chapter 3

1. Thomas DT, Erdman KA, Burke LM. American College of Sports Medicine joint position statement. Nutrition and athletic performance. *Med Sci Sports Exerc.* 2016;48(3):543-568.
2. Hawley JA, Leckey JJ. Carbohydrate dependence during prolonged, intense endurance exercise. *Sports Med.* 2015;45 Suppl 1:S5-12.
3. Williams C, Rollo I. Carbohydrate nutrition and team sport performance. *Sports Med.* 2015;45 Suppl 1:S13-22.
4. Couto PG, Bertuzzi R, de Souza CC, et al. High carbohydrate diet induces faster final sprint and overall 10,000-m times of young runners. *Pediatr Exerc Sci.* 2015;27(3):355-363.
5. Balsom PD, Wood K, Olsson P, Ekblom B. Carbohydrate intake and multiple sprint sports: with special reference to football (soccer). *Int J Sports Med.* 1999;20(1):48-52.
6. Souglis AG, Chryssanthopoulos CI, Travlos AK, et al. The effect of high vs. low carbohydrate diets on distances covered in soccer. *J Strength Cond Res.* 2013;27(8):2235-2247.
7. Larson DE, Hesslink RL, Hrovat MI, Fishman RS, Systrom DM. Dietary effects on exercising muscle metabolism and performance by 31P-MRS. *J Appl Physiol (1985).* 1994;77(3):1108-1115.
8. Burke LM, Hawley JA, Wong SH, Jeukendrup AE. Carbohydrates for training and competition. *J Sports Sci.* 2011;29 Suppl 1:S17-27.
9. Achten J, Halson SL, Moseley L, Rayson MP, Casey A, Jeukendrup AE. Higher dietary carbohydrate content during intensified running training results in better maintenance of performance and mood state. *J Appl Physiol (1985).* 2004;96(4):1331-1340.
10. Brouns F, Saris WH. Diet manipulation and related metabolic changes in competitive cyclists. Paper presented at American College of Sports Medicine Annual Meeting 1990.
11. Brewer J, Williams C, Patton A. The influence of high carbohydrate diets on endurance running performance. *Eur J Appl Physiol Occup Physiol.* 1988;57(6):698-706.
12. Costill DL, Sherman WM, Fink WJ, Maresh C, Witten M, Miller JM. The role of dietary carbohydrates in muscle glycogen resynthesis after strenuous running. *Am J Clin Nutr.* 1981;34(9):1831-1836.
13. Jenkins DJ, Kendall CW, Augustin LS, et al. Glycemic index: overview of implications in health and disease. *Am J Clin Nutr.* 2002;76(1):266S-273S.
14. Augustin LS, Kendall CW, Jenkins DJ, et al. Glycemic index, glycemic load and glycemic response: an international scientific consensus summit from the International Carbohydrate Quality Consortium (ICQC). *Nutr Metab Cardiovasc Dis.* 2015;25(9):795-815.
15. Lis D, Stellingwerff T, Kitic CM, Ahuja KD, Fell J. No effects of a short-term gluten-free diet on performance in nonceliac athletes. *Med Sci Sports Exerc.* 2015;47(12):2563-2570.
16. Biesiekierski JR, Peters SL, Newnham ED, Rosella O, Muir JG, Gibson PR. No effects of gluten in patients with self-reported non-celiac gluten sensitivity after dietary reduction of fermentable, poorly absorbed, short-chain carbohydrates. *Gastroenterology.* 2013;145(2):320-328 e321-323.
17. Eswaran S, Farida JP, Green J, Miller JD, Chey WD. Nutrition in the management of gastrointestinal diseases and disorders: the evidence for the low FODMAP diet. *Curr Opin Pharmacol.* 2017;37:151-157.
18. Ireton-Jones C. The low FODMAP diet: fundamental therapy in the management of irritable bowel syndrome. *Curr Opin Clin Nutr Metab Care.* 2017;20(5):414-419.
19. Lis D, Ahuja KD, Stellingwerff T, Kitic CM, Fell J. Case study: utilizing a low FODMAP diet to combat exercise-induced gastrointestinal symptoms. *Int J Sport Nutr Exerc Metab.* 2016;26(5):481-487.
20. Lis DM, Stellingwerff T, Kitic CM, Fell JW, Ahuja KDK. Low FODMAP: a preliminary strategy to reduce gastrointestinal distress in athletes. *Med Sci Sports Exerc.* 2018;50(1):116-123.

Chapter 4

1. Yngve A. A Historical perspective of the understanding of the link between diet and coronary heart disease. *Am J Lifestyle Med.* 2009;3(1 Suppl.):35S-38S.

2. Romijn J, Coyle EF, Sidossis LS, et al. Regulation of endogenous fat and carbohydrate metabolism in relation to exercise intensity and duration. *Am J Physiol.* 1993;265(28):E380-E391.

3. Romijn JA, Coyle EF, Sidossis LS, Rosenblatt J, Wolfe RR. Substrate metabolism during different exercise intensities in endurance-trained women. *J Appl Physiol.* 2000;88(5):1707-1714.

4. Larson-Meyer DE, Borkhsenious ON, Gullett JC, et al. Effect of dietary fat on serum and intramyocellular lipids and running performance. *Med Sci Sports Exerc.* 2008;40(5):892-902.

5. Larson-Meyer DE, Newcomer BR, Hunter GR. Influence of endurance running and recovery diet on intramyocellular lipid content in women: a 1H NMR study. *Am J Physiol Endocrinol Metab.* 2002;282(1):E95-E106.

6. Decombaz J, Schmitt B, Ith M, et al. Postexercise fat intake repletes intramyocellular lipids but no faster in trained than in sedentary subjects. *Am J Physiol Regul Integr Comp Physiol.* 2001;281(3):R760-769.

7. Dugan A. Americans still avoid fat more than carbs. Gallup website. http://news.gallup.com/poll/174176/americans-avoid-fat-carbs.aspx. Published July 29, 2014. Accessed March 14, 2018.

8. Zehnder M, Christ ER, Ith M, et al. Intramyocellular lipid stores increase markedly in athletes after 1.5 days lipid supplementation and are utilized during exercise in proportion to their content. *Eur J Appl Physiol.* 2006;98(4):341-354.

9. Burke LM, Kiens B. "Fat adaptation" for athletic performance: the nail in the coffin? *J Appl Physiol (1985).* 2006;100(1):7-8.

10. Chang CK, Borer K, Lin PJ. Low-carbohydrate-high-fat diet: can it help exercise performance? *J Hum Kinet.* 2017;56:81-92.

11. Volek JS, Freidenreich DJ, Saenz C, et al. Metabolic characteristics of keto-adapted ultra-endurance runners. *Metabolism.* 2016;65(3):100-110.

12. Burke LM, Ross ML, Garvican-Lewis LA, et al. Low carbohydrate, high fat diet impairs exercise economy and negates the performance benefit from intensified training in elite race walkers. *J Physiol.* 2017;595(9):2785-2807.

13. Havemann L, West SJ, Goedecke JH, et al. Fat adaptation followed by carbohydrate loading compromises high-intensity sprint performance. *J Appl Physiol (1985).* 2006;100(1):194-202.

14. Burke LM, Hawley JA, Angus DJ, et al. Adaptations to short-term high-fat diet persist during exercise despite high carbohydrate availability. *Med Sci Sports Exerc.* 2002;34(1):83-91.

15. Venkatraman JT, Leddy J, Pendergast DR. Dietary fats and immune status in athletes: clinical implications. *Med Sci Sports Exerc.* 2000;32(7):S389-395.

16. Crist DM, Hill JM. Diet and insulinlike growth factor I in relation to body composition in women with exercise-induced hypothalamic amenorrhea. *J Am Coll Nutr.* 1990;9(3):200-204.

17. Deuster PA, Kyle SB, Moser PB, Vigersky RA, Singh A, Schoomaker EB. Nutritional intakes and status of highly trained amenorrheic and eumenorrheic women runners. *Fertil Steril.* 1986;46(4):636-643.

18. Laughlin GA, Yen SS. Nutritional and endocrine-metabolic aberrations in amenorrheic athletes. *J Clin Endocrinol Metab.* 1996;81(12):4301-4309.

19. Brown RC, Cox CM. Effects of high fat versus high carbohydrate diets on plasma lipids and lipoproteins in endurance athletes. *Med Sci Sports Exerc.* 1998;30(12):1677-1683.

20. Muoio DM, Leddy JJ, Horvath PJ, Awad AB, Pendergast DR. Effect of dietary fat on metabolic adjustments to maximal VO_2 and endurance in runners. *Med Sci Sports Exerc.* 1994;26(1):81-88.

21. Lissner L, Heitmann BL. Dietary fat and obesity: evidence from epidemiology. *Eur J Clin Nutr.* 1995;49(2):79-90.

22. Larson DE, Hunter GR, Williams MJ, Kekes-Szabo T, Nyikos I, Goran MI. Dietary fat in relation to body fat and intraabdominal adipose tissue: a cross-sectional analysis. *Am J Clin Nutr.* 1996;64(5):677-684.

23. Larson DE, Tataranni PA, Ferraro RT, Ravussin E. Ad libitum food intake on a "cafeteria diet" in Native American women: relations with body composition and 24-h energy expenditure. *Am J Clin Nutr.* 1995;62(5):911-917.

24. Spencer EA, Appleby PN, Davey GK, Key TJ. Diet and body mass index in 38000 EPIC-Oxford meat-eaters, fish-eaters, vegetarians and vegans. *Int J Obes Relat Metab Disord.* 2003;27(6):728-734.

25. Willett WC. Is dietary fat a major determinant of body fat? *Am J Clin Nutr.* 1998;67(3 Suppl):556S-562S.

26. Leibel R, Hirsch J, Appel B, Checani G. Energy intake required to maintain body weight is not affected by wide variation in diet composition. *Am. J. Clin. Nutr.* 1992;55:350-355.

27. Prentice AM. Manipulation of dietary fat and energy density and subsequent effects on substrate flux and food intake. *Am. J. Clin. Nutr .* 1998;67(3 Suppl):535S-541S.

28. Pendergast DR, Leddy JJ, Venkatraman JT. A perspective on fat intake in athletes. *J Am Coll Nutr.* 2000;19(3):345-350.

29. Trumbo P, Schlicker S, Yates AA, Poos M, Food, Nutrition Board of the Institute of Medicine, The National Academies. Dietary reference intakes for energy, carbohydrate, fiber, fat, fatty acids, cholesterol, protein and amino acids. *J Am Diet Assoc.* 2002;102(11):1621-1630.

30. Thomas DT, Erdman KA, Burke LM. American College of Sports Medicine joint position statement. Nutrition and athletic performance. *Med Sci Sports Exerc.* 2016;48(3):543-568.

31. Ornish D, Brown S, Scherwitz L, et al. Can lifestyle changes reverse coronary heart disease? The Lifestyle Heart Trial. *The Lancet.* 1990;336:129-133.

32. Barnard ND, Katcher HI, Jenkins DJ, Cohen J, Turner-McGrievy G. Vegetarian and vegan diets in type 2 diabetes management. *Nutr Rev.* 2009;67(5):255-263.

33. Barnard ND, Cohen J, Jenkins DJ, et al. A low-fat vegan diet and a conventional diabetes diet in the treatment of type 2 diabetes: a randomized, controlled, 74-wk clinical trial. *Am J Clin Nutr.* 2009;89(5):1588S-1596S.

34. Gould KL, Ornish D, Kirkeeide R, et al. Improved stenosis geometry by quantitative coronary arteriography after vigorous risk factor modification. *Am J Cardiol.* 1992;69(9):845-853.

35. Gould KL, Ornish D, Scherwitz L, et al. Changes in myocardial perfusion abnormalities by positron emission tomography after long-term, intense risk factor modification. *JAMA.* 1995;274(11):894-901.

36. Hu FB, Willett WC. Optimal diets for prevention of coronary heart disease. *JAMA.* 2002;288(20):2569-2578.

37. Hu FB, Stampfer MJ, Manson JE, et al. Dietary fat intake and the risk of coronary heart disease in women. *N Engl J Med.* 1997;337(21):1491-1499.

38. U.S. Department of Health and Human Services and U.S. Department of Agriculture. 2015-2020 dietary guidelines for Americans. 8th Edition. Office of Disease Prevention and Health Promotion website. https://health.gov/dietaryguidelines/2015. Published December 2015. Accessed March 14 2018.

39. American Diabetes Association. Standards of medical care in diabetes–2014. *Diabetes Care.* 2014;37 Suppl 1:S14-80.

40. Eckel RH, Jakicic JM, Ard JD, et al. 2013 AHA/ACC guideline on lifestyle management to reduce cardiovascular risk: a report of the American College of Cardiology/American Heart Association Task Force on Practice Guidelines. *J Am Coll Cardiol.* 2014;63(25 Pt B):2960-2984.

41. Final determination regarding partially hydrogenated oils (removing trans fat). U.S. Food and Drug Administration website. www.fda.gov/Food/IngredientsPackagingLabeling/FoodAdditivesIngredients/ucm449162.htm. Published June 2015. Updated June 18, 2018.

42. Fretts AM, Mozaffarian D, Siscovick DS, et al. Plasma phospholipid saturated fatty acids and incident atrial fibrillation: the Cardiovascular Health Study. *J Am Heart Assoc.* 2014;3(3):e000889.

43. Geppert J, Kraft V, Demmelmair H, Koletzko B. Docosahexaenoic acid supplementation in vegetarians effectively increases omega-3 index: a randomized trial. *Lipids.* 2005;40(8):807-814.

44. Conquer JA, Holub BJ. Supplementation with an algae source of docosahexaenoic acid increases (n-3) fatty acid status and alters selected risk factors for heart disease in vegetarian subjects. *J Nutr.* 1996;126(12):3032-3039.

45. Williams CM, Burdge G. Long-chain n-3 PUFA: plant v. marine sources. *Proc Nutr Soc.* 2006;65(1):42-50.

46. Rosato V, Temple NJ, La Vecchia C, Castellan G, Tavani A, Guercio V. Mediterranean diet and cardiovascular disease: a systematic review and meta-analysis of observational studies. *Eur J Nutr.* 2017.

47. Melina V, Craig W, Levin S. Position of the Academy of Nutrition and Dietetics: vegetarian diets. *J Acad Nutr Diet.* 2016;116(12):1970-1980.

48. Da Boit M, Hunter AM, Gray SR. Fit with good fat? The role of n-3 polyunsaturated fatty acids on exercise performance. *Metabolism.* 2017;66:45-54.

49. Bloomer RJ, Larson DE, Fisher-Wellman KH, Galpin AJ, Schilling BK. Effect of eicosapentaenoic and docosahexaenoic acid on resting and exercise-induced inflammatory and oxidative stress biomarkers: a randomized, placebo controlled, cross-over study. *Lipids Health Dis.* 2009;8:36.

50. Jakeman JR, Lambrick DM, Wooley B, Babraj JA, Faulkner JA. Effect of an acute dose of omega-3 fish oil following exercise-induced muscle damage. *Eur J Appl Physiol.* 2017;117(3):575-582.

51. Saunders AV, Davis BC, Garg ML. Omega-3 polyunsaturated fatty acids and vegetarian diets. *Med J Aust.* 2013;199(4 Suppl):S22-26.

52. Aragon A, Schoenfeld B, Wildman R et al. International society of sports nutrition position stand: diets and body composition. J Int Soc Sports Nutr. 2017;14(1). doi:10.1186/s12970-017-0174-y

Chapter 5

1. Simopoulos AP. Opening address. Nutrition and fitness from the first Olympiad in 776 BC to 393 AD and the concept of positive health. *Am J Clin Nutr.* 1989;49(5 Suppl):921-926.

2. Manore M, Thompson J. *Sport Nutrition for Health and Performance.* Champaign, IL: Human Kinetics; 2000.

3. Otten JJ, Hellwig JP, Meyers LD. *The Dietary Reference Intakes: The Essential Guide to Nutrient Requirements.* Washington, DC: Food and Nutrition Board, Institutes of Medicine; 2006.

4. Drummond MJ, Fry CS, Glynn EL, et al. Rapamycin administration in humans blocks the contraction-induced increase in skeletal muscle protein synthesis. *J Physiol.* 2009;587(Pt 7):1535-1546.

5. Drummond MJ, Dreyer HC, Fry CS, Glynn EL, Rasmussen BB. Nutritional and contractile regulation of human skeletal muscle protein synthesis and mTORC1 signaling. *J Appl Physiol (1985).* 2009;106(4):1374-1384.

6. Young VR, Pellett PL. Plant proteins in relation to human protein and amino acid nutrition. *Am J Clin Nutr.* 1994;59(5 Suppl):1203S-1212S.

7. Woolf PJ, Fu LL, Basu A. vProtein: identifying optimal amino acid complements from plant-based foods. *PLoS One.* 2011;6(4):e18836.

8. Thomas DT, Erdman KA, Burke LM. American College of Sports Medicine joint position statement. Nutrition and athletic performance. *Med Sci Sports Exerc.* 2016;48(3):543-568.

9. Tarnopolsky M. Protein requirements for endurance athletes. *Nutrition.* 2004;20(7-8):662-668.

10. Breen L, Churchward-Venne TA. Leucine: a nutrient 'trigger' for muscle anabolism, but what more? *J Physiol.* 2012;590(9):2065-2066.

11. Phillips SM, Van Loon LJ. Dietary protein for athletes: from requirements to optimum adaptation. *J sports sci.* 2011;29 Suppl 1:S29-38.

12. Lemon PW, Mullin JP. Effect of initial muscle glycogen levels on protein catabolism during exercise. *J Appl Physiol Respir Environ Exerc Physiol.* 1980;48(4):624-629.

13. Gontzea I, Sutzescu R, Dumitrache S. Influence of adaptation to physical effort on nitrogen-balance in man. *Nutr Rep Int.* 1975;11(3):231-236.

14. Melina V, Craig W, Levin S. Position of the Academy of Nutrition and Dietetics: vegetarian diets. *J Acad Nutr Diet.* 2016;116(12):1970-1980.

15. Young VR. Soy protein in relation to human protein and amino acid nutrition. *J Am Diet Assoc.* 1991;91(7):828-835.

16. Simon MS. The impossible burger: inside the strange science of the fake meat that bleeds. Wired website. www.wired.com/story/the-impossible-burger/2017. Published September 20, 2017. Accessed November 14, 2018.

17. Tarnopolsky MA, Atkinson SA, MacDougall JD, Chesley A, Phillips S, Schwarcz HP. Evaluation of protein requirements for trained strength athletes. *J Appl Physiol (1985).* 1992;73(5):1986-1995.

18. Morton RW, Murphy KT, McKellar SR, et al. A systematic review, meta-analysis and meta-regression of the effect of protein supplementation on resistance training-induced gains in muscle mass and strength in healthy adults. *Br J Sports Med.* 2018;52(6):376-384.

19. Messina M, Lynch H, Dickinson JM, Reed KE. No difference between the effects of supplementing with soy protein versus animal protein on gains in muscle mass and strength in response to resistance exercise. *Int J Sport Nutr Exerc Metab.* 2018:1-36.

20. Marckmann P, Osther P, Pedersen AN, Jespersen B. High-protein diets and renal health. *J Ren Nutr.* 2015;25(1):1-5.

21. Reddy ST, Wang CY, Sakhaee K, Brinkley L, Pak CY. Effect of low-carbohydrate high-protein diets on acid-base balance, stone-forming propensity, and calcium metabolism. *Am J Kidney Dis.* 2002;40(2):265-274.

22. Mamerow MM, Mettler JA, English KL, et al. Dietary protein distribution positively influences 24-h muscle protein synthesis in healthy adults. *J nutr.* 2014;144(6):876-880.

23. Paddon-Jones D, Leidy H. Dietary protein and muscle in older persons. *Curr Opin Clin Nutr Metab Care.* 2014;17(1):5-11.

24. Babault N, Paizis C, Deley G, et al. Pea proteins oral supplementation promotes muscle thickness gains during resistance training: a double-blind, randomized, placebo-controlled clinical trial vs. whey protein. *J Int Soc Sports Nutr.* 2015;12(1):3.

25. Kanda A, Nakayama K, Sanbongi C, Nagata M, Ikegami S, Itoh H. Effects of whey, caseinate, or milk protein ingestion on muscle protein synthesis after exercise. *Nutrients.* 2016;8(6).

26. Fraser RZ, Shitut M, Agrawal P, Mendes O, Klapholz S. Safety evaluation of soy leghemoglobin protein preparation derived from pichia pastoris, intended for use as a flavor catalyst in plant-based meat. *Int J Toxicol.* 2018;37(3):241-262.

Chapter 6

1. Marsh AG, Sanchez TV, Michelsen O, Chaffee FL, Fagal SM. Vegetarian lifestyle and bone mineral density. *Am J Clin Nutr.* 1988;48(3 Suppl):837-841.

2. Ambroszkiewicz J, Klemarczyk W, Gajewska J, Chelchowska M, Franek E, Laskowska-Klita T. The influence of vegan diet on bone mineral density and biochemical bone turnover markers. *Pediatr Endocrinol Diabetes Metab.* 2010;16(3):201-204.

3. Chiu JF, Lan SJ, Yang CY, et al. Long-term vegetarian diet and bone mineral density in postmenopausal Taiwanese women. *Calcif Tissue Int.* 1997;60(3):245-249.

4. Lau EM, Kwok T, Woo J, Ho SC. Bone mineral density in Chinese elderly female vegetarians, vegans, lacto-vegetarians and omnivores. *Eur J Clin Nutr.* 1998;52(1):60-64.

5. Weaver CM. Nutrition and bone health. *Oral Dis.* 2017;23(4):412-415.

6. Laurent M, Gielen E, Claessens F, Boonen S, Vanderschueren D. Osteoporosis in older men: recent advances in pathophysiology and treatment. *Best Pract Res Clin Endocrinol Metab.* 2013;27(4):527-539.

7. Raisz LG. Pathogenesis of osteoporosis: concepts, conflicts, and prospects. *J Clin Invest.* 2005;115(12):3318-3325.

8. Gaffney CD, Pagano MJ, Kuker AP, Stember DS, Stahl PJ. Osteoporosis and low bone mineral density in men with testosterone deficiency syndrome. *Sex Med Rev.* 2015;3(4):298-315.

9. Nordin BE. Calcium and osteoporosis. *Nutrition.* 1997;13(7-8):664-686.

10. Otten JJ, Hellwig JP, Meyers LD. *The Dietary Reference Intakes: The Essential Guide to Nutrient Requirements.* Washington, DC: Food and Nutrition Board, Institutes of Medicine; 2006.

11. Kok DJ, Iestra JA, Doorenbos CJ, Papapoulos SE. The effects of dietary excesses in animal protein and in sodium on the composition and the crystallization kinetics of calcium oxalate monohydrate in urines of healthy men. *J Clin Endocrinol Metab.* 1990;71(4):861-867.

12. Mangels AR. Bone nutrients for vegetarians. *Am J Clin Nutr.* 2014;100 Suppl 1:469S-475S.

13. Alexy U, Remer T, Manz F, Neu CM, Schoenau E. Long-term protein intake and dietary potential renal acid load are associated with bone modeling and remodeling at the proximal radius in healthy children. *Am J Clin Nutr.* 2005;82(5):1107-1114.

14. Weaver CM, Gordon CM, Janz KF, et al. The National Osteoporosis Foundation's position statement on peak bone mass development and lifestyle factors: a systematic review and implementation recommendations. *Osteoporos Int.* 2016;27(4):1281-1386.

15. Thomas DT, Erdman KA, Burke LM. American College of Sports Medicine joint position statement. Nutrition and athletic performance. *Med Sci Sports Exerc.* 2016;48(3):543-568.

16. Tenforde AS, Sayres LC, Sainani KL, Fredericson M. Evaluating the relationship of calcium and vitamin D in the prevention of stress fracture injuries in the young athlete: a review of the literature. *PM R.* 2010;2(10):945-949.

17. United States Department of Agriculture. Choose MyPlate website. www.choosemyplate.gov. Published 2015. Accessed 1 March, 2019

18. Melina V, Craig W, Levin S. Position of the Academy of Nutrition and Dietetics: vegetarian diets. *J Acad Nutr Diet.* 2016;116(12):1970-1980.

19. Heaney RP, Dowell MS, Rafferty K, Bierman J. Bioavailability of the calcium in fortified soy imitation milk, with some observations on method. *Am J Clin Nutr.* 2000;71(5):1166-1169.

20. Weaver CM, Plawecki KL. Dietary calcium: adequacy of a vegetarian diet. *Am J Clin Nutr.* 1994;59(5 Suppl):1238S-1241S.

21. Weaver CM, Proulx WR, Heaney R. Choices for achieving adequate dietary calcium with a vegetarian diet. *Am J Clin Nutr.* 1999;70(3 Suppl):543S-548S.

22. Heaney RP, Rafferty K, Dowell MS, Bierman J. Calcium fortification systems differ in bioavailability. *J Am Diet Assoc.* 2005;105(5):807-809.

23. Kohlenberg-Mueller K, Raschka L. Calcium balance in young adults on a vegan and lacto-vegetarian diet. *J Bone Miner Metab.* 2003;21(1):28-33.

24. Minihane AM, Fairweather-Tait SJ. Effect of calcium supplementation on daily nonheme-iron absorption and long-term iron status. *Am J Clin Nutr.* 1998;68(1):96-102.

25. Hallberg L. Does calcium interfere with iron absorption? *Am J Clin Nutr.* 1998;68(1):3-4.

26. Heaney RP, Dowell MS, Hale CA, Bendich A. Calcium absorption varies within the reference range for serum 25-hydroxyvitamin D. *J Am Coll Nutr.* 2003;22(2):142-146.

27. Weaver CM, Alexander DD, Boushey CJ, et al. Calcium plus vitamin D supplementation and risk of fractures: an updated meta-analysis from the National Osteoporosis Foundation. *Osteoporos Int.* 2016;27(1):367-376.

28. Hossein-nezhad A, Holick MF. Vitamin D for health: a global perspective. *Mayo Clin Proc.* 2013;88(7):720-755.

29. Ruohola JP, Laaksi I, Ylikomi T, et al. Association between serum 25(OH)D concentrations and bone stress fractures in Finnish young men. *J Bone Miner Res.* 2006;21(9):1483-1488.

30. Miller JR, Dunn KW, Ciliberti LJ Jr., Patel RD, Swanson BA. Association of vitamin D with stress fractures: a retrospective cohort study. *J Foot Ankle Surg.* 2016;55(1):117-120.

31. Larson-Meyer E. Vitamin D supplementation in athletes. *Nestle Nutrition Institute workshop series.* 2013;75:109-121.

32. Cannell JJ, Hollis BW, Zasloff M, Heaney RP. Diagnosis and treatment of vitamin D deficiency. *Expert Opin Pharmacother.* 2008;9(1):107-118.

33. Crowe FL, Steur M, Allen NE, Appleby PN, Travis RC, Key TJ. Plasma concentrations of 25-hydroxyvitamin D in meat eaters, fish eaters, vegetarians and vegans: results from the EPIC-Oxford study. *Public Health Nutr.* 2011;14(2):340-346.

34. Chan J, Jaceldo-Siegl K, Fraser GE. Serum 25-hydroxyvitamin D status of vegetarians, partial vegetarians, and nonvegetarians: the Adventist Health Study-2. *Am J Clin Nutr.* 2009;89(5):1686S-1692S.

35. Holick MF, Binkley NC, Bischoff-Ferrari HA, et al. Evaluation, treatment, and prevention of vitamin D deficiency: an Endocrine Society clinical practice guideline. *J Clin Endocrinol Metab.* 2011;96(7):1911-1930.

36. Logan VF, Gray AR, Peddie MC, Harper MJ, Houghton LA. Long-term vitamin D3 supplementation is more effective than vitamin D2 in maintaining serum 25-hydroxyvitamin D status over the winter months. *Br J Nutr.* 2013;109(6):1082-1088.

37. Carpenter TO, DeLucia MC, Zhang JH, et al. A randomized controlled study of effects of dietary magnesium oxide supplementation on bone mineral content in healthy girls. *J Clin Endocrinol Metab.* 2006;91(12):4866-4872.

38. Ryder KM, Shorr RI, Bush AJ, et al. Magnesium intake from food and supplements is associated with bone mineral density in healthy older white subjects. *J Am Geriatr Soc.* 2005;53(11):1875-1880.

39. Rude RK, Singer FR, Gruber HE. Skeletal and hormonal effects of magnesium deficiency. *J Am Coll Nutr.* 2009;28(2):131-141.

40. Nielsen FH, Lukaski HC. Update on the relationship between magnesium and exercise. *Magnes Res.* 2006;19(3):180-189.

41. Nieman DC, Underwood BC, Sherman KM, et al. Dietary status of Seventh-Day Adventist vegetarian and non-vegetarian elderly women. *J Am Diet Assoc.* 1989;89(12):1763-1769.

42. Rizzo NS, Jaceldo-Siegl K, Sabate J, Fraser GE. Nutrient profiles of vegetarian and nonvegetarian dietary patterns. *J Acad Nutr Diet.* 2013;113(12):1610-1619.

43. Palmer CA, Gilbert JA. Position of the Academy of Nutrition and Dietetics: the impact of fluoride on health. *J Acad Nutr Diet.* 2012;112(9):1443-1453.

44. Haguenauer D, Welch V, Shea B, Tugwell P, Adachi JD, Wells G. Fluoride for the treatment of postmenopausal osteoporotic fractures: a meta-analysis. *Osteoporos Int.* 2000;11(9):727-738.

45. U.S. Department of Health and Human Services Federal Panel on Community Water Fluoridation. U.S. Public Health Service recommendation for fluoride concentration in drinking water for the prevention of dental caries. *Public Health Rep.* 2015;130(4):318-331.

46. Calvo MS, Tucker KL. Is phosphorus intake that exceeds dietary requirements a risk factor in bone health? *Ann N Y Acad Sci.* 2013;1301:29-35.

47. Wyshak G. Teenaged girls, carbonated beverage consumption, and bone fractures. *Arch Pediatr Adolesc Med.* 2000;154(6):610-613.

48. Tucker KL, Morita K, Qiao N, Hannan MT, Cupples LA, Kiel DP. Colas, but not other carbonated beverages, are associated with low bone mineral density in older women: The Framingham Osteoporosis Study. *Am J Clin Nutr.* 2006;84(4):936-942.

49. Calvo MS, Kumar R, Heath H. Persistently elevated parathyroid hormone secretion and action in young women after four weeks of ingesting high phosphorus, low calcium diets. *J Clin Endocrinol Metab.* 1990;70(5):1334-1340.

50. Kristensen M, Jensen M, Kudsk J, Henriksen M, Molgaard C. Short-term effects on bone turnover of replacing milk with cola beverages: a 10-day interventional study in young men. *Osteoporos Int.* 2005;16(12):1803-1808.

51. Feskanich D, Weber P, Willett WC, Rockett H, Booth SL, Colditz GA. Vitamin K intake and hip fractures in women: a prospective study. *Am J Clin Nutr.* 1999;69(1):74-79.

52. Kalkwarf HJ, Khoury JC, Bean J, Elliot JG. Vitamin K, bone turnover, and bone mass in girls. *Am J Clin Nutr.* 2004;80(4):1075-1080.

53. O'Connor E, Molgaard C, Michaelsen KF, Jakobsen J, Lamberg-Allardt CJ, Cashman KD. Serum percentage undercarboxylated osteocalcin, a sensitive measure of vitamin K status, and its relationship to bone health indices in Danish girls. *Br J Nutr.* 2007;97(4):661-666.

54. Hamidi MS, Gajic-Veljanoski O, Cheung AM. Vitamin K and bone health. *J Clin Densitom.* 2013;16(4):409-413.

55. Dhonukshe-Rutten RA, van Dusseldorp M, Schneede J, de Groot LC, van Staveren WA. Low bone mineral density and bone mineral content are associated with low cobalamin status in adolescents. *Eur J Nutr.* 2005;44(6):341-347.

56. Dhonukshe-Rutten RA, Pluijm SM, de Groot LC, Lips P, Smit JH, van Staveren WA. Homocysteine and vitamin B12 status relate to bone turnover markers, broadband ultrasound attenuation, and fractures in healthy elderly people. *J Bone Miner Res.* 2005;20(6):921-929.

57. Herrmann W, Obeid R, Schorr H, et al. Enhanced bone metabolism in vegetarians–the role of vitamin B12 deficiency. *Clin Chem Lab Med.* 2009;47(11):1381-1387.

58. Bauer DC, Browner WS, Cauley JA, et al. Factors associated with appendicular bone mass in older women. The Study of Osteoporotic Fractures Research Group. *Ann Intern Med.* 1993;118(9):657-665.

59. Barrett-Connor E, Chang JC, Edelstein SL. Coffee-associated osteoporosis offset by daily milk consumption. The Rancho Bernardo Study. *JAMA.* 1994;271(4):280-283.

60. Conlisk AJ, Galuska DA. Is caffeine associated with bone mineral density in young adult women? *Prev Med.* 2000;31(5):562-568.

61. Weaver CM, Alekel DL, Ward WE, Ronis MJ. Flavonoid intake and bone health. *J Nutr Gerontol Geriatr.* 2012;31(3):239-253.

62. Hardcastle AC, Aucott L, Reid DM, Macdonald HM. Associations between dietary flavonoid intakes and bone health in a Scottish population. *J Bone Miner Res.* 2011;26(5):941-947.

63. Zhang X, Shu XO, Li H, et al. Prospective cohort study of soy food consumption and risk of bone fracture among postmenopausal women. *Arch Intern Med.* 2005;165(16):1890-1895.

64. Taku K, Melby MK, Takebayashi J, et al. Effect of soy isoflavone extract supplements on bone mineral density in menopausal women: meta-analysis of randomized controlled trials. *Asia Pac J Clin Nutr.* 2010;19(1):33-42.

65. Hooshmand S, Kern M, Metti D, et al. The effect of two doses of dried plum on bone density and bone biomarkers in osteopenic postmenopausal women: a randomized, controlled trial. *Osteoporos Int.* 2016;27(7):2271-2279.

66. Hooshmand S, Arjmandi BH. Viewpoint: dried plum, an emerging functional food that may effectively improve bone health. *Ageing Res Rev.* 2009;8(2):122-127.

67. Hooshmand S, Chai SC, Saadat RL, Payton ME, Brummel-Smith K, Arjmandi BH. Comparative effects of dried plum and dried apple on bone in postmenopausal women. *Br J Nutr.* 2011;106(6):923-930.

68. Marsh AG, Sanchez TV, Midkelsen O, Keiser J, Mayor G. Cortical bone density of adult lacto-ovo-vegetarian and omnivorous women. *J Am Diet Assoc.* 1980;76(2):148-151.

69. Marsh AG, Sanchez TV, Chaffee FL, Mayor GH, Mickelsen O. Bone mineral mass in adult lacto-ovo-vegetarian and omnivorous males. *Am J Clin Nutr.* 1983;37(3):453-456.

70. Ho-Pham LT, Nguyen ND, Nguyen TV. Effect of vegetarian diets on bone mineral density: a Bayesian meta-analysis. *Am J Clin Nutr.* 2009;90(4):943-950.

71. Ambroszkiewicz J, Chelchowska M, Szamotulska K, et al. The assessment of bone regulatory pathways, bone turnover, and bone mineral density in vegetarian and omnivorous children. *Nutrients.* 2018;10(2).

72. Tucker KL. Vegetarian diets and bone status. *Am J Clin Nutr.* 2014;100 Suppl 1:329S-335S.

73. Fontana L, Shew JL, Holloszy JO, Villareal DT. Low bone mass in subjects on a long-term raw vegetarian diet. Arch Intern Med. 2005;165(6):684-689.

74. Ackerman KE, Cano Sokoloff N, G DENM, Clarke HM, Lee H, Misra M. Fractures in Relation to Menstrual Status and Bone Parameters in Young Athletes. Med Sci Sports Exerc. 2015;47(8):1577-1586.

75. Chakkalakal DA. Alcohol-induced bone loss and deficient bone repair. Alcohol Clin Exp Res. 2005;29(12):2077-2090.

76. Peterson BA, Klesges RC, Kaufman EM, Cooper TV, Vukadinovich CM. The effects of an educational intervention on calcium intake and bone mineral content in young women with low calcium intake. Am J Health Promot. 2000;14(3):149-156.

77. Tylavsky FA, Anderson JJ. Dietary factors in bone health of elderly lactoovovegetarian and omnivorous women. Am J Clin Nutr. 1988;48(3 Suppl):842-849.

78. Dawson-Hughes B. Racial/ethnic considerations in making recommendations for vitamin D for adult and elderly men and women. Am J Clin Nutr. 2004;80(Suppl 6):1763S-1766S.

79. Monsen ER, Balintfy JL. Calculating dietary iron bioavailability: refinement and computerization. *J. Am. Diet. Assoc.* 1982;80(4):307-311.

Chapter 7

1. Melina V, Craig W, Levin S. Position of the Academy of Nutrition and Dietetics: vegetarian diets. *J Acad Nutr Diet.* 2016;116(12):1970-1980.

2. Rizzo NS, Jaceldo-Siegl K, Sabate J, Fraser GE. Nutrient profiles of vegetarian and nonvegetarian dietary patterns. *J Acad Nutr Diet.* 2013;113(12):1610-1619.

3. Cámara-Martos F, Amaro-López MA. Influence of dietary factors on calcium bioavailability: a brief review. *Biol Trace Elem Res.* 2002;89:43-52.

4. Haider L, Schwingshackl L, Hoffmann G, Ekmekcioglu C. The effect of vegetarian diets on iron status in adults: a systematic review and meta-analysis. *Crit Rev Food Sci Nutr.* 2017;58(8):1359-1374.

5. Otten JJ, Hellwig JP, Meyers LD. *The Dietary Reference Intakes: The Essential Guide to Nutrient Requirements.* Washington, DC: Food and Nutrition Board, Institutes of Medicine; 2006.

6. Hallberg L, Hulthén L. Prediction of dietary iron absorption: an algorithm for calculating absorption and bioavailability of dietary iron. *Am J Clin Nutr.* 2000;71:1147-1160.

7. Hinton PS. Iron and the endurance athlete. *Appl Physiol Nutr Metab.* 2014;39(9):1012-1018.

8. Nachtigall D, Nielsen P, Fischer R, Engelhardt R, Gabbe EE. Iron deficiency in distance runners. A reinvestigation using Fe-labelling and non-invasive liver iron quantification. *Int. J. Sports Med.* 1996;17(7):473-479.

9. Rudzki SJ, Hazard H, Collinson D. Gastrointestinal blood loss in triathletes: it's etiology and relationship to sports anaemia. *Aust. J. Sci. Med. Sport.* 1995;27(1):3-8.

10. Thalmann M, Sodeck GH, Kavouras S, et al. Proton pump inhibition prevents gastrointestinal bleeding in ultramarathon runners: a randomised, double blinded, placebo controlled study. *Br J Sports Med.* 2006;40(4):359-362; discussion 362.

11. Larson DC, Fisher R. Management of exercise-induced gastrointestinal problems. *Phys Sportsmed.* 1987;15(9):112-126.

12. Davies NM. Toxicity of nonsteroidal anti-inflammatory drugs in the large intestine. *Dis Colon Rectum.* 1995;38(12):1311-1321.

13. Eichner ER. Runner's macrocytosis: a clue to footstrike hemolysis. Runner's anemia as a benefit versus runner's hemolysis as a detriment. *Am J Med.* 1985;78(2):321-325.

14. Telford RD, Sly GJ, Hahn AG, Cunningham RB, Bryant C, Smith JA. Footstrike is the major cause of hemolysis during running. *J Appl Physiol (1985).* 2003;94(1):38-42.

15. Waller MF, Haymes EM. The effects of heat and exercise on sweat iron loss. *Med Sci Sports Exerc.* 1996;28(2):197-203.

16. DeRuisseau KC, Cheuvront SN, Haymes EM, Sharp RG. Sweat iron and zinc losses during prolonged exercise. *Int J Sport Nutr Exerc Metab.* 2002;12(4):428-437.

17. Weaver CM, Rajaram S. Exercise and iron status. *J Nutr.* 1992;122(3 Suppl):782-787.

18. DellaValle DM, Glahn RP, Shaff JE, O'Brien KO. Iron absorption from an intrinsically labeled lentil meal is low but upregulated in women with poor iron status. *J nutr.* 2015;145(10):2253-2257.

19. Brutsaert TD, Hernandez-Cordero S, Rivera J, Viola T, Hughes G, Haas JD. Iron supplementation improves progressive fatigue resistance during dynamic knee extensor exercise in iron-depleted, nonanemic women. *Am. J. Clin. Nutr.* 2003;77(2):441-448.

20. Burden RJ, Morton K, Richards T, Whyte GP, Pedlar CR. Is iron treatment beneficial in, iron-deficient but non-anaemic (IDNA) endurance athletes? A systematic review and meta-analysis. *Br J Sports Med.* 2015;49(21):1389-1397.

21. Hinton PS, Giordano C, Brownlie T, Haas JD. Iron supplementation improves endurance after training in iron-depleted, nonanemic women. *J Appl Physiol (1985).* 2000;88(3):1103-1111.

22. Hinton PS, Sinclair LM. Iron supplementation maintains ventilatory threshold and improves energetic efficiency in iron-deficient nonanemic athletes. *Eur J Clin Nutr.* 2007;61(1):30-39.

23. Dellavalle DM, Haas JD. Iron status is associated with endurance performance and training in female rowers. *Med Sci Sports Exerc.* 2012;44(8):1552-1559.

24. Brownlie T 4th, Utermohlen V, Hinton PS, Haas JD. Tissue iron deficiency without anemia impairs adaptation in endurance capacity after aerobic training in previously untrained women. *Am J Clin Nutr.* 2004;79(3):437-443.

25. Murray-Kolb LE, Beard JL. Iron treatment normalizes cognitive functioning in young women. *Am J Clin Nutr.* 2007;85(3):778-787.

26. World Health Organization. The prevalence of anaemia in 2011. Geneva: World Health Organization; 2015. https://www.who.int/nutrition/publications/micronutrients/global_prevalence_anaemia_2011/en/, accessed 3 February 2019

27. Thomas DT, Erdman KA, Burke LM. American College of Sports Medicine joint position statement. Nutrition and athletic performance. *Med Sci Sports Exerc.* 2016;48(3):543-568.

28. Woolf K, St Thomas MM, Hahn N, Vaughan LA, Carlson AG, Hinton P. Iron status in highly active and sedentary young women. *Int J Sport Nutr Exerc Metab.* 2009;19(5):519-535.

29. Haider LM, Schwingshackl L, Hoffmann G, Ekmekcioglu C. The effect of vegetarian diets on iron status in adults: A systematic review and meta-analysis. *Crit Rev Food Sci Nutr.* 2016:1-16.

30. Snyder A, Dvorak L, Roepke J. Influence of dietary iron source on measures of iron status among female runners. *Med Sci Sports Exerc.* 1989;21(1):7-10.

31. Ball MJ, Bartlett MA. Dietary intake and iron status of Australian vegetarian women. *Am J Clin Nutr.* 1999;70(3):353-358.

32. Haddad EH, Berk LS, Kettering JD, Hubbard RW, Peters WR. Dietary intake and biochemical, hematologic, and immune status of vegans compared with nonvegetarians. *Am J Clin Nutr.* 1999;70(3 Suppl):586S-593S.

33. Larsson CL, Johansson GK. Dietary intake and nutritional status of young vegans and omnivores in Sweden. *Am J Clin Nutr.* 2002;76(1):100-106.

34. Collings R, Harvey LJ, Hooper L, et al. The absorption of iron from whole diets: a systematic review. *Am J Clin Nutr.* 2013;98(1):65-81.

35. Simon MS. The Impossible Burger: inside the strange science of the fake meat that bleeds. Wired website. www.wired.com/story/the-impossible-burger. Published September 20, 2017. Accessed October 2, 2018.

36. Hallberg L, Brune M, Rossander L. The role of vitamin C in iron absorption. *Int J Vitam Nutr Res Suppl.* 1989;30:103-108.

37. Monsen ER, Balintfy JL. Calculating dietary iron bioavailability: refinement and computerization. *J. Am. Diet. Assoc.* 1982;80(4):307-311.

38. Salovaara S, Sandberg AS, Andlid T. Organic acids influence iron uptake in the human epithelial cell line Caco-2. *J Agric Food Chem.* 2002;50(21):6233-6238.

39. Olivares M, Pizarro F, Hertrampf E, Fuenmayor G, Estevez E. Iron absorption from wheat flour: effects of lemonade and chamomile infusion. *Nutrition.* 2007;23(4):296-300.

40. Kandiah J. Impact of tofu or tofu + orange juice on hematological indices of lacto-ovo vegetarian females. *Plant Foods Hum Nutr.* 2002;57(2):197-204.

41. Schumacher YO, Schmid A, Grathwohl D, Bultermann D, Berg A. Hematological indices and iron status in athletes of various sports and performances. *Med. Sci. Sports Exerc.* 2002;34(5):869-875.

42. Beard JL. Weekly iron intervention: the case for intermittent iron supplementation. *Am J Clin Nutr.* 1998;68(2):209-212.

43. Herbert V. Everyone should be tested for iron disorders. *J Am Diet Assoc.* 1992;92(12):1502-1509.

44. Zoller H, Vogel W. Iron supplementation in athletes–first do no harm. *Nutrition.* 2004;20(7-8):615-619.

45. Ambroszkiewicz J, Klemarczyk W, Mazur J, et al. Serum Hepcidin and Soluble Transferrin Receptor in the Assessment of Iron Metabolism in Children on a Vegetarian Diet. Biol Trace Elem Res. 2017;180(2):182-190.

46. Peeling P, Sim M, Badenhorst CE, et al. Iron status and the acute post-exercise hepcidin response in athletes. PLoS One. 2014;9(3):e93002.

Chapter 8

1. Williams MH, Rawson ES, Branch JD. *Nutrition for Health, Fitness & Sport.* New York: McGrawHill Education; 2017.

2. Otten JJ, Hellwig JP, Meyers LD. *The Dietary Reference Intakes: The Essential Guide to Nutrient Requirements.* Washington, DC: Food and Nutrition Board, Institutes of Medicine; 2006.

3. Thomas DT, Erdman KA, Burke LM. American College of Sports Medicine joint position statement. Nutrition and athletic performance. *Med Sci Sports Exerc.* 2016;48(3):543-568.

4. Micheletti A, Rossi R, Rufini S. Zinc status in athletes: relation to diet and exercise. *Sports Med.* 2001;31(8):577-582.

5. Lukaski HC. Magnesium, zinc, and chromium nutrition and athletic performance. *Can J Appl Physiol.* 2001;26 Suppl:S13-22.

6. McClung JP, Gaffney-Stomberg E, Lee JJ. Female athletes: a population at risk of vitamin and mineral deficiencies affecting health and performance. *J Trace Elem Med Biol.* 2014;28(4):388-392.

7. Cade JE, Burley VJ, Greenwood DC, UK Women's Cohort Study Steering Group. The UK Women's Cohort Study: comparison of vegetarians, fish-eaters and meat-eaters. *Public Health Nutr.* 2004;7(7):871-878.

8. Davey GK, Spencer EA, Appleby PN, Allen NE, Knox KH, Key TJ. EPIC-Oxford: lifestyle characteristics and nutrient intakes in a cohort of 33 883 meat-eaters and 31 546 non meat-eaters in the UK. *Public Health Nutr.* 2003;6(3):259-269.

9. Melina V, Craig W, Levin S. Position of the Academy of Nutrition and Dietetics: vegetarian diets. *J Acad Nutr Diet.* 2016;116(12):1970-1980.

10. Thakur VS, Deb G, Babcook MA, Gupta S. Plant phytochemicals as epigenetic modulators: role in cancer chemoprevention. *AAPS J.* 2014;16(1):151-163.

11. De Luca LM, Ross SA. Beta-carotene increases lung cancer incidence in cigarette smokers. *Nutr Rev.* 1996;54(6):178-180.

12. Lange H, Suryapranata H, De Luca G, et al. Folate therapy and in-stent restenosis after coronary stenting. *N Engl J Med.* 2004;350(26):2673-2681.

13. Omenn GS, Goodman GE, Thornquist MD, et al. Effects of a combination of beta-carotene and vitamin A on lung cancer and cardiovascular disease. *N Engl J Med.* 1996;334(18):1150-1155.

14. Bjelakovic G, Nikolova D, Gluud LL, Simonetti RG, Gluud C. Mortality in randomized trials of antioxidant supplements for primary and secondary prevention: systematic review and meta-analysis. *JAMA.* 2007;297(8):842-857.

15. Steinmetz KA, Potter JD. Vegetables, fruit, and cancer. I. Epidemiology. *Cancer Causes Control.* 1991;2(5):325-357.

16. Aboussaleh Y, Capone R, Bilali HE. Mediterranean food consumption patterns: low environmental impacts and significant health-nutrition benefits. *Proc Nutr Soc.* 2017;76(4):543-548.

17. Aune D, Giovannucci E, Boffetta P, et al. Fruit and vegetable intake and the risk of cardiovascular disease, total cancer and all-cause mortality-a systematic review and dose-response meta-analysis of prospective studies. *Int J Epidemiol.* 2017;46(3):1029-1056.

18. Powers S, Nelson WB, Larson-Meyer E. Antioxidant and vitamin D supplements for athletes: sense or nonsense? *J Sports Sci.* 2011;29 Suppl 1:S47-55.

19. Powers SK, DeRuisseau KC, Quindry J, Hamilton KL. Dietary antioxidants and exercise. *J Sports Sci.* 2004;22(1):81-94.

20. Urso ML, Clarkson PM. Oxidative stress, exercise, and antioxidant supplementation. *Toxicology.* 2003;189(1-2):41-54.

21. Krajcovicova-Kudlackova M, Ursinyova M, Blazicek P, et al. Free radical disease prevention and nutrition. *Bratisl Lek Listy.* 2003;104(2):64-68.

22. Steinmetz KA, Potter JD. Vegetables, fruit, and cancer. II. Mechanisms. *Cancer Causes Control.* 1991;2(6):427-442.

23. Rauma AL, Mykkanen H. Antioxidant status in vegetarians versus omnivores. *Nutrition.* 2000;16(2):111-119.

24. Trapp D, Knez W, Sinclair W. Could a vegetarian diet reduce exercise-induced oxidative stress? A review of the literature. *J Sports Sci.* 2010;28(12):1261-1268.

25. Morillas-Ruiz JM, Villegas Garcia JA, Lopez FJ, Vidal-Guevara ML, Zafrilla P. Effects of polyphenolic antioxidants on exercise-induced oxidative stress. *Clin Nutr.* 2006;25(3):444-453.

26. Connolly DA, McHugh MP, Padilla-Zakour OI, Carlson L, Sayers SP. Efficacy of a tart cherry juice blend in preventing the symptoms of muscle damage. *Br J Sports Med.* 2006;40(8):679-683; discussion 683.

27. Bell PG, McHugh MP, Stevenson E, Howatson G. The role of cherries in exercise and health. *Scand J Med Sci Sports.* 2014;24(3):477-490.

28. Coelho Rabello Lima L, Oliveira Assumpcao C, Prestes J, Sergio Denadai B. Consumption of cherries as a strategy to attenuate exercise-induced muscle damage and inflammation in humans. *Nutr Hosp.* 2015;32(5):1885-1893.

29. Ammar A, Turki M, Hammouda O, et al. Effects of pomegranate juice supplementation on oxidative stress biomarkers following weightlifting exercise. *Nutrients.* 2017;9(8).

30. Trombold JR, Reinfeld AS, Casler JR, Coyle EF. The effect of pomegranate juice supplementation on strength and soreness after eccentric exercise. *J Strength Cond Res.* 2011;25(7):1782-1788.

31. Hutchison AT, Flieller EB, Dillon KJ, Leverett BD. Black currant nectar reduces muscle damage and inflammation following a bout of high-intensity eccentric contractions. *J Diet Suppl.* 2016;13(1):1-15.

32. Woolf K, Manore MM. B-vitamins and exercise: does exercise alter requirements? *Int J Sport Nutr Exerc Metab.* 2006;16(5):453-484.

33. Manore MM. Effect of physical activity on thiamine, riboflavin, and vitamin B-6 requirements. *Am J Clin Nutr.* 2000;72(2 Suppl):598S-606S.

34. Soares MJ, Satyanarayana K, Bamji MS, Jacob CM, Ramana YV, Rao SS. The effect of exercise on the riboflavin status of adult men. *Br J Nutr.* 1993;69(2):541-551.

35. Larsson CL, Johansson GK. Dietary intake and nutritional status of young vegans and omnivores in Sweden. *Am J Clin Nutr.* 2002;76(1):100-106.

36. Majchrzak D, Singer I, Manner M, et al. B-vitamin status and concentrations of homocysteine in Austrian omnivores, vegetarians and vegans. *Ann Nutr Metab.* 2006;50(6):485-491.

37. Waldmann A, Koschizke JW, Leitzmann C, Hahn A. Dietary intakes and lifestyle factors of a vegan population in Germany: results from the German Vegan Study. *Eur J Clin Nutr.* 2003;57(8):947-955.

38. Hoffman MD, Valentino TR, Stuempfle KJ, Hassid BV. A placebo-controlled trial of riboflavin for enhancement of ultramarathon recovery. *Sports Med Open.* 2017;3(1):14.

39. Herrmann W, Geisel J. Vegetarian lifestyle and monitoring of vitamin B-12 status. *Clin Chim Acta.* 2002;326(1-2):47-59.

40. Pawlak R, Parrott SJ, Raj S, Cullum-Dugan D, Lucus D. How prevalent is vitamin B(12) deficiency among vegetarians? *Nutr Rev.* 2013;71(2):110-117.

41. Herrmann W, Schorr H, Obeid R, Geisel J. Vitamin B-12 status, particularly holotranscobalamin II and methylmalonic acid concentrations, and hyperhomocysteinemia in vegetarians. *Am J Clin Nutr.* 2003;78(1):131-136.

42. Lee Y, Krawinkel M. The nutritional status of iron, folate, and vitamin B-12 of Buddhist vegetarians. *Asia Pac J Clin Nutr.* 2011;20(1):42-49.

43. Watanabe F, Yabuta Y, Bito T, Teng F. Vitamin B(1)(2)-containing plant food sources for vegetarians. *Nutrients.* 2014;6(5):1861-1873.

44. Krajcovicova-Kudlackova M, Valachovicova M, Blazicek P. Seasonal folate serum concentrations at different nutrition. *Cent Eur J Public Health.* 2013;21(1):36-38.

45. Rousseau AS, Robin S, Roussel AM, Ducros V, Margaritis I. Plasma homocysteine is related to folate intake but not training status. *Nutr Metab Cardiovasc Dis.* 2005;15(2):125-133.

46. Peake JM. Vitamin C: effects of exercise and requirements with training. *Int J Sport Nutr Exerc Metab.* 2003;13(2):125-151.

47. Peters EM, Goetzsche JM, Grobbelaar B, Noakes TD. Vitamin C supplementation reduces the incidence of postrace symptoms of upper-respiratory-tract infection in ultramarathon runners. *Am J Clin Nutr.* 1993;57(2):170-174.

48. Hemila H, Chalker E. Vitamin C for preventing and treating the common cold. *Cochrane Database Syst Rev.* 2013(1):CD000980.

49. Nieman DC, Henson DA, McAnulty SR, et al. Influence of vitamin C supplementation on oxidative and immune changes after an ultramarathon. *J Appl Physiol (1985).* 2002;92(5):1970-1977.

50. Goldfarb AH, Patrick SW, Bryer S, You T. Vitamin C supplementation affects oxidative-stress blood markers in response to a 30-minute run at 75% VO2max. *Int J Sport Nutr Exerc Metab.* 2005;15(3):279-290.

51. Gomez-Cabrera MC, Domenech E, Romagnoli M, et al. Oral administration of vitamin C decreases muscle mitochondrial biogenesis and hampers training-induced adaptations in endurance performance. *Am J Clin Nutr.* 2008;87(1):142-149.

52. Steinmetz KA, Potter JD. Vegetables, fruit, and cancer prevention: a review. *J Am Diet Assoc.* 1996;96(10):1027-1039.

53. Eisenhauer B, Natoli S, Liew G, Flood VM. Lutein and zeaxanthin-food sources, bioavailability and dietary variety in age-related macular degeneration protection. *Nutrients.* 2017;9(2).

54. van Leeuwen R, Boekhoorn S, Vingerling JR, et al. Dietary intake of antioxidants and risk of age-related macular degeneration. *JAMA.* 2005;294(24):3101-3107.

55. Desai CK, Huang J, Lokhandwala A, Fernandez A, Riaz IB, Alpert JS. The role of vitamin supplementation in the prevention of cardiovascular disease events. *Clin Cardiol.* 2014;37(9):576-581.

56. Knekt P, Ritz J, Pereira MA, et al. Antioxidant vitamins and coronary heart disease risk: a pooled analysis of 9 cohorts. *Am J Clin Nutr.* 2004;80(6):1508-1520.

57. Stepanyan V, Crowe M, Haleagrahara N, Bowden B. Effects of vitamin E supplementation on exercise-induced oxidative stress: a meta-analysis. *Appl Physiol Nutr Metab.* 2014;39(9):1029-1037.

58. Braakhuis AJ, Hopkins WG. Impact of dietary antioxidants on sport performance: a review. *Sports Med.* 2015;45(7):939-955.

59. Ilavazhagan G, Bansal A, Prasad D, et al. Effect of vitamin E supplementation on hypoxia-induced oxidative damage in male albino rats. *Aviat Space Environ Med.* 2001;72(10):899-903.

60. Simon-Schnass I, Pabst H. Influence of vitamin E on physical performance. *Int J Vitam Nutr Res.* 1988;58(1):49-54.

61. Hunt JR, Matthys LA, Johnson LK. Zinc absorption, mineral balance, and blood lipids in women consuming controlled lactoovovegetarian and omnivorous diets for 8 wk. *Am J Clin Nutr.* 1998;67(3):421-430.

62. Hunt JR. Bioavailability of iron, zinc, and other trace minerals from vegetarian diets. *Am J Clin Nutr.* 2003;78(3 Suppl):633S-639S.

63. Platel K, Srinivasan K. Bioavailability of micronutrients from plant foods: an update. *Crit Rev Food Sci Nutr.* 2016;56(10):1608-1619.

64. Manore MM, Helleksen JM, Merkel J, Skinner JS. Longitudinal changes in zinc status in untrained men: effects of two different 12-week exercise training programs and zinc supplementation. *J Am Diet Assoc.* 1993;93(10):1165-1168.

65. Micheletti A, Rossi R, Rufini S. Zinc status in athletes: relation to diet and exercise. *Sports Med.* 2001;31(8):577-582.

66. Lukaski HC. Vitamin and mineral status: effects on physical performance. *Nutrition.* 2004;20(7-8):632-644.

67. Singh A, Moses FM, Deuster PA. Vitamin and mineral status in physically active men: effects of a high-potency supplement. *Am J Clin Nutr.* 1992;55(1):1-7.

68. Lukaski HC. Low dietary zinc decreases erythrocyte carbonic anhydrase activities and impairs cardiorespiratory function in men during exercise. *Am J Clin Nutr.* 2005;81(5):1045-1051.

69. Davidsson L. Are vegetarians an 'at risk group' for iodine deficiency? *Br J Nutr.* 1999;81(1):3-4.

70. Krajcovicova-Kudlackova M, Buckova K, Klimes I, Sebokova E. Iodine deficiency in vegetarians and vegans. *Ann Nutr Metab.* 2003;47(5):183-185.

71. Kristensen NB, Madsen ML, Hansen TH, et al. Intake of macro- and micronutrients in Danish vegans. *Nutr J.* 2015;14:115.

72. Lightowler HJ, Davies GJ. Iodine intake and iodine deficiency in vegans as assessed by the duplicate-portion technique and urinary iodine excretion. *Br J Nutr.* 1998;80(6):529-535.

73. Yeliosof O, Silverman LA. Veganism as a cause of iodine deficient hypothyroidism. *J Pediatr Endocrinol Metab.* 2018.

74. Elorinne AL, Alfthan G, Erlund I, et al. Food and nutrient intake and nutritional status of Finnish vegans and non-vegetarians. *PLoS One.* 2016;11(2):e0148235.

75. Crohn D. Perchlorate controversy calls for improving iodine nutrition. *Vegetarian Nutrition Update.* 2005;XIV:6-7.

76. Kadrabova J, Madaric A, Kovacikova Z, Ginter E. Selenium status, plasma zinc, copper, and magnesium in vegetarians. *Biol Trace Elem Res.* 1995;50(1):13-24.

77. Wapnir RA. Copper absorption and bioavailability. *Am J Clin Nutr.* 1998;67(5 Suppl):1054S-1060S.

78. Resina A, Fedi S, Gatteschi L, et al. Comparison of some serum copper parameters in trained runners and control subjects. *Int J Sports Med.* 1990;11(1):58-60.

79. Lukaski HC. Micronutrients (magnesium, zinc, and copper): are mineral supplements needed for athletes? *Int J Sport Nutr.* 1995;5 Suppl:S74-83.

80. Maynar M, Llerena F, Bartolome I, et al. Seric concentrations of copper, chromium, manganesum, nickel and selenium in aerobic, anaerobic and mixed professional sportsmen. *J Int Soc Sports Nutr.* 2018;15:8.

81. Wang L, Zhang J, Wang J, He W, Huang H. Effects of high-intensity training and resumed training on macroelement and microelement of elite basketball athletes. *Biol Trace Elem Res.* 2012;149(2):148-154.

82. Maughan RJ, Shirreffs SM. IOC Consensus Conference on Nutrition in Sport, 25-27 October 2010, International Olympic Committee, Lausanne, Switzerland. *J Sports Sci.* 2011;29 Suppl 1:S1.

83. Maughan RJ, Burke LM, Dvorak J, et al. IOC Consensus Statement: dietary supplements and the high-performance athlete. *Int J Sport Nutr Exerc Metab.* 2018;28(2):104-125.

84. Peeling P, Binnie MJ, Goods PSR, Sim M, Burke LM. Evidence-based supplements for the enhancement of athletic performance. *Int J Sport Nutr Exerc Metab.* 2018;28(2):178-187.

85. Rawson ES, Miles MP, Larson-Meyer DE. Dietary supplements for health, adaptation, and recovery in athletes. *Int J Sport Nutr Exerc Metab.* 2018;28(2):188-199.

86. Remer T, Neubert A, Manz F. Increased risk of iodine deficiency with vegetarian nutrition. *Br J Nutr.* 1999;81(1):45-49.

Chapter 9

1. Thomas DT, Erdman KA, Burke LM. American College of Sports Medicine joint position statement. Nutrition and athletic performance. *Med Sci Sports Exerc.* 2016;48(3):543-568.

2. Sherman WM, Brodowicz G, Wright DA, Allen WK, Simonsen J, Dernbach A. Effects of 4 h preexercise carbohydrate feedings on cycling performance. *Med Sci Sports Exerc.* 1989;21(5):598-604.

3. Wright DA, Sherman WM, Dernbach AR. Carbohydrate feedings before, during, or in combination improve cycling endurance performance. *J Appl Physiol (1985).* 1991;71(3):1082-1088.

4. Schabort EJ, Bosch AN, Weltan SM, Noakes TD. The effect of a preexercise meal on time to fatigue during prolonged cycling exercise. *Med Sci Sports Exerc.* 1999;31(3):464-471.

5. Maffucci DM, McMurray RG. Towards optimizing the timing of the pre-exercise meal. *Int J Sport Nutr Exerc Metab.* 2000;10(2):103-113.

6. Jeukendrup AE, Killer SC. The myths surrounding pre-exercise carbohydrate feeding. *Ann Nutr Metab.* 2010;57 Suppl 2:18-25.

7. Lis D, Ahuja KD, Stellingwerff T, Kitic CM, Fell J. Case study: utilizing a low FODMAP diet to combat exercise-induced gastrointestinal symptoms. *Int J Sport Nutr Exerc Metab.* 2016;26(5):481-487.

8. Lis D, Ahuja KD, Stellingwerff T, Kitic CM, Fell J. Food avoidance in athletes: FODMAP foods on the list. *Appl Physiol Nutr Metab.* 2016;41(9):1002-1004.

9. Lis DM, Stellingwerff T, Kitic CM, Fell JW, Ahuja KDK. Low FODMAP: a preliminary strategy to reduce gastrointestinal distress in athletes. *Med Sci Sports Exerc.* 2018;50(1):116-123.

10. Kirwan JP, Cyr-Campbell D, Campbell WW, Scheiber J, Evans WJ. Effects of moderate and high glycemic index meals on metabolism and exercise performance. *Metabolism.* 2001;50(7):849-855.

11. Siu PM, Wong SH. Use of the glycemic index: effects on feeding patterns and exercise performance. *J Physiol Anthropol Appl Human Sci.* 2004;23(1):1-6.

12. Thomas DE, Brotherhood JR, Brand JC. Carbohydrate feeding before exercise: effect of glycemic index. *Int J Sports Med.* 1991;12(2):180-186.

13. Philp A, Hargreaves M, Baar K. More than a store: regulatory roles for glycogen in skeletal muscle adaptation to exercise. *Am J Physiol Endocrinol Metab.* 2012;302(11):E1343-1351.

14. Bartlett JD, Hawley JA, Morton JP. Carbohydrate availability and exercise training adaptation: too much of a good thing? *Eur J Sport Sci.* 2015;15(1):3-12.

15. Williams C, Brewer J, Walker M. The effect of a high carbohydrate diet on running performance during a 30-km treadmill time trial. *Eur J Appl Physiol Occup Physiol.* 1992;65(1):18-24.

16. Balsom PD, Wood K, Olsson P, Ekblom B. Carbohydrate intake and multiple sprint sports: with special reference to football (soccer). *Int J Sports Med.* 1999;20(1):48-52.

17. Goforth HW Jr., Laurent D, Prusaczyk WK, Schneider KE, Petersen KF, Shulman GI. Effects of depletion exercise and light training on muscle glycogen supercompensation in men. *Am J Physiol Endocrinol Metab.* 2003;285(6):E1304-1311.

18. Fairchild TJ, Fletcher S, Steele P, Goodman C, Dawson B, Fournier PA. Rapid carbohydrate loading after a short bout of near maximal-intensity exercise. *Med Sci Sports Exerc.* 2002;34(6):980-986.

19. Baker LB, Rollo I, Stein KW, Jeukendrup AE. Acute effects of carbohydrate supplementation on intermittent sports performance. *Nutrients.* 2015;7(7):5733-5763.

20. Currell K, Conway S, Jeukendrup AE. Carbohydrate ingestion improves performance of a new reliable test of soccer performance. *Int J Sport Nutr Exerc Metab.* 2009;19(1):34-46.

21. Vergauwen L, Brouns F, Hespel P. Carbohydrate supplementation improves stroke performance in tennis. *Med Sci Sports Exerc.* 1998;30(8):1289-1295.

22. Chryssanthopoulos C, Williams C, Nowitz A, Kotsiopoulou C, Vleck V. The effect of a high carbohydrate meal on endurance running capacity. *Int J Sport Nutr Exerc Metab.* 2002;12(2):157-171.

23. Jeukendrup AE. Oral carbohydrate rinse: placebo or beneficial? *Curr Sports Med Rep.* 2013;12(4):222-227.

24. Burke LM, Maughan RJ. The Governor has a sweet tooth - mouth sensing of nutrients to enhance sports performance. *Eur J Sport Sci.* 2015;15(1):29-40.

25. Krings BM, Peterson TJ, Shepherd BD, McAllister MJ, Smith JW. Effects of carbohydrate ingestion and carbohydrate mouth rinse on repeat sprint performance. *Int J Sport Nutr Exerc Metab.* 2017;27(3):204-212.

26. Fallowfield JL, Williams C, Booth J, Choo BH, Growns S. Effect of water ingestion on endurance capacity during prolonged running. *J Sports Sci.* 1996;14(6):497-502.

27. Below PR, Mora-Rodriguez R, Gonzalez-Alonso J, Coyle EF. Fluid and carbohydrate ingestion independently improve performance during 1 h of intense exercise. *Med Sci Sports Exerc.* 1995;27(2):200-210.

28. Hew-Butler T, Rosner MH, Fowkes-Godek S, et al. Statement of the 3rd International Exercise-Associated Hyponatremia Consensus Development Conference, Carlsbad, California, 2015. *Br J Sports Med.* 2015;49(22):1432-1446.

29. Almond CS, Shin AY, Fortescue EB, et al. Hyponatremia among runners in the Boston Marathon. *N Engl J Med.* 2005;352(15):1550-1556.

30. Shirreffs SM, Sawka MN. Fluid and electrolyte needs for training, competition, and recovery. *J Sports Sci.* 2011;29 Suppl 1:S39-46.

31. Jentjens RL, Shaw C, Birtles T, Waring RH, Harding LK, Jeukendrup AE. Oxidation of combined ingestion of glucose and sucrose during exercise. *Metabolism.* 2005;54(5):610-618.

32. Jeukendrup AE. Carbohydrate and exercise performance: the role of multiple transportable carbohydrates. *Curr Opin Clin Nutr Metab Care.* 2010;13(4):452-457.

33. Luetkemeier MJ, Hanisko JM, Aho KM. Skin tattoos alter sweat rate and Na+ concentration. *Med Sci Sports Exerc.* 2017;49(7):1432-1436.

34. Kreider RB, Rasmussen CJ, Lancaster SL, Kerksick C, Greenwood M. Honey: an alternative sports gel. *Strength Cond J.* 2002;24(1):50-51.

35. Robergs RA, McMinn SB, Mermier C, Leadbetter G, Ruby B, Quinn C. Blood glucose and glucoregulatory hormone responses to solid and liquid carbohydrate ingestion during exercise. *Int J Sport Nutr.* 1998;8(1):70-83.

36. Gisolfi CV, Duchman SM. Guidelines for optimal replacement beverages for different athletic events. *Med Sci Sports Exerc.* 1992;24(6):679-687.

37. Broad EM, Burke LM, Cox GR, Heeley P, Riley M. Body weight changes and voluntary fluid intakes during training and competition sessions in team sports. *Int J Sport Nutr.* 1996;6(3):307-320.

38. Maughan RJ, Watson P, Cordery PA, et al. A randomized trial to assess the potential of different beverages to affect hydration status: development of a beverage hydration index. *Am J Clin Nutr.* 2016;103(3):717-723.

39. Ivy JL, Goforth HW Jr., Damon BM, McCauley TR, Parsons EC, Price TB. Early postexercise muscle glycogen recovery is enhanced with a carbohydrate-protein supplement. *J Appl Physiol (1985).* 2002;93(4):1337-1344.

40. Messina M, Lynch H, Dickinson JM, Reed KE. No difference between the effects of supplementing with soy protein versus animal protein on gains in muscle mass and strength in response to resistance exercise. *Int J Sport Nutr Exerc Metab.* 2018:1-36.

41. Larson-Meyer DE, Borkhsenious ON, Gullett JC, et al. Effect of dietary fat on serum and intramyocellular lipids and running performance. *Med Sci Sports Exerc.* 2008;40(5):892-902.

42. Johannsen NM, Lind E, King DS, Sharp RL. Effect of preexercise electrolyte ingestion on fluid balance in men and women. Med Sci Sports Exerc. 2009;41(11):2017-2025.

43. Phillips SM. The science of muscle hypertrophy: making dietary protein count. Proc Nutr Soc. 2011;70(1):100-103.

44. Phillips SM, Van Loon LJ. Dietary protein for athletes: from requirements to optimum adaptation. J sports sci. 2011;29 Suppl 1:S29-38

Chapter 10

1. Maughan RJ, Burke LM, Dvorak J, et al. IOC consensus statement: dietary supplements and the high-performance athlete. *Int J Sport Nutr Exerc Metab.* 2018;28(2):104-125.

2. Maughan R. Dietary supplements and the high-performance athlete. *Int J Sport Nutr Exerc Metab.* 2018;28(2):101.

3. Peeling P, Binnie MJ, Goods PSR, Sim M, Burke LM. Evidence-based supplements for the enhancement of athletic performance. *Int J Sport Nutr Exerc Metab.* 2018;28(2):178-187.

4. Thomas DT, Erdman KA, Burke LM. American College of Sports Medicine Joint Position Statement. Nutrition and athletic performance. *Med Sci Sports Exerc.* 2016;48(3):543-568.

5. Rawson ES, Miles MP, Larson-Meyer DE. Dietary supplements for health, adaptation, and recovery in athletes. *Int J Sport Nutr Exerc Metab.* 2018;28(2):188-199.

6. National Institutes of Health Office of Dietary Supplements. Dietary Supplement Health and Education Act of 1994. https://ods.od.nih.gov/About/DSHEA_Wording.aspx. Accessed July 26 2018

7. Denham BE. Athlete Information sources about dietary supplements: a review of extant research. *Int J Sport Nutr Exerc Metab.* 2017;27(4):325-334.

8. Can you trust supplements? *Harv Women's Health Watch.* 1998;November(4-5).

9. Walker EP. Abbott Pulls Meridia from Market. MedPage Today website. www.medpagetoday.com/productalert/prescriptions/22633. Published October 8, 2010. Assessed July 26 2018

10. Outram S, Stewart B. Doping through supplement use: a review of the available empirical data. *Int J Sport Nutr Exerc Metab.* 2015;25(1):54-59.

11. Larson-Meyer DE, Hunter GR, Trowbridge CA, et al. The effect of creatine supplementation on muscle strength and body composition during off-season training in female soccer players. *J Strength Cond Res.* 2000;14(4):434-442.

12. Larson-Meyer DE, Woolf K, Burke L. Assessment of nutrient status in athletes and the need for supplementation. *Int J Sport Nutr Exerc Metab.* 2018;28(2):139-158.

13. International Olympic Committee Expert Group on Dietary Supplements in Athletes. *Int J Sport Nutr Exerc Metab.* 2018;28(2):102-103.

14. Garthe I, Maughan RJ. Athletes and supplements: prevalence and perspectives. *Int J Sport Nutr Exerc Metab.* 2018;28(2):126-138.

15. Burke LM, Peeling P. Methodologies for investigating performance changes with supplement use. *Int J Sport Nutr Exerc Metab.* 2018;28(2):159-169.

16. Geller AI, Shehab N, Weidle NJ, et al. Emergency department visits for adverse events related to dietary supplements. *N Engl J Med.* 2015;373(16):1531-1540.

17. Rawson ES, Conti MP, Miles MP. Creatine supplementation does not reduce muscle damage or enhance recovery from resistance exercise. *J Strength Cond Res.* 2007;21(4):1208-1213.

18. Balsom PD, Soderlund K, Ekblom B. Creatine in humans with special reference to creatine supplementation. *Sports Med.* 1994;18(4):268-280.

19. Delanghe J, De Slypere JP, De Buyzere M, Robbrecht J, Wieme R, Vermeulen A. Normal reference values for creatine, creatinine, and carnitine are lower in vegetarians. *Clin Chem.* 1989;35(8):1802-1803.

20. Shomrat A, Weinstein Y, Katz A. Effect of creatine feeding on maximal exercise performance in vegetarians. *Eur J Appl Physiol.* 2000;82(4):321-325.

21. Novakova K, Kummer O, Bouitbir J, et al. Effect of L-carnitine supplementation on the body carnitine pool, skeletal muscle energy metabolism and physical performance in male vegetarians. *Eur J Nutr.* 2016;55(1):207-217.

22. Harris RC, Soderlund K, Hultman E. Elevation of creatine in resting and exercised muscle of normal subjects by creatine supplementation. *Clin Sci.* 1992;83(3):367-374.

23. Lukaszuk JM, Robertson RJ, Arch JE, et al. Effect of creatine supplementation and a lacto-ovo-vegetarian diet on muscle creatine concentration. *Int J Sport Nutr Exerc Metab.* 2002;12(3):336-348.

24. Burke DG, Chilibeck PD, Parise G, Candow DG, Mahoney D, Tarnopolsky M. Effect of creatine and weight training on muscle creatine and performance in vegetarians. *Med Sci Sports Exerc.* 2003;35(11):1946-1955.

25. Clarys P, Zinzen E, Hebbelinck M. The effect of oral creatine supplementation on torque production in a vegetarian and non-vegetarian population: a double blind study. *Veg Nutr: Int J.* 1997;1:100-105.

26. Terjung RL, Clarkson P, Eichner ER, et al. American College of Sports Medicine roundtable. The physiological and health effects of oral creatine supplementation. *Med Sci Sports Exerc.* 2000;32(3):706-717.

27. Stephens FB, Constantin-Teodosiu D, Greenhaff PL. New insights concerning the role of carnitine in the regulation of fuel metabolism in skeletal muscle. *J Physiol.* 2007;581(Pt 2):431-444.

28. Davis A, Davis P, Phinney S. Plasma and urinary carnitine of obese subjects on very-low-calorie diets. *J Am Coll Nutr.* 1990;9:261-4.

29. Spriet LL. Exercise and sport performance with low doses of caffeine. *Sports Med.* 2014;44 Suppl 2:S175-184.

30. Graham EE, Spriet LL. Caffeine and exercise performance. *Gatorade Sports Science Exchange.* 1996;9(1).

31. Armstrong LE. Caffeine, body fluid-electrolyte balance, and exercise performance. *Int J Sport Nutr Exerc Metab.* 2002;12(2):189-206.

32. Bailey SJ, Winyard P, Vanhatalo A, et al. Dietary nitrate supplementation reduces the O2 cost of low-intensity exercise and enhances tolerance to high-intensity exercise in humans. *J Appl Physiol (1985).* 2009;107(4):1144-1155.

33. Webb AJ, Patel N, Loukogeorgakis S, et al. Acute blood pressure lowering, vasoprotective, and antiplatelet properties of dietary nitrate via bioconversion to nitrite. *Hypertension.* 2008;51(3):784-790.

34. Jones AM. Influence of dietary nitrate on the physiological determinants of exercise performance: a critical review. *Appl Physiol Nutr Metab.* 2014;39(9):1019-1028.

35. Flueck JL, Bogdanova A, Mettler S, Perret C. Is beetroot juice more effective than sodium nitrate? The effects of equimolar nitrate dosages of nitrate-rich beetroot juice and sodium nitrate on oxygen consumption during exercise. *Appl Physiol Nutr Metab.* 2016;41(4):421-429.

36. Murphy M, Eliot K, Heuertz RM, Weiss E. Whole beetroot consumption acutely improves running performance. *J Acad Nutr Diet.* 2012;112(4):548-552.

37. Jonvik KL, Nyakayiru J, Pinckaers PJ, Senden JM, van Loon LJ, Verdijk LB. Nitrate-rich vegetables increase plasma nitrate and nitrite concentrations and lower blood pressure in healthy adults. *J Nutr.* 2016;146(5):986-993.

38. Bryan NS, Alexander DD, Coughlin JR, Milkowski AL, Boffetta P. Ingested nitrate and nitrite and stomach cancer risk: an updated review. *Food Chem. Toxicol.* 2012;50(10):3646-3665.

39. Jonvik KL, Nyakayiru J, van Dijk JW, Wardenaar FC, van Loon LJ, Verdijk LB. Habitual dietary nitrate intake in highly trained athletes. *Int J Sport Nutr Exerc Metab.* 2017;27(2):148-157.

40. Saunders B, Elliott-Sale K, Artioli GG, et al. Beta-alanine supplementation to improve exercise capacity and performance: a systematic review and meta-analysis. *Br J Sports Med.* 2017;51(8):658-669.

41. Horswill CA, Costill DL, Fink WJ, et al. Influence of sodium bicarbonate on sprint performance: relationship to dosage. *Med Sci Sports Exerc.* 1988;20(6):566-569.

42. Williams MH, Rawson ES, Branch JD. Vitamins: the organic regulators. In: *Nutrition for Health, Fitness and Sport.* 11th ed. New York, NY: McGrawHill Education; 2017.

43. Pelletier DM, Lacerte G, Goulet ED. Effects of quercetin supplementation on endurance performance and maximal oxygen consumption: a meta-analysis. *Int J Sport Nutr Exerc Metab.* 2013;23(1):73-82.

Chapter 11

1. Bentley S. Exercise-induced muscle cramp. Proposed mechanisms and management. *Sports Med.* 1996;21(6):409-420.
2. Miller KC, Stone MS, Huxel KC, Edwards JE. Exercise-associated muscle cramps: causes, treatment, and prevention. *Sports Health.* 2010;2(4):279-283.
3. Miller KC. Rethinking the cause of exercise-associated muscle cramping: moving beyond dehydration and electrolyte losses. *Curr Sports Med Rep.* 2015;14(5):353-354.
4. Miller KC. Plasma potassium concentration and content changes after banana ingestion in exercised men. *J Athl Train.* 2012;47(6):648-654.
5. Miller KC. Myths and misconceptions about exercise-associated muscle cramping. *ACSM s Health Fit J.* 2016;20(2):37-39.
6. Miller KC. Electrolyte and plasma responses after pickle juice, mustard, and deionized water ingestion in dehydrated humans. *J Athl Train.* 2014;49(3):360-367.
7. Schwellnus MP. Cause of exercise associated muscle cramps (EAMC)—altered neuromuscular control, dehydration or electrolyte depletion? *Br J Sports Med.* 2009;43(6):401-408.
8. Schwellnus MP, Derman EW, Noakes TD. Aetiology of skeletal muscle 'cramps' during exercise: a novel hypothesis. *J Sports Sci.* 1997;15(3):277-285.
9. Schwellnus MP, Allie S, Derman W, Collins M. Increased running speed and pre-race muscle damage as risk factors for exercise-associated muscle cramps in a 56 km ultramarathon: a prospective cohort study. *Br J Sports Med.* 2011;45(14):1132-1136.
10. Lee R, Nieman DC. *Nutritional Assessment.* 6th ed. New York, NY: McGraw Hill; 2013.
11. Sulzer NU, Schwellnus MP, Noakes TD. Serum electrolytes in Ironman triathletes with exercise-associated muscle cramping. *Med Sci Sports Exerc.* 2005;37(7):1081-1085.
12. Jung AP, Bishop PA, Al-Nawwas A, Dale RB. Influence of hydration and electrolyte supplementation on incidence and time to onset of exercise-associated muscle cramps. *J Athl Train.* 2005;40(2):71-75.
13. Craighead DH, Shank SW, Gottschall JS, et al. Ingestion of transient receptor potential channel agonists attenuates exercise-induced muscle cramps. *Muscle Nerve.* 2017;56(3):379-385.
14. Schwellnus MP, Drew N, Collins M. Increased running speed and previous cramps rather than dehydration or serum sodium changes predict exercise-associated muscle cramping: a prospective cohort study in 210 Ironman triathletes. *Br J Sports Med.* 2011;45(8):650-656.
15. Schwellnus MP, Nicol J, Laubscher R, Noakes TD. Serum electrolyte concentrations and hydration status are not associated with exercise associated muscle cramping (EAMC) in distance runners. *Br J Sports Med.* 2004;38(4):488-492.
16. Summers KM, Snodgrass SJ, Callister R. Predictors of calf cramping in rugby league. *J Strength Cond Res.* 2014;28(3):774-783.
17. Williamson SI, Johnson RW, Hudkins PG, Strate SM. Exertional cramps: a prospective study of biochemical and anthropometric variables in bicycle riders. *Cycling Science.* 1993;5(1):15-20.
18. Stofan JR, Zachwieja JJ, Horswill CA, Murray R, Anderson SA, Eichner ER. Sweat and sodium losses in NCAA football players: a precursor to heat cramps? *Int J Sport Nutr Exerc Metab.* 2005;15(6):641-652.
19. Bergeron MF. Heat cramps during tennis: a case report. *Int J Sport Nutr.* 1996;6(1):62-68.
20. Bergeron MF. Heat cramps: fluid and electrolyte challenges during tennis in the heat. *J Sci Med Sport.* 2003;6(1):19-27.
21. Clark N. *Nancy Clark's Sports Nutrition Guidebook.* 5th ed. Champaign, IL: Human Kinetics; 2014.

22. Jackson S, Coleman King S, Zhao L. Prevalence of excess sodium intake in the United States–NHANES, 2009-2012. Centers for Disease Control and Prevention website. www.cdc.gov/mmwr/preview/mmwrhtml/mm6452a1.htm?s_cid=mm6452a1_w. Published January 8, 2016. Accessed August 13, 2018.

23. Luetkemeier MJ, Hanisko JM, Aho KM. Skin tattoos alter sweat rate and Na+ concentration. *Med Sci Sports Exerc.* 2017;49(7):1432-1436.

24. Murray D, Miller KC, Edwards JE. Does a reduction in serum sodium concentration or serum potassium concentration increase the prevalence of exercise-associated muscle cramps? *J Sport Rehabil.* 2016;25(3):301-304.

25. McKenney MA, Miller KC, Deal JE, Garden-Robinson JA, Rhee YS. Plasma and electrolyte changes in exercising humans after ingestion of multiple boluses of pickle juice. *J Athl Train.* 2015;50(2):141-146.

26. Scientific Report of the 2015 Dietary Guidelines Advisory Committee. Office of Disease Prevention and Health Promotion website. http://health.gov/dietaryguidelines/2015-scientific-report. Published February 2015. Accessed September 5, 2018.

27. Lennon-Edwards S, Allman BR, Schellhardt TA, Ferreira CR, Farquhar WB, Edwards DG. Lower potassium intake is associated with increased wave reflection in young healthy adults. *Nutr J.* 2014;13:39. doi: 10.1186/1475-2891-13-39.

28. Lanham-New SA. The balance of bone health: tipping the scales in favor of potassium-rich, bicarbonate-rich foods. *J nutr.* 2008;138(1):172S-177S.

29. Zhou K, West HM, Zhang J, Xu L, Li W. Interventions for leg cramps in pregnancy. *Cochrane Database Syst Rev.* 2015(8):CD010655.

30. Thomas DT, Erdman KA, Burke LM. American College of Sports Medicine joint position statement. Nutrition and athletic performance. *Med Sci Sports Exerc.* 2016;48(3):543-568.

31. Litman RS, Rosenberg H. Malignant hyperthermia: update on susceptibility testing. *JAMA.* 2005;293(23):2918-2924.

32. Bye AM, Kan AE. Cramps following exercise. *Aust Paediatr J.* 1988;24(4):258-259.

33. Fredericson M, Kim BJ, Date ES. Disabling foot cramping in a runner secondary to paramyotonia congenita: a case report. *Foot Ankle Int.* 2004;25(7):510-512.

34. Pinzon EG, Larrabee M. Chronic overuse sports injuries. Practical Pain Management website. www.practicalpainmanagement.com/pain/acute/sports-overuse/chronic-overuse-sports-injuries. 2012;6(4). Accessed November 5, 2018.

35. Deng T, Lyon CJ, Bergin S, Caligiuri MA, Hsueh WA. Obesity, inflammation, and cancer. *Annu Rev Pathol.* 2016;11:421-449.

36. Gardener SL, Rainey-Smith SR, Martins RN. Diet and inflammation in Alzheimer's disease and related chronic diseases: a review. *J Alzheimers Dis.* 2016;50(2):301-334.

37. Tsoupras A, Lordan R, Zabetakis I. Inflammation, not cholesterol, is a cause of chronic disease. *Nutrients.* 2018;10(5). doi: 10.3390/nu10050604.

38. Ricker MA, Haas WC. Anti-inflammatory diet in clinical practice: a review. *Nutr Clin Pract.* 2017;32(3):318-325.

39. Geppert J, Kraft V, Demmelmair H, Koletzko B. Docosahexaenoic acid supplementation in vegetarians effectively increases omega-3 index: a randomized trial. *Lipids.* 2005;40(8):807-814.

40. Jungbauer A, Medjakovic S. Anti-inflammatory properties of culinary herbs and spices that ameliorate the effects of metabolic syndrome. *Maturitas.* 2012;71(3):227-239.

41. Sears B. Anti-inflammatory diets. *J Am Coll Nutr.* 2015;34 Suppl 1:14-21.

42. Grimble RF, Tappia PS. Modulation of pro-inflammatory cytokine biology by unsaturated fatty acids. *Z Ernahrungswiss.* 1998;37 Suppl 1:57-65.

43. Bloomer RJ, Larson DE, Fisher-Wellman KH, Galpin AJ, Schilling BK. Effect of eicosapentaenoic and docosahexaenoic acid on resting and exercise-induced inflammatory and oxidative stress biomarkers: a randomized, placebo controlled, cross-over study. *Lipids Health Dis.* 2009;8:36. doi: 10.1186/1476-511X-8-36.

44. Adam O, Beringer C, Kless T, et al. Anti-inflammatory effects of a low arachidonic acid diet and fish oil in patients with rheumatoid arthritis. *Rheumatol Int.* 2003;23(1):27-36.

45. Berbert AA, Kondo CRM, Almendra CL, Matsuo T, Dichi I. Supplementation of fish oil and olive oil in patients with rheumatoid arthritis. *Nutrition.* 2005;21(2):131-136.

46. Messina V, Melina V, Mangels AR. A new food guide for North American vegetarians. *J Am Diet Assoc.* 2003;103(6):771-775.

47. Larson-Meyer E. Vitamin D supplementation in athletes. *Nestle Nutrition Institute workshop series.* 2013;75:109-121.

48. Moore ME, Piazza A, McCartney Y, Lynch MA. Evidence that vitamin D3 reverses age-related inflammatory changes in the rat hippocampus. *Biochem Soc Trans.* 2005;33(Pt 4):573-577.

49. Willis KS, Smith DT, Broughton KS, Larson-Meyer DE. Vitamin D status and biomarkers of inflammation in runners. *Open Access J Sports Med.* 2012;3:35-42.

50. Barcal JN, Thomas JT, Hollis BW, Austin KJ, Alexander BM, Larson-Meyer DE. Vitamin D and weight cycling: impact on injury, illness, and inflammation in collegiate wrestlers. *Nutrients.* 2016;8(12). pii: E775.

51. Lewis RM, Redzic M, Thomas DT. The effects of season-long vitamin D supplementation on collegiate swimmers and divers. *Int J Sport Nutr Exerc Metab.* 2013;23(5):431-440.

52. Wyon MA, Koutedakis Y, Wolman R, Nevill AM, Allen N. The influence of winter vitamin D supplementation on muscle function and injury occurrence in elite ballet dancers: a controlled study. *J Sci Med Sport.* 2014;17(1):8-12.

53. Rebolledo BJ, Bernard JA, Werner BC, et al. The Association of Vitamin D Status in Lower Extremity Muscle Strains and Core Muscle Injuries at the National Football League Combine. *Arthroscopy.* 2018;34(4):1280-1285.

54. Barker T, Martins TB, Hill HR, et al. Vitamin D sufficiency associates with an increase in anti-inflammatory cytokines after intense exercise in humans. *Cytokine.* 2014;65(2):134-137.

55. Hossein-nezhad A, Holick MF. Vitamin D for health: a global perspective. *Mayo Clinic Proceedings.* 2013;88(7):720-755.

56. Holick MF, Binkley NC, Bischoff-Ferrari HA, et al. Evaluation, treatment, and prevention of vitamin D deficiency: an Endocrine Society clinical practice guideline. J Clin Endocrinol Metab. 2011;96(7):1911-1930

57. Fisher ND, Hurwitz S, Hollenberg NK. Habitual flavonoid intake and endothelial function in healthy humans. *J Am Coll Nutr.* 2012;31(4):275-279.

58. Patel RK, Brouner J, Spendiff O. Dark chocolate supplementation reduces the oxygen cost of moderate intensity cycling. *J Int Soc Sports Nutr.* 2015;12:47.

59. Totsch SK, Meir RY, Quinn TL, Lopez SA, Gower BA, Sorge RE. Effects of a standard American diet and an anti-inflammatory diet in male and female mice. *Eur J Pain.* 2018;22(7):1203-1213.

60. Rawson ES, Miles MP, Larson-Meyer DE. Dietary supplements for health, adaptation, and recovery in athletes. *Int J Sport Nutr Exerc Metab.* 2018;28(2):188-199.

61. Bell PG, McHugh MP, Stevenson E, Howatson G. The role of cherries in exercise and health. *Scand J Med Sci Sports.* 2014;24(3):477-490.

62. Coelho Rabello Lima L, Oliveira Assumpcao C, Prestes J, Sergio Denadai B. Consumption of cherries as a strategy to attenuate exercise-induced muscle damage and inflammation in humans. *Nutr Hosp.* 2015;32(5):1885-1893.

63. Ahmed S, Anuntiyo J, Malemud CJ, Haqqi TM. Biological basis for the use of botanicals in osteoarthritis and rheumatoid arthritis: a review. *Evid Based Complement Alternat Med.* 2005;2(3):301-308.

64. Richter EA, Kiens B, Raben A, Tvede N, Pedersen BK. Immune parameters in male athletes after a lacto-ovo vegetarian diet and a mixed Western diet. *Med Sci Sports Exerc.* 1991;23(5):517-521.

65. Riso P, Visioli F, Grande S, et al. Effect of a tomato-based drink on markers of inflammation, immunomodulation, and oxidative stress. *J Agric Food Chem.* 2006;54(7):2563-2566.

66. Beauchamp GK, Keast RS, Morel D, et al. Phytochemistry: ibuprofen-like activity in extra-virgin olive oil. *Nature*. 2005;437(7055):45-46.

67. Ahmed S, Wang N, Hafeez BB, Cheruvu VK, Haqqi TM. Punica granatum L. extract inhibits IL-1beta-induced expression of matrix metalloproteinases by inhibiting the activation of MAP kinases and NF-kappaB in human chondrocytes in vitro. *J nutr*. 2005;135(9):2096-2102.

68. Schmid B, Ludtke R, Selbmann HK, et al. Efficacy and tolerability of a standardized willow bark extract in patients with osteoarthritis: randomized placebo-controlled, double blind clinical trial. *Phytother Res*. 2001;15(4):344-350.

69. Bergeron MF. Muscle cramps during exercise - is it fatigue or electrolyte deficit? *Curr Sport Med Rep*. 2008;7(4):S50-S55.

Chapter 12

1. A brief history of USDA food guides. United States Department of Agriculture website. www.choosemyplate.gov/brief-history-usda-food-guides. Published June, 2011. Accessed July 7 2018.

2. Choose MyPlate. United States Department of Agriculture website. www.choosemyplate.gov. Published 2015. Accessed July 7, 208.

3. Messina V, Melina V, Mangels AR. A new food guide for North American vegetarians. *J Am Diet Assoc*. 2003;103(6):771-775.

4. Houtkooper L. Food selection for endurance sports. *Med Sci Sports Exerc*. 1992;24(9 Suppl):S349-359.

5. Vegan version of USDA MyPlate now available as full-color handout and coloring page. The Vegetarian Resource Group blog. www.vrg.org/blog/2011/08/01/vegan-version-of-usda-myplate-now-available-as-full-color-handout-and-coloring-page. Published August 1, 2011. Accessed July 7, 2018.

6. Athlete's Plate. United States Olympic Committee Sports Dietitians, University of Colorado Sports Nutrition Graduate Program. teamusa.org; 2006.

7. Tips for vegetarians. USDA ChooseMyPlate website. www.choosemyplate.gov/tips-vegetarians. Updated March 7, 2018. Accessed July 7, 2018.

8. Wang Y, Ho CT. Polyphenolic chemistry of tea and coffee: a century of progress. *J Agric Food Chem*. 2009;57(18):8109-8114.

9. Gokcen BB, Sanlier N. Coffee consumption and disease correlations. *Crit Rev Food Sci Nutr*. 2017;1-13. doi: 10.1080/10408398.

10. Nieber K. The impact of coffee on health. *Planta Med*. 2017;83(16):1256-1263.

11. Denke MA. Nutritional and health benefits of beer. *Am J Med Sci*. 2000;320(5):320-326.

12. Arranz S, Chiva-Blanch G, Valderas-Martinez P, et al. Wine, beer, alcohol and polyphenols on cardiovascular disease and cancer. *Nutrients*. 2012;4(7):759-781.

13. Maughan RJ, Watson P, Cordery PA, et al. A randomized trial to assess the potential of different beverages to affect hydration status: development of a beverage hydration index. *Am J Clin Nutr*. 2016;103(3):717-723.

14. Yacoubou J. Vegetarian Journal's guide to food ingredients. The Vegetarian Resource Group website. www.vrg.org/ingredients. Published 2017. Accessed July 7 2018.

15. Satija A, Bhupathiraju SN, Rimm EB, et al. Plant-based dietary patterns and incidence of type 2 diabetes in US men and women: results from three prospective cohort studies. *PLoS Med*. 2016;13(6):e1002039.

Chapter 13

1. Manore MM, Larson-Meyer DE, Lindsay AR, Hongu N, Houtkooper L. Dynamic energy balance: an integrated framework for discussing diet and physical activity in obesity prevention-is it more than eating less and exercising more? *Nutrients*. 2017;9(8). doi: 10.3390/nu9080905.

2. Manore MM. Weight management in the performance athlete. *Nestle Nutrition Institute workshop series*. 2013;75:123-133.

3. Schwartz MW, Seeley RJ, Zeltser LM, et al. Obesity pathogenesis: An Endocrine Society scientific statement. *Endocr Rev.* 2017;38(4):267-296.

4. Larson DE, Rising R, Ferraro RT, Ravussin E. Spontaneous overfeeding with a 'cafeteria diet' in men: effects on 24-hour energy expenditure and substrate oxidation. *Int J Obes Relat Metab Disord.* 1995;19(5):331-337.

5. Larson DE, Tataranni PA, Ferraro RT, Ravussin E. Ad libitum food intake on a 'cafeteria diet' in Native American women: relations with body composition and 24-h energy expenditure. *Am J Clin Nutr.* 1995;62(5):911-917.

6. Could those common symptoms be thyroid trouble? Fatigue, brain fog, and weight gain are telltale signs that may be mistaken for other conditions. *Harv Health Lett.* 2014;39(3):6.

7. Carl RL, Johnson MD, Martin TJ, Council on Sports Medicine and Fitness. Promotion of healthy weight-control practices in young athletes. *Pediatrics.* 2017;140(3).

8. Thomas DT, Erdman KA, Burke LM. American College of Sports Medicine joint position statement. Nutrition and athletic performance. *Med Sci Sports Exerc.* 2016;48(3):543-568.

9. Garthe I, Raastad T, Refsnes PE, Koivisto A, Sundgot-Borgen J. Effect of two different weight-loss rates on body composition and strength and power-related performance in elite athletes. *Int J Sport Nutr Exerc Metab.* 2011;21(2):97-104.

10. Rhyu HS, Cho SY. The effect of weight loss by ketogenic diet on the body composition, performance-related physical fitness factors and cytokines of taekwondo athletes. *J Exerc Rehabil.* 2014;10(5):326-331.

11. Tinsley GM, Willoughby DS. Fat-free mass changes during ketogenic diets and the potential role of resistance training. *Int J Sport Nutr Exerc Metab.* 2016;26(1):78-92.

12. Mujika I. Case study: long-term low carbohydrate, high fat diet impairs performance and subjective wellbeing in a world-class vegetarian long-distance triathlete. *Int J Sport Nutr Exerc Metab.* 2018:1-6. doi: 10.1123/ijsnem.2018-0124.

13. Hector AJ, Phillips SM. Protein recommendations for weight loss in elite athletes: a focus on body composition and performance. *Int J Sport Nutr Exerc Metab.* 2018;28(2):170-177.

14. Mettler S, Mitchell N, Tipton KD. Increased protein intake reduces lean body mass loss during weight loss in athletes. *Med Sci Sports Exerc.* 2010;42(2):326-337.

15. Crovetti R, Porrini M, Santangelo A, Testolin G. The influence of thermic effect of food on satiety. *Eur J Clin Nutr.* 1998;52(7):482-488.

16. Prentice AM. Manipulation of dietary fat and energy density and subsequent effects on substrate flux and food intake. *Am J Clin Nutr.* 1998;67(3 Suppl):535S-541S.

17. Turner-McGrievy GM, Davidson CR, Wingard EE, Wilcox S, Frongillo EA. Comparative effectiveness of plant-based diets for weight loss: a randomized controlled trial of five different diets. *Nutrition.* 2015;31(2):350-358.

18. Young LR, Nestle M. Expanding portion sizes in the US marketplace: implications for nutrition counseling. *J Am Diet Assoc.* 2003;103(2):231-234.

19. Wyatt HR, Grunwald GK, Mosca CL, Klem ML, Wing RR, Hill JO. Long-term weight loss and breakfast in subjects in the National Weight Control Registry. *Obes Res.* 2002;10(2):78-82.

20. Rolls BJ, Drewnowski A, Ledikwe JH. Changing the energy density of the diet as a strategy for weight management. *J Am Diet Assoc.* 2005;105(5):S98-S103.

21. Rolls BJ, Roe LS, Beach AM, Kris-Etherton PVM. Provision of foods differing in energy density affects long-term weight loss. *Obes Res.* 2005;13(6):1052-1060.

22. DellaValle DM, Roe LS, Rolls BJ. Does the consumption of caloric and non-caloric beverages with a meal affect energy intake? *Appetite.* 2005;44(2):187-193.

23. Suter PM, Schutz Y, Jequier E. The effect of ethanol on fat storage in healthy subjects. *N Engl J Med.* 1992;326(15):983-987.

24. Tremblay A, St-Pierre S. The hyperphagic effect of a high-fat diet and alcohol intake persists after control for energy density. *Am J Clin Nutr.* 1996;63(4):479-482.

25. Burke LM, Collier GR, Broad EM, et al. Effect of alcohol intake on muscle glycogen storage after prolonged exercise. *J Appl Physiol (1985).* 2003;95(3):983-990.

26. Leeman M, Ostman E, Bjorck I. Vinegar dressing and cold storage of potatoes lowers

postprandial glycaemic and insulinaemic responses in healthy subjects. *Eur J Clin Nutr.* 2005;59(11):1266-1271.

27. Ostman E, Granfeldt Y, Persson L, Bjorck I. Vinegar supplementation lowers glucose and insulin responses and increases satiety after a bread meal in healthy subjects. *Eur J Clin Nutr.* 2005;59(9):983-988.

28. Kohn JB. Is vinegar an effective treatment for glycemic control or weight loss? *J Acad Nutr Diet.* 2015;115(7):1188.

29. Hamilton MT, Healy GN, Dunstan DW, Zderic TW, Owen N. Too little exercise and too much sitting: inactivity physiology and the need for new recommendations on sedentary behavior. *Curr Cardiovasc Risk Rep.* 2008;2(4):292-298.

30. Booth AO, Huggins CE, Wattanapenpaiboon N, Nowson CA. Effect of increasing dietary calcium through supplements and dairy food on body weight and body composition: a meta-analysis of randomised controlled trials. *Br J Nutr.* 2015;114(7):1013-1025.

31. He RR, Chen L, Lin BH, Matsui Y, Yao XS, Kurihara H. Beneficial effects of oolong tea consumption on diet-induced overweight and obese subjects. *Chin J Integr Med.* 2009;15(1):34-41.

32. Westerterp-Plantenga MS, Lejeune MP, Kovacs EM. Body weight loss and weight maintenance in relation to habitual caffeine intake and green tea supplementation. *Obes Res.* 2005;13(7):1195-1204.

33. Yajima H, Noguchi T, Ikeshima E, et al. Prevention of diet-induced obesity by dietary isomerized hop extract containing isohumulones, in rodents. *Int J Obes (Lond).* 2005;29(8):991-997.

34. Dostalek P, Karabin M, Jelinek L. Hop phytochemicals and their potential role in metabolic syndrome prevention and therapy. *Molecules.* 2017;22(10).

35. Phillips SM, Van Loon LJ. Dietary protein for athletes: from requirements to optimum adaptation. *J Sports Sci.* 2011;29 Suppl 1:S29-38.

36. Butterfield GE, Lemon PW, Kleiner S, Stone M. Roundtable: methods of weight gain in athletes. *Sports Science Exchange. RG 21.* 1995;5:1-4.

37. Hill PB, Wynder EL. Effect of a vegetarian diet and dexamethasone on plasma prolactin, testosterone and dehydroepiandrosterone in men and women. *Cancer Lett.* 1979;7(5):273-282.

38. Raben A, Kiens B, Richter EA, et al. Serum sex hormones and endurance performance after a lacto-ovo vegetarian and a mixed diet. *Med Sci Sports Exerc.* 1992;24(11):1290-1297.

39. Reed MJ, Cheng RW, Simmonds M, Richmond W, James VH. Dietary lipids: an additional regulator of plasma levels of sex hormone binding globulin. *J Clin Endocrinol Metab.* 1987;64(5):1083-1085.

40. Key TJ, Roe L, Thorogood M, Moore JW, Clark GM, Wang DY. Testosterone, sex hormone-binding globulin, calculated free testosterone, and oestradiol in male vegans and omnivores. *Br J Nutr.* 1990;64(1):111-119.

41. Hill P, Wynder E, Garbaczewski L, Garnes H, Walker AR, Helman P. Plasma hormones and lipids in men at different risk for coronary heart disease. *Am J Clin Nutr.* 1980;33(5):1010-1018.

42. Allen NE, Appleby PN, Davey GK, Key TJ. Hormones and diet: low insulin-like growth factor-I but normal bioavailable androgens in vegan men. *Br J Cancer.* 2000;83(1):95-97.

43. Key TJ, Fraser GE, Thorogood M, et al. Mortality in vegetarians and nonvegetarians: detailed findings from a collaborative analysis of 5 prospective studies. *Am J Clin Nutr.* 1999;70(3 Suppl):516S-524S.

44. Houston ME. Gaining weight: the scientific basis of increasing skeletal muscle mass. *Can J Appl Physiol.* 1999;24(4):305-316.

45. Grandjean A. Nutritional requirements to increase lean mass. *Clin Sports Med.* 1999;18(3):623-632.

46. Garthe I, Raastad T, Sundgot-Borgen J. Long-term effect of nutritional counselling on desired gain in body mass and lean body mass in elite athletes. *Appl Physiol Nutr Metab.* 2011;36(4):547-554.

47. Ravussin E, Lillioja S, Knowler WC, et al. Reduced rate of energy expenditure as a risk factor for body-weight gain. N Engl J Med. 1988;318(8):467-472.

48. Zurlo F, Lillioja S, Esposito-Del Puente A, et al. Low ratio of fat to carbohydrate oxidation as predictor of weight gain: study of 24-h RQ. Am J Physiol. 1990;259(5 Pt 1):E650-657.

49. Kim SJ, de Souza RJ, Choo VL, et al. Effects of dietary pulse consumption on body weight: a systematic review and meta-analysis of randomized controlled trials. Am J Clin Nutr. 2016;103(5):1213-1223.

Chapter 14

1. Schwendel BH, Morel PC, Wester TJ, et al. Fatty acid profile differs between organic and conventionally produced cow milk independent of season or milking time. *J Dairy Sci.* 2015;98(3):1411-1425.

2. Unlu NZ, Bohn T, Clinton SK, Schwartz SJ. Carotenoid absorption from salad and salsa by humans is enhanced by the addition of avocado or avocado oil. *J Nutr.* 2005;135(3):431-436.

3. Kim JE, Gordon SL, Ferruzzi MG, Campbell WW. Effects of egg consumption on carotenoid absorption from co-consumed, raw vegetables. *Am J Clin Nutr.* 2015;102(1):75-83.

4. Position of the American Dietetic Association: vegetarian diets–technical support paper. *J Am Diet Assoc.* 1988;88(3):352-355.

INDEX

Note: The italicized *f* and *t* following page numbers refer to figures and tables, respectively.

ABOUT THE AUTHORS

Enette Larson-Meyer, PhD, RD, CSSD, FACSM, is a professor at the University of Wyoming and is a well-respected researcher in the area of sports and exercise metabolism. Her research centers on how nutrition influences the health and performance of active individuals at all stages of the life cycle and at all levels of performance—from the casual exerciser to the elite athlete.

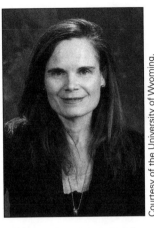

Courtesy of the University of Wyoming.

Larson-Meyer is the author of *Vegetarian Sports Nutrition* (Human Kinetics, 2007) and has also authored over 80 scientific journal articles and book chapters. She served on the 2011 International Olympic Committee (IOC) Sports Nutrition Consensus Panel and on the IOC Consensus Panel for Supplementation in the Elite Athlete (2017-2018). She is a board certified specialist in sports dietetics, is a former sports dietitian for the University of Alabama at Birmingham, and is active in SCAN (the sports, cardiovascular, and wellness nutrition practice group of the Academy of Nutrition and Dietetics) and the American College of Sports Medicine, where she serves as an associate editor for medicine and science in sports and exercise. She is also a past chair of both SCAN and the vegetarian nutrition (VN) practice group of the Academy of Nutrition and Dietetics. Personal interests include trail running, flat water kayaking, Irish step dancing, yoga, and being the number-one fan of her two vegetarian and one semi-vegetarian athletes.

Matt Ruscigno, MPH, RD, is a leading expert in plant-based nutrition and has followed a vegan diet for more than 20 years. He has a nutritional science degree from Pennsylvania State University, a public health nutrition master's degree from Loma Linda University, and certification as a registered dietitian. He is a coauthor of the *No Meat Athlete* book with Matt Frazier and *Appetite for Reduction* with Isa Moskowitz and is lead author of *Cacao, Superfoods for Life*. He is the past chair of the vegetarian nutrition (VN) practice group of the Academy of Nutrition and Dietetics and currently is the chief nutrition officer at Nutrinic, a

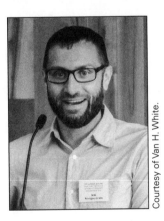

Courtesy of Van H. White.

start-up health-care company using plant-based nutrition for the prevention of cardiovascular diseases. Recreationally, he has raced ultramarathons, Ironman races, and 24-hour mountain bike races, and he has bike toured over 15,000 miles. He is a long-time resident of Los Angeles, California.

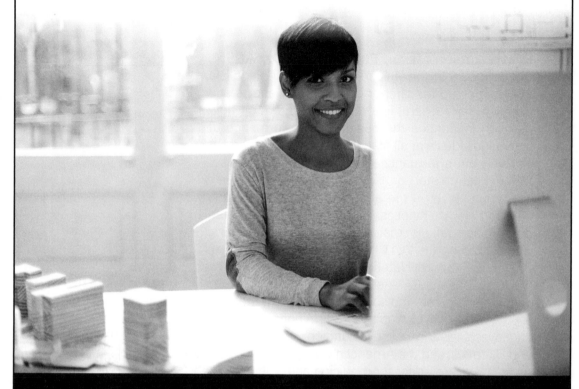
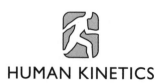